GERIATRIC SECRETS

Third Edition

Mary Ann Forciea, MD
Clinical Associate Professor of Medicine
Division of Geriatric Medicine
University of Pennsylvania Health System
Philadelphia, Pennsylvania

Edna P. Schwab, MD
Department of Medicine, Division of Geriatric Medicine
University of Pennsylvania School of Medicine
Hospital of the University of Pennsylvania
Veterans Administration Medical Center
Presbyterian Medical Center
Philadelphia, Pennsylvania

Donna Brady Raziano, MD, MBA
Medical Director of Case Management
Internal Medicine/Geriatrics
Temple University Health System Discharge Planning Center
Philadelphia, Pennsylvania

Risa Lavizzo-Mourey, MD, MBA
President and Chief Executive Officer
Robert Wood Johnson Foundation
Princeton, New Jersey

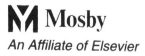 Mosby
An Affiliate of Elsevier

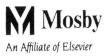

Mosby

An Affiliate of Elsevier

The Curtis Center
Independence Square West
Philadelphia, Pennsylvania 19106

Note to the reader: Although the techniques, ideas, and information in this book have been carefully reviewed for correctness, the authors, editor, and publisher cannot accept any legal responsibility for any errors or omissions that may be made. Neither the publisher nor the editor makes any guarantee, expressed or implied, with respect to the material contained herein.

Library of Congress Control Number: 2003114344

GERIATRIC SECRETS, 3rd edition

Permissions may be sought directly from Elsevier's Health Sciences Rights Department in Philadelphia, PA, USA: phone: (+1) 215 239 3804, fax: (+1) 215 239 3805, e-mail: healthpermissions@elsevier.com. You may also complete your request on-line via the Elsevier homepage (http://www.elsevier.com), by selecting 'Customer Support' and then 'Obtaining Permissions'.

ISBN-13: 978-1-56053-597-3
ISBN-10: 1-56053-597-0

Printed in the United States
Transferred to Digital Printing, 2011

GERIATRIC SECRETS

Third Edition

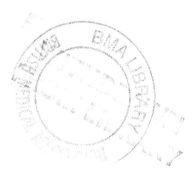

CONTENTS

I. OVERVIEW

II. SYMPTOMS

III. OFFICE CARE OF THE GERIATRIC PATIENT

CONTRIBUTORS

Janet L. Abrahm, MD
Associate Professor, Department of Medicine and Anesthesia, Harvard Medical School; Dana-Farber Cancer Institute; Brigham and Women's Hospital, Boston, Massachusetts

Steven E. Arnold, MD
Departments of Psychiatry and Neurology, University of Pennsylvania School of Medicine; Hospital of the University of Pennsylvania, Philadelphia, Pennsylvania

Marie A. Bernard, MD
Professor, Donald W. Reynolds Department of Geriatric Medicine, University of Oklahoma College of Medicine, Oklahoma City, Oklahoma

Douglas C. Bigelow, MD
Associate Professor, Director of Otology and Neurotology, Department of Otorhinolaryngology, University of Pennsylvania, Philadelphia, Pennsylvania

John Bruza, MD
Department of Medicine, Division of Geriatric Medicine, University of Pennsylvania Health System, Philadelphia, Pennsylvania

John D. Cacciamani, MD, MBA
Chief Medical Officer, Department of Internal Medicine, Temple University Hospital, Philadelphia, Pennsylvania

Angela C. Cafiero, PharmD, CGP
Assistant Professor of Clinical Pharmacy, Department of Pharmacy Practice and Pharmacy Administration, University of the Sciences in Philadelphia/Philadelphia College of Pharmacy, Philadelphia, Pennsylvania

Elizabeth Capezuti, PhD, RN, FAAN
Associate Professor, Division of Nursing, School of Education, New York University, New York, New York

Lesley Carson, MD
Department of Medicine, Division of Geriatric Medicine, University of Pennsylvania School of Medicine; Hospital of the University of Pennsylvania; Presbyterian Medical Center, Philadelphia, Pennsylvania

David Cassarett, MD, MA
Assistant Professor, Department of Medicine, Philadelphia Veterans Administration Medical Center/University of Pennsylvania, Philadelphia, Pennsylvania

Christopher M. Clark, MD
Associate Professor, Department of Neurology, University of Pennsylvania; Hospital of the University of Pennsylvania, Philadelphia, Pennsylvania

Grace A. Cordts, MD, MS, MPH
Faculty, Internal Medicine, York Health System, York, Pennsylvania

Valerie T. Cotter, MSN, CRNP
Associate Director, Adult Health and Gerontology Nurse Practitioner Program, School of Nursing; Education Director, Alzheimer's Disease Center, University of Pennsylvania; Memory Disorders Clinic, University of Pennsylvania, Philadelphia, Pennsylvania

Hollis Day, MD, MS
Department of Medicine, Division of Geriatric Medicine, University of Pennsylvania School of Medicine, Philadelphia, Pennsylvania

Susan C. Day, MD, MPH
Clinical Associate Professor, University of Pennsylvania; Presbyterian Medical Center; University of Pennsylvania Health System, Philadelphia, Pennsylvania

George W. Drach, MD
Professor, Department of Surgery/Urology, University of Pennsylvania; Hospital of the University of Pennsylvania, Philadelphia, Pennsylvania

Brian M. Drachman, MD
Clinical Assistant Professor, Department of Medicine, Division of Cardiology, University of Pennsylvania Health System/Presbyterian Medical Center, Philadelphia, Pennsylvania

William F. Edwards, MSN, APRN, BC, CDRNP
Geriatric Nurse Practitioner, Department of Medicine, Division of Geriatric Medicine, University of Pennsylvania; Hospital of the University of Pennsylvania, Philadelphia, Pennsylvania

Kathleen L. Egan, PhD
Director, Geriatrics Education, Department of Medicine, Division of Geriatric Medicine, University of Pennsylvania, Philadelphia, Pennsylvania

Mary Ann Forciea, MD
Clinical Associate Professor of Medicine, Division of Geriatric Medicine, University of Pennsylvania Health System, Philadelphia, Pennsylvania

Mary L. Fornek, RN, BSN, MBA, CIC
Veterans Administration Medical Center, Philadelphia, Pennsylvania

Robert J. Goldman, MD
Assistant Professor, Department of Rehabilitation Medicine, University of Pennsylvania; Presbyterian Hospital, Philadelphia, Pennsylvania

Nalaka S. Gooneratne, MD, MSc
Assistant Professor, Department of Medicine, Division of Geriatric Medicine, University of Pennsylvania, Philadelphia, Pennsylvania

Raquel E. Gur, MD, PhD
Professor, Department of Psychiatry, University of Pennsylvania; Hospital of the University of Pennsylvania, Philadelphia, Pennsylvania

Ruben C. Gur, PhD
Professor, Department of Psychiatry, University of Pennsylvania; Hospital of the University of Pennsylvania, Philadelphia, Pennsylvania

Arthur E. Helfand, DPM, DABPPH
Professor Emeritus, School of Podiatric Medicine, Community, Health, Aging and Health Policy, Temple University; Honorary Staff, Thomas Jefferson University Hospital, Philadelphia, Pennsylvania

Kelly Henning, MD
Veterans Administration Medical Center, Philadelphia, Pennsylvania

Howard Hurtig, MD
Professor and Vice Chair, Department of Neurology; Codirector, Parkinson's Disease and Movement Disorders at Pennsylvania Hospital, University of Pennsylvania Health System, Philadelphia, Pennsylvania

Jerry C. Johnson, MD
Professor, Department of Medicine; Chief, Division of Geriatric Medicine, University of Pennsylvania, Philadelphia, Pennsylvania

Michael C. Jung
University of Pennsylvania, Philadelphia, Pennsylvania

Fran E. Kaiser, MD
Clinical Professor of Medicine, University of Texas Southwestern Medical Center, Dallas, Texas; Adjunct Professor of Medicine, St. Louis University, St. Louis, Missouri

Jennifer M. Kapo, MD
Instructor, Department of Medicine, Division of Geriatric Medicine, University of Pennsylvania, Philadelphia, Pennsylvania

Jason H. T. Karlawski, MD
Assistant Professor, Department of Medicine, University of Pennsylvania, Philadelphia, Pennsylvania

William Kavesh, MD, MPH
Director, Geriatric Clinic, Philadelphia Veterans Administration Hospital; Clinical Assistant Professor, Department of Medicine, Division of Geriatric Medicine, University of Pennsylvania School of Medicine, Philadelphia, Pennsylvania

Tatyana Kemarskaya, MD
Assistant Professor, School of Medicine, Department of Geriatrics, University of Medicine and Dentistry of New Jersey; Kennedy Health System, Stratford, New Jersey

Bruce Kinosian, MD
Department of Medicine, Division of Geriatric Medicine, University of Pennsylvania Health System, Philadelphia, Pennsylvania

Glenn W. Knox, MD
Department of Surgery, University of Florida Health Science Center; Baptist-St. Vincent's Medical Center, Jacksonville, Florida

Matthew M. Kurtz, PhD
Assistant Clinical Professor, Department of Psychiatry, Yale School of Medicine, New Haven, Connecticut; Neurophysiologist, Schizophrenia Rehabilitation Program, Institute of Living, Hartford, Connecticut

Risa Lavizzo-Mourey, MD, MBA
President and Chief Executive, Robert Wood Johnson Foundation, Princeton, New Jersey

Thomas E. Lawrence, MD
Clinical Assistant Professor, Department of Medicine, Division of Geriatric Medicine, University of Pennsylvania Health System, Philadelphia, Pennsylvania

Elizabeth R. Mackenzie, PhD
Project Director, Department of Psychiatry; Lecturer, Graduate Program in Folklore and Folklife, University of Pennsylvania; Center for Mental Health Policy and Services Research, University of Pennsylvania Health System, Philadelphia, Pennsylvania

Marjorie Marenberg, MD, PhD
Department of Medicine, Division of Geriatric Medicine, University of Pennsylvania School of Medicine, Philadelphia, Pennsylvania

David S. Miller, MD
Chief of Older Adult Psychiatry, Friends Hospital, Philadelphia, Pennsylvania

Paul J. Moberg, PhD
Associate Professor, Department of Psychiatry, University of Pennsylvania, Philadelphia, Pennsylvania

Daniel F. Motter, MPT
Philadelphia College of Osteopathic Medicine, Philadelphia, Pennsylvania

Roberta A. Newton, PhD
Professor of Physical Therapy, Adjunct Clinical Professor of Medicine, Institute on Aging; School of Medicine, Temple University, Philadelphia, Pennsylvania

David W. Oslin, MD
Assistant Professor, Department of Psychiatry, University of Pennsylvania, Philadelphia, Pennsylvania

Sheila Pasupathy, BA
Program Manager, Geriatrics Education, Division of Geriatric Medicine, University of Pennsylvania, Philadelphia, Pennsylvania

Robert J. Pignolo, MD, PhD
Assistant Professor, Department of Medicine, Division of Geriatric Medicine, University of Pennsylvania School of Medicine; Hospital of the University of Pennsylvania; Presbyterian Medical Center; Philadelphia Veterans Administration Medical Center, Philadelphia, Pennsylvania

Donna Brady Raziano, MD, MBA
Medical Director of Case Management, Internal Medicine/Geriatrics, Temple University Health System Discharge Planning Center, Philadelphia, Pennsylvania

Jane Bonner Reitmeyer, MSW, LSW
Social Worker, Department of Medicine, Division of Geriatric Medicine, University of Pennsylvania School of Medicine, Philadelphia, Pennsylvania

Ann Slaughter, DDS, MPH
Assistant Professor, Department of Community Oral Health, University of Pennsylvania School of Dental Medicine, Philadelphia, Pennsylvania

Dina H. Salman, PharmD
Clinical Pharmacist, Ambulatory Care, Department of Pharmacy, The Medical Center of Central Georgia, Macon, Georgia

Edna P. Schwab, MD
Department of Medicine, Division of Geriatric Medicine, University of Pennsylvania School of Medicine; Hospital of the University of Pennsylvania; Veterans Administration Medical Center; Presbyterian Medical Center, Philadelphia, Pennsylvania

Charles Spencer, MD, PhD
Assistant Professor, Department of Medicine, Division of Geriatric Medicine, University of Pennsylvania School of Medicine; Philadelphia Veterans Administration Medical Center, Hospital of the University of Pennsylvania, Philadelphia, Pennsylvania

Janet DeBerry Steinberg, OD, FAAO
Department of Medicine, Division of Geriatrics, University of Pennsylvania School of Medicine, Philadelphia, Pennsylvania

Joel E. Streim, MD
Associate Professor, Department of Psychiatry, University of Pennsylvania; Philadelphia Veterans Administration Medical Center, Philadelphia, Pennsylvania

Dana Suskind-Liu, MD
Department of Pediatric Otolaryngology, Louisiana State University Medical Center, New Orleans, Louisiana

Jennifer Tija, MD, MSCE
Instructor, Department of Medicine, Division of Geriatric Medicine, University of Pennsylvania School of Medicine; Hospital of the University of Pennsylvania, Philadelphia, Pennsylvania

Joan Weinryb, MD, CMD
Clinical Assistant Professor, Department of Medicine, University of Pennsylvania; Hospital of the University of Pennsylvania; Presbyterian Medical Center, Philadelphia, Pennsylvania

Jeff Wick, MD
University of Pennsylvania School of Medicine, Philadelphia, Pennsylvania

Jean Yudin, MSN, RN, CS
Department of Medicine, Division of Geriatric Medicine, University of Pennsylvania School of Medicine, Philadelphia, Pennsylvania

Ross R Zimmer, MD
Clinical Assistant Professor, Department of Medicine, Division of Cardiology, University of Pennsylvania Health System; Presbyterian Medical Center, Philadelphia, Pennsylvania

PREFACE

Geriatric Secrets is designed for medical students and other health care professionals who are learning the principles of geriatric practice. We use a direct approach familiar to students, the question-answer format, because of its ability to cut to the chase. Now more than ever, students must assimilate large amounts of information quickly and effectively. The Socratic approach is an efficient method of imparting information. We attempted to make the book reader-friendly. Where possible, we encouraged the use of summary tables and bullets rather than long passages of text.

This third edition has been expanded to include new sections on vision, hearing, and dental issues. We have also included a chapter on peripheral vascular disease and its complications as well as chapters on pharmacotherapy and spirituality.

Consider *Geriatric Secrets* a handbook, not a textbook. It provides an overview of the salient issues in the practice of geriatrics rather than a comprehensive or exhaustive discussion. Within these constraints, we have tried to emphasize the art of geriatrics—the personal touch, the team approach, the clinical challenges, and the tremendous satisfaction of improving the quality of someone's life, however briefly. Chapter 1 focuses on the art of practicing geriatrics and introduces some of the patients who have taught us the real "secrets" of geriatrics.

Next to the satisfaction of practicing geriatrics, our greatest pleasure comes from teaching it. For many reasons, too few students are exposed to geriatric medicine early enough and often enough to experience its rewards. We take pleasure in the fact that the impact of this book will be felt not only by the students who learn directly from its pages, but also by the clinicians of tomorrow who will benefit from the educational programs of the Division of Geriatric Medicine at the University of Pennsylvania. Royalties from the sale of the book will be donated to the Division as well as to the Carrie Steele-Pitts Home, a residential facility for abused, abandoned, and neglected children.

Finally, we gratefully acknowledge those whose contributions helped us turn a concept into a book, the authors for providing content, and the project team, Sheila Pasupathy and Daniel Motter, for making it happen.

Mary Ann Forciea, MD
Edna Schwab, MD
Donna Brady Raziano, MD, MBA
Risa Lavizzo-Mourey, MD, MBA

Note: The views expressed in this publication do not represent the policies of the Robert Wood Johnson Foundation.

I. Overview

1. THE ART AND PRACTICE OF GERIATRICS

Risa Lavizzo-Mourey, MD, MBA, Edna P. Schwab, MD,
Donna Brady Raziano, MD, MBA, and Mary Ann Forciea, MD

Most of this book focuses on the practice of geriatrics. It strives to impart the basics of geriatric medicine by using a direct approach—questions and answers. However, the art of caring for older patients is as important as the clinical facts, albeit less appreciated. The principles that underlie the art and inherent satisfaction of practicing geriatrics are the "Geriatric Secrets" revealed in this chapter. As with all health care, the real secrets reside in the patients. Although every patient is unique, the commonality among them often defines the approach and direction of a specialty or a discipline. Sometimes the commonality is as simple as a particular disease. In the case of geriatrics, the commonalities are more complex, going beyond age, specific diseases, or particular organ systems. This chapter introduces a few of our patients who, over the years, defined the art and practice of geriatrics for us.

Complex Medicine—Mr. H.

Geriatric patients have multiple chronic diseases, along with all the sequelae and treatments that chronic conditions entail. Chronic disease, coupled with a vulnerability to acute illness and disability, means that geriatric clinical situations are rarely simple. As clinicians, mostly we are taught to make the diagnosis, to find the malady, and to cure it. In geriatrics there rarely is one diagnosis; the average is four. The diagnoses may be related, sharing organ systems or pathophysiology, but just as often coexisting conditions merely fulfill the dictum that common diseases occur commonly together. Whichever the case, multiple chronic diseases interact, adding ambiguity and complications. As a result, geriatric clinical situations are almost always challenging, requiring knowledge, judgment, and good problem-solving skills.

Mr. H. illustrates this point. A 92-year-old retired engineer, Mr. H. moved in with his son and daughter-in-law after the death of his wife. Mr. H. is limited in mobility by coronary artery disease and severe osteoarthritis of both knees. Despite his mobility limitations, Mr. H. leads an active intellectual and social life through telephone conversations and visits from neighbors.

One winter, Mr. H. developed a severe respiratory tract infection. A chest x-ray revealed multiple smooth pulmonary nodules, which almost certainly represented multiple metastases. His respiratory tract infection resolved. Mr. H. and his family discussed diagnostic and therapeutic options with the geriatrics team. Mr. H. decided not to pursue further evaluation of the metastases.

Eighteen months later, Mr. H. continues to be pain-free. He is unable to leave his room due to his dyspnea but still plays a vital role in his family and neighborhood.

In caring for patients with multiple illnesses, the key is to facilitate patients or their surrogates in determining which symptoms are the most burdensome. The impact of treatment on "critical" symptoms must be evaluated, both in terms of efficacy and potential side effects. To Mr. H., dyspnea was familiar and tolerable. He had adjusted his lifestyle to this limitation and was not frightened by the thought of progression of breathlessness. He was terrified by the prospect of pain or nausea. In his family meetings, he finally concluded that he wished no disruption of his life unless pain intervened. The geriatrics team and Mr. H.'s family were able to focus on Mr. H.'s view of his life and to design a program of care that responded to his wishes.

Differentiating Aging from Disease—Mr. I.

Shakespeare characterized old age as a second childhood: "sans eyes, sans teeth, sans everything."

The body changes with aging, and many organs and organ systems become more limited in their capacity to carry out prescribed functions. However, the losses conjured by Shakespeare's words generally result from disease, not normal aging. Differentiating the consequences of normal aging from disease so that disease can be treated or managed is a fundamental principle of geriatrics. For example, the ratio of type I to type II muscle fibers changes with age, but does not cause debilitating muscle atrophy. Sleep patterns change—less deep sleep and increased ratios of REM to non-REM sleep. Yet daytime somnolence, insomnia, and early awaking, while common complaints among the elderly, are not a part of normal aging. Part of the art of geriatrics is not only knowing the difference between normal aging and disease, but also being able to convince patients of the difference.

Mr. I. could not hear as well as he did as a young man. He saw it as an inevitable consequence of aging and was prepared to accept the attendant inconveniences. It was his wife who insisted that he "look into it." She complained about the blaring television and was growing tired of repeating herself or arguing about what had been said. Mr. I.'s hearing loss was severe and asymmetric, involving low- as well as high-frequency ranges. Presbycusis, commonly seen in elders (see Chapter 11), typically involves high frequencies. Mr. I.'s problem was not normal aging and was treatable with a hearing aid.

Convincing Mr. I. that he had a treatable problem meant correcting a lot of misconceptions without creating unrealistically high expectations. After he got a hearing aid, his hearing improved but was not perfect. He admits to being more comfortable in social situations and is amazed at how isolated he had become. In accepting the treatment, he improved his quality of life and taught his physicians the value of pursuing treatable diseases in old age.

Limited Physiologic Reserve—Miss O.

Conceptually, older people often tolerate illness and other threats to homeostasis poorly, because they have limited "physiologic reserve." An 80-year-old's minute ventilation may be adequate at rest, but he or she does not have the reserve necessary to handle two flights of stairs in the setting of a viral upper respiratory infection. Physiologic changes in most organ systems contribute to the diminished reserve observed in the elderly. For example, lean body mass decreases with age, as does muscle strength. Cardiac output with exertion decreases with age. Cognitive functioning, with the exception of executive functions, attenuates. All of these examples can have clinical consequences, particularly when older adults are stressed with an acute illness. Anticipating the consequences of limited physiologic reserves is fundamental to practicing high-quality geriatrics. For example, decreased muscle strength is associated with rapid deconditioning and necessitates attention to ambulation and physical therapy, even during relatively brief illnesses.

Miss O. was the patient who first peaked our interest in this aspect of geriatrics. She was in her 80s, mildly demented, but still independent in all activities of daily living. Her sister, with whom she shared an apartment, brought her to the emergency department because of her obtunded state. According to the sister, Miss O. had been "fine" two days earlier save for a slight fever and foul-smelling urine. Over 48 hours the patient's oral intake progressively worsened, and lethargy developed. On admission to the hospital her serum sodium was 178 mg/dl. That such severe hypernatremia could develop so rapidly seemed improbable at the time, yet we now appreciate that the patient had virtually no reserve and was severely stressed physiologically. Her total body water at baseline was compromised by several factors, including her small size and age-related decreases. Her acute illness, pyelonephritis, exacerbated the dehydration by causing mild diabetes insipidus. Although one cannot be sure that she did not have the infection for longer than two days (but was afebrile), the severity of the dehydration, the devastating effect on her mental status, and the complete reversal of symptoms with hydration left an indelible impression of the need to anticipate the clinical consequences of limited physiologic reserve.

The Interdisciplinary Team Approach—Mrs. W.

All too often the uninitiated believe geriatrics to be overwhelming and depressing. Many patients are frail and often have social problems in addition to complex illnesses. To be sure, providing care to such patients in the context of a busy, single-discipline office practice is daunting. Geriatrics is inherently interdisciplinary. To provide comprehensive care (see later section), a well-functioning, interdisciplinary team is critical.

An interdisciplinary team usually has members with defined but fluid roles that, to some degree, frequently overlap. For example, both nurse practitioner and physician may provide primary care, with the nurse taking responsibility for assessment of functional status or other factors, depending on the availability of physical or occupational therapy. Similarly, case management may fall to nursing, social work, or, in complicated situations, medicine. The hallmarks of a well-functioning cooperative team are flexibility, mutual respect, and the ability to stay focused on the patient's needs and goals.

Mrs. W. is a 68-year-old woman with insulin-dependent diabetes mellitus of 30 years' duration; complications involve almost every organ system. She requires chronic intermittent bladder catheterization because of autonomic nervous system dysfunction. She cannot perform this task for herself because of peripheral neuropathy involving her fingers. She requires help in drawing up her insulin because of the neuropathy and decreased vision. At a routine office visit, review of her diabetic diary revealed marked deterioration in glucose control. Careful questioning made clear that Mrs. W. is no longer certain about guidelines for adjusting her insulin doses to changes in blood sugar level.

A team meeting is followed by a meeting of the team with the patient and her family. The family meeting includes an update of Mrs. W.'s current complications and their impact on her daily life. The medical team members develop new medication schedules and guidelines. Mrs. W. agrees to allow her family to assist in her care and in the adjustment of her insulin doses. Family members volunteer to be trained in insulin administration and in bladder catheterization; team nurses conduct the training sessions. Home health aides are recruited by the team social worker to assist the patient in personal hygiene while the family members are at work.

One month later, the patient and family are much more satisfied with Mrs. W.'s daily life. Her diary reveals much improved glycemic control. The entire team as well as the patient and her family participated in a series of changes in Mrs. W.'s daily routine. A crisis that would have required hospitalization for serious hyper- or hypoglycemia was almost certainly averted; the quality of Mrs. W.'s daily life improved.

Care Across the Continuum—Mrs. Z.

Geriatricians and the teams of care to which those geriatricians belong care for patients in a variety of sites: the office, the hospital, the long-term care facility, and the patient's home. The constancy of the relationship between the patient, family, and geriatric team can be a powerful asset during diagnosis and treatment of an illness.

Mrs. Z. is an 88-year-old retired bookkeeper who lives with her daughter. She has been "shy" all her life: she has little social contact outside her family and dislikes crowds. Her daughter convinced her to seek medical care for long-term arthritis of both knees. She established an ongoing relationship with the geriatrician and the practice nurse. One Sunday morning, Mrs. Z. trips on a bathroom rug, falls to the floor, and is unable to rise. Mrs. Z. is taken to the ER, where a hip fracture is diagnosed. Despite severe pain, she refuses surgery and becomes increasingly agitated with efforts to obtain consent for surgery. Her geriatrician arrives, is able to calm her (draws the curtains to create privacy, sits down next to her, and speaks quietly), and she agrees to surgery. She tolerates hip replacement well, but has postoperative problems with anticoagulation and heart failure. The geriatrician and orthopedist work together to manage these problems and speak daily with the family. The patient is transferred to a skilled nursing facility for rehabilitation after reassurance that "her" doctor will continue to see her during rehabilitation. The geriatrician continues to provide medical care for the patient; the home care nurse practitioner meets the patient in the nursing home. After 1 month, the patient is discharged to home. She can stand but cannot leave the house. The home care team oversees home physical therapy and therapy for her congestive failure. After 3 months, the patient is able to travel by car and returns to the office for ongoing care.

The continuing presence of a familiar physician and other team members allowed Mrs. Z. to accept necessary care. That continuity also facilitates management of new problems and medications (such as anticoagulation) in a safer fashion.

Family Involvement—Mrs. K.

Geriatrics is a family-oriented specialty. The geriatrician frequently relies on an older person's family to implement the care plan, to be a surrogate decision-maker, and in many ways to function as a member of the team. Yet the family member's unique role and perspective must be preserved. Similarly, geriatricians are faced with the challenge of keeping the patient's interests paramount when day-to-day interactions frequently involve communication only with family members. The rewards of becoming closely involved not only with a patient but also with his or her family are among the most significant in geriatric practice—particularly when the "family" extends beyond the usual definition. Although a geriatrician's interactions with family members are complex, four dimensions seem universal: emotional support, decision making, provision of care, and education.

Education is the foundation on which a sound relationship with the family is built. The willingness to take the time to explain the cause of a clinical event, the next stage of the illness, alternative treatment, and the contents of articles that appear in the newspapers or other lay publications is consistently mentioned by both patients and families as key determinants of their satisfaction or dissatisfaction with physicians. A family that is attempting to cope with a frail elder who may be deteriorating functionally and cognitively is filled with anxiety because they do not know what to expect or when. By educating the family, the clinician not only builds rapport but also gains a critical member of the care team. Family members and other caregivers are the first-line decision-makers in any changing clinical situation. The family decides when to call the physician as well as whether to carry out the physician's suggestion, seek an alternative healer, or do nothing at all. Moreover, the geriatrician frequently must make a medical judgment based on the information provided by family members. Confidence in the accuracy and reliability of this information makes decision making easier.

In their roles as caregivers, family members interact with geriatricians in two other ways: as surrogate decision-makers and as potential patients. When an elderly person is cognitively impaired, it is often the family who participates in medical decision making rather than the patient. The challenge of keeping the patient's interests paramount while meeting the family's needs can be accomplished only through open communication between the family and geriatric team. When effective, such communication produces gratifying rapport, respect, and closeness. Moreover, it forms the basis for providing ongoing emotional support to the family and offers insight into when more intensive intervention is needed to preserve the caregiver's health and well-being.

Mrs. K is an 87-year-old retired nurse who was recently admitted to a nursing home following a hospitalization for mental status change. A subdural hematoma was surgically drained, but her mental status has still not returned to baseline. A temporary nasogastric tube has been in place about 2 weeks. Her past medical history is significant for dementia for 6 years. Her only living family is her daughter, who has durable power of attorney. The daughter reports that Mrs. K "did not want to be kept alive with tubes." Her nursing home course has had its pitfalls surrounding her nasogastric tube, including recurrent occlusion, a vasovagal event during insertion, and diarrhea. The latter has caused skin integrity breakdown. The geriatrician initiates a family and staff meeting. The doctor explained the complications from the feeding tube. A discussion about her wishes and prognosis takes place. The decision is made to discontinue tube feedings and provide care focused on Mrs. K's comfort.

The Role of Culture in the Picture of Geriatrics—Mr. M.

Culture is the set of shared beliefs, values, and morals that guide individual behaviors. Culture plays an important role in the way every individual interacts with the health care system. With the elderly, it is often a critical element in the physician-patient relationship. The unprecedented advances in technology and medicine that have shaped much of present-day American culture contrast starkly with the environment that influenced many of our elders' values. Moreover, many of America's present-day elders are immigrants or first-generation descendants of immigrants, making them much closer to a set of values that may be quite different from the dominant values of the U.S. today. Most elderly patients were teenagers during the late 1930s and early 1940s, and many immigrated to the United States under political or economic duress. African-American elders endured the humiliation of segregation. Although we take antibiotics, chemotherapy, and sophisticated diagnostic procedures, such as magnetic resonance imaging (MRI), for granted, rest and good air were the predominant treatment for almost every ailment when most elderly patients were growing up. They were adults when the first antibiotics became available and are all too familiar with the devastation that diseases such as polio can cause. Now most Americans receive more than 13 years of formal education, whereas most elderly people had on average only eight years of formal education. Seventy years ago, health education classes were not a standard part of the curriculum. The basic concepts of biology and human physiology that we take for granted in explaining medical conditions to our patients are not necessarily a part of our older patients' fund of knowledge. An elder's understanding of disease and illness may be rooted in religion rather than biology. Every effort should be made to learn the elderly patient's perspectives and values and to give them careful consideration in explanations, conversations, and care planning.

Mr. M. is an 86-year-old African-American man who grew up in the rural southeastern part of the United States. Despite little formal education, he is articulate and extremely skilled in social interactions. He is quite vocal about his major regrets in life, the most prominent being the missed opportunity to go to college. Mr. M.'s two clinical problems were hypertension and hearing loss. The hypertension was easily controlled, but over several years the hearing loss became more disabling. Audiometry revealed classic presbycusis, yet Mr. M. adamantly refused a hearing aid. As his disability from the hearing loss progressed and attempts to persuade him to use a hearing aid were repeatedly spurned, an exploration of his health beliefs was initiated. Surprisingly, this worldly gentleman believed that all illness was punishment from God. Once the hearing loss was discussed in the context of a disease caused by God's wrath rather than neuronal loss, we were able to identify the ways in which a hearing aid could be useful. Mr. M. illustrates a vital lesson: the sharing of many values, such as love of education, does not necessarily mean that one shares all values, including a belief in the biomedical model.

Bioethics

Geriatricians often grapple with thorny ethical dilemmas. The difficult decision-making surrounding end-of-life choices often gets media attention. However, other decisions—such as the timing of nursing home placement, whether to proceed with surgical therapy, or whether to place a feeding tube when an elderly person seems unwilling or unable to eat—are equally difficult. The geriatrician's role is complex. The tasks may shift from educator to advisor to sounding board. However, the critical and unwavering role always must be as patient advocate. Older patients can find themselves particularly vulnerable and therefore need the security of knowing that someone always will be their advocate. Because ethical issues surrounding treatment choices are likely to touch most older people, geriatricians must be comfortable in discussing such issues with their patients. Discussions should occur in the context of the patient's cultural values. Some patients who come from family-centered cultures may prefer to involve family members in the decision-making process, whereas patients from Western cultures are generally comfortable making decisions autonomously.

Mrs. L is a 77-year-old, mildly demented woman who has resided in an assisted living facility for the past year and a half. She was widowed 5 years ago and has a daughter, Sarah, who visits weekly. Mrs. L's son was killed accidentally in childhood, and she suffered for 5 years with depression. At present, Mrs. L is well liked and is able to participate in activities. Unfortunately, her daughter was fatally killed in a car accident last month. The staff and her distant relatives are fearful to disclose her daughter's death because she "won't be able to handle it." Mrs. L keeps asking for Sarah. The geriatrician identifies the problematic situation and consults the family.

They discuss not only their fears but also their overwhelming desire to be honest with Mrs. L. At a family meeting they inform Mrs. L of Sarah's death. Mrs. L cries but is consoled by family. The staff is told about the meeting and instructed to be prepared to comfort her as needed.

Ethical issues call on all of the other principles of the art and practice of geriatrics. The geriatrician must be knowledgeable about the complexity of medical care in older patients and able to base prognostications on a clear differentiation between disease and aging; know when to use the other members of an interdisciplinary team; and, above all, discuss such complex issues in the context of the patient's culture and family. Failure to do so can be devastating to the therapeutic relationship and to compliance with recommendations. Success in these efforts can lead to improved quality of life for patients and caregivers and more satisfaction for ourselves.

2. BIOLOGY OF AGING

Robert J. Pignolo, MD, PhD, and Mary Ann Forciea, MD

1. What is the difference between gerontology and geriatrics?

Gerontology takes its name from the Greek *geront* for "old man" and was first proposed by Elie Metchnikoff as a new science in 1903. Gerontology has been alternatively described as the study of aging or the scientific study of old age and today includes scientific investigations on processes of aging, clinical studies of mature adults, humanities-related perspectives on aging, and applications of the current knowledge base to benefit aged individuals. Scientists who study aging are called **gerontologists**.

The term **geriatrics** was first used by the American physician Ignatz Nascher in noting similarities with the specialty of pediatrics. Geriatrics is the discipline of medicine that focuses on prevention, diagnosis, treatment, and long-term care in older adults. The adjective form has been associated with many other medical professions, including geriatric social work, geriatric nursing, geriatric dentistry, and geriatric psychiatry, to denote added training and expertise relevant to older individuals. Although any of these professionals may be called a **geriatrician**, the name is generally reserved for a physician who specializes in geriatric medicine.

2. Is aging (senescence) universal?

Aging refers to all time-related processes that occur in the life of an organism, including those that contribute beneficial, neutral, and deteriorative effects. Although used interchangeably with the term *aging*, **senescence** specifically refers to deteriorative changes during postmaturational life that increase vulnerability and decrease the likelihood of survival.

There is no evidence that prokaryotes (bacteria) undergo senescence. Populations of single-celled eukaryotic organisms, such as budding yeast, are also immortal; however, individual cells within the population have a limited life span as measured by the number of bud generations or cell divisions. In multicellular organisms, senescence is thought to occur in species that have a germ line separate from a somatic (body) line, in those with a distinction between parent and smaller offspring, or, more precisely, in those that undergo somatic cell differentiation (by which cells become specialized during growth and development of the organism).

Senescence has been described among different species as rapid, gradual, or negligible. Rapid senescence occurs abruptly with deteriorative changes after maturation in short-lived invertebrates such as nematodes and flies or soon after reproduction in species such as annual plants and Pacific salmon. Gradual senescence progresses slowly but persistently after maturation in all placental mammals, including humans. Negligible senescence is exhibited by long-lived species such as clams, trees, fish, and reptiles, in which there is no clear evidence for postmaturational increases in mortality rate. However, measurements necessary to corroborate the occurrence of senescence are complicated and often confounded by predation, infection, and other environmental factors that predispose species to very high accidental death rates. Senescence is thought to occur largely as the result of **primary aging processes**; that is, aging in the relative absence of disease or injury.

3. How have median length of life, life expectancy, and maximum life span changed over the past century and through history?

The **median length of life** is the age at which there are as many individuals with shorter life spans as there are individuals with longer life spans. **Life expectancy** is the expectation of a certain mean length of life at birth or at any age, calculated from the *current mortality conditions in a population*. For example, the life expectancy for a hypothetical group of 65-year-olds would be based on the currently observed age-specific death rates among individuals age 65, 66, and so on, up to the greatest age attained in the prevailing population. **Maximum life span** is the age of the longest-lived survivors of a cohort or population; for humans, it is operationally considered to be the oldest age reached by one in 100 million people. Protection from premature death, rather than changes in aging processes, underlie the survival increases reflected by median life span and life expectancy. Reduction in the high rate of infant deaths by improvements in sanitation, nutrition, and immunization account for much of the protection from premature death by environmental hazards and infectious diseases seen early in the 19th century. Median life span and life expectancy are thus influenced by many factors and are thought not to reflect primary aging processes.

Despite some challenges to the contrary, maximum life span has been considered an index of the rate of aging of a population and the maximum life span of a species tends to be inversely related to its rate of aging. For example, rats, with a maximum life span of about 5 years, are thought to age more rapidly than dogs, with a maximum life span of about 20 years. Any factor that increases the maximum life span of a species is considered to have influenced primary aging processes. Maximum human life span is greater than 115 years, with reliably reported ages of 121 years for Jeanne Calment, who died in France in 1996, and 112 years for Antonio Todde, who died in Sardinia (Italy) in 2002, two weeks before his 113th birthday.

Although the median length of life and life expectancy for humans have markedly increased over the past 100 years, there has been little, if any, change in maximum life span. In fact, over long periods of history maximum human life span has been relatively constant.

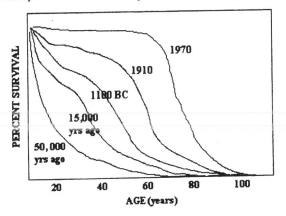

Human survivorship through history.

4. List common characteristics of aging. Discuss their limitations in describing primary aging processes.

Organisms exhibit a spectrum of morphologic and physiologic changes with age, some of which may be deleterious and cause functional decline. These changes may be due to aging processes, disease processes, toxic exposures, compensatory responses to injury or physiological deficits, or some combination of the preceding. A challenge of basic gerontologic research is to determine which of the many characteristics of aged individuals directly or indirectly relate to aging per se and constitute *primary* aging processes.

CHARACTERISTICS OF AGING	EXAMPLES
Increased mortality after maturation	Survival curves showing exponential increase in mortality with age
Changes in biochemical composition of tissues	Increases in lipofuscin or age pigment Increased cross-linking in extracellular matrix molecules such as collagen

(Cont'd.)

CHARACTERISTICS OF AGING	EXAMPLES
Progressive, deteriorative physiologic changes	Declines in glomerular filtration rate, maximal heart rate, vital capacity
Decreased ability to adaptively respond to environmental changes	Decreased "first past" hepatic metabolism Blunted maximal cardiac responses to exercise
Increasing incidence of many diseases	Ischemic heart disease, type II diabetes, osteoporosis, Alzheimer's disease

These "characteristics" of aging, although widely found, have exceptions that call into question their relevance to primary aging processes. For example, human age-specific mortality rates in many cases do not continue to increase exponentially at very advanced ages. Alterations in biochemical composition of tissues, deteriorative physiologic changes, and maladaptive responses to environmental challenges are quite heterogeneous from organ to organ within a specific individual and also from individual to individual. It is in this context that the terms *usual* and *successful* aging have been proposed as descriptors for those without discernible disease who exhibit an aging characteristic to a degree similar to most individuals of the same age (usual) or who minimally or do not exhibit an aging characteristic (successful). Although mortality rates for many diseases increase with age and parallel the exponential increase in mortality with age, at least one estimate predicts that elimination of atherosclerosis and cancer as causes of death would add only about 10 years to average life span and would not affect maximum life span potential.

5. Suggest a scheme for categorizing theories of aging.

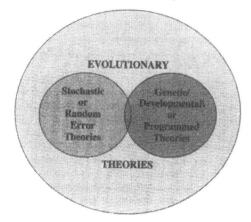

Possible relationship between the major groups of aging theories.

Theories of aging can broadly be divided into **stochastic (random error)** theories, **developmental-genetic** or **programmed** theories, and **evolutionary** theories. Stochastic theories hold that aging is caused by the accumulation of random damage to important molecules that eventually leads to physiologic decline. Developmental-genetic theories consider the process of aging as part of the genetically programmed continuum of development and maturation. Evolutionary theories propose that selective pressures influence potentially deleterious processes associated with aging only if they hinder reproductive success. Other aging theories attempt to reconcile stochastic theories with aspects of genetic/developmental theories in order to explain the regulation of maximum life span. However, there is still no single well-accepted theory that adequately unifies all or even most of the observations made in aging organisms. In addition, these theories are not necessarily mutually exclusive and their relative contributions may vary with tissue type, species, or biologic age.

6. Describe the currently plausible stochastic (random error) theories of aging.

STOCHASTIC (RANDOM ERROR) THEORIES	EXAMPLES
Somatic mutation	Ionizing radiation shortens life span
DNA repair	Decreased DNA repair capacity among shorter-lived species
Cross-linking	Altered extracellular matrix components impair cellular function
Glycosylation	Abnormal eye lens protein
Free radical	Higher levels of free radical metabolizing enzymes in longer-lived species

Examples of random error theories include the **somatic mutation theory**, which states that genetic damage from environmental insults, predominantly radiation, produces mutations in DNA such that inactivation of loci eventually causes failure in critical functions. Major support for this theory comes from the observation that ionizing radiation shortens life span; however, this exposure tends to cause an increase in initial mortality related to damage such as increased neoplastic disease and glomerulosclerosis. The **DNA repair theory** proposes that the inability to repair DNA damage is responsible for age-related detrimental effects. The direct correlation between species-specific DNA repair capacity and maximum life span potential lends some proof to this notion. The **cross-linking theory** asserts that altered macromolecules (e.g., protein) can impair normal cellular function and that accumulation of erroneous molecules eventually disrupts essential processes. Most of the evidence for this theory comes from studies of cross-linked extracellular matrix components, like collagen and elastin, which account for more than 20% of a mammal's body weight and are important for processes such as diffusion of essential molecules. Another type of cross-linking involves the nonenzymatic reaction of glucose with the amino acids of protein. This so-called **glycosylation theory** invokes a similar mechanism of error accumulation as above. Examples of glycosylated proteins include collagen and the eye lens protein crystallin.

Probably the best-known stochastic theory, especially among the lay public, is the **free radical theory** of aging. This theory proposes that most aging changes are due to molecular damage created by highly reactive chemical species that contain an unpaired electron. In normal aerobic metabolism, numerous single electron transfers take place that generate oxygen-derived free radicals. Although there are both enzymatic and nonenzymatic defenses against reactive oxygen species, some radicals do escape neutralization and react with cellular components. This theory is supported by the inverse relationship between free radical production and maximum life span potential as well as the presence of higher levels of free radical metabolizing enzymes in longer-lived species. However, efforts to increase life span in experimental animals with dietary antioxidants have not yet demonstrated a significant effect on median or maximum life span.

7. Describe the currently plausible developmental-genetic or programmed theories of aging.

Developmental-genetic theories are supported by the high conservation of maximum life span seen between species, by the similarity of attained age between monozygotic twins compared with dizygotic twins or nontwin siblings, by examples of exceptional longevity within families, and by the presence of subsets of aging features in human genetic diseases of premature aging (see below). The **neuroendocrine theory** regards functional decrements in neurons and associated hormones (e.g., the hypothalamic-pituitary-adrenal axis) as central to the aging process. Altered neuroendocrine control is an attractive programmed theory since early development, growth, puberty, reproduction, metabolism, and other elements of normal physiology are tightly regulated by hormonal axes. Decline in female reproductive capacity and alterations in growth hormone secretion are examples of age-related decrements in endocrine function. The contribution of this theory to aging in higher vertebrates lacking complex neuroendocrine systems is less clear. The **immunologic theory** is based on observations that the immune system declines with age as evidenced by a decreased response of T cells to growth signals, reduced resistance to infection, and autoimmune phenomena in which antibodies against self (autoantibodies) are produced. Again, complex immune systems are not found in all organisms that share similar aging phenotypes. The **rate of living** or **metabolic theory** held that life span across species would be inversely proportional to metabolic rate and that smaller mammals tended to have higher metabolic rates (adjusted for size) and shorter life spans than larger animals. This theory has largely been disproved by the identification of mammals that have both long lives and high metabolic rates (e.g., bats) or short lives and low metabolic rates (e.g., marsupials).

8. Discuss how evolution may influence aging.

The **evolutionary theory** of aging proposes that in species where the germ line is separate from somatic tissue, the risk of mortality increases with time after reproduction. This theory is based on the supposition that selective pressure to retain genes with a positive effect on reproductive fitness occurs in *young* individuals. Thus genes that confer early beneficial effects on reproduction will be selected by evolution, even if they may account for deleterious effects in later life, after reproduction and care of the young after birth. However, there is strong selective pressure to retain genes that diminish vulnerability in the young and old alike, that would both increase reproductive success and produce increases in longevity. Evidence in favor of the evolutionary theory comes from studies in flies and lower mammals, in which either intentionally or by examples of reduced predation in nature, respectively, the decreased need for early, rapid, and prolific reproduction caused extended life spans. Similarly, the exceptional longevity of birds and turtles, relative to comparably sized mammals, is though to be related to the selection of genes that favor later reproduction, independent of predator-free environments.

9. Describe the major hereditary syndromes of premature aging or progeroid syndromes.

Although no single genetic disorder recapitulates all of the commonly recognized manifestations of aging, several appear to approximate multiple aspects or segments of aging phenomena and are thus referred to as **segmental progeroid syndromes**.

Hutchinson-Gilford syndrome (progeria or "progeria of childhood") is characterized by profound growth retardation, sparse hair and subcutaneous fat, skin atrophy, atherosclerosis, and death at a median age of 12 by myocardial infarction or congestive heart failure.

Individuals with **Werner syndrome** ("progeria of adulthood") develop premature graying and loss of hair, thinning of the dermis, loss of subcutaneous fat, bilateral cataracts, osteoporosis, and arteriosclerosis as young adults. They have an increased incidence of cancer, especially sarcomas, and typically die in their mid-forties of degenerative vascular disease or neoplasia. The gene responsible for Werner syndrome has been identified as a helicase that unwinds double stranded nucleic acids and is likely the cause for several chromosomal abnormalities including DNA deletions. Interestingly, this helicase is one of a family of such unwinding enzymes (called RecQ) that together are responsible for at least three different syndromes which to varying degrees are marked by the onset of features resembling aging.

Down syndrome (DS) is distinguished by premature graying and loss of hair, hypogonadism, altered distribution of subcutaneous fat, short stature, hypotonia, premature lipofuscin deposits, cataracts, and neurodegeneration. High mortality rates secondary to infections and certain malignancies may be related to immune dysfunction. Mental retardation is also common in affected individuals. The trisomy on chromosome 21 is thought to account for a 50% increase in expression of some of the 50–100 genes located on the duplicated long arm, including one of the genes for the free radical scavenger superoxide dismutase (SOD1) and the gene that codes for the β-amyloid precursor protein (βPP). Thus, part of the DS phenotype may be caused by excessive oxidative stress as the result of increased hydrogen peroxide, the product of initial superoxide radical quenching catalyzed by SOD. The high prevalence of dementia in DS patients over age 40 (~95%) may potentially be explained by overexpression of βPP, as the amyloid found in brain plaques and blood vessels of DS patients is also found in patients with Alzheimer's disease.

10. What is cellular senescence? How may it contribute to processes associated with aging?

Cellular (replicative) senescence refers to the limited in vitro proliferative life span of somatic cells when placed in culture. This finite potential to divide has been interpreted as a manifestation of aging at the cellular level in those cell types that in vivo require the ability to proliferate as part of their function (e.g., fibroblasts during wound healing). Normal (nontumor) cells cease to proliferate after about 40–60 divisions but continue to exist in a metabolically active state with some characteristics of cells from aged individuals. Replicative senescence has served as a model to study the relationship between cellular aging and the molecular control of cell growth, differentiation, and neoplastic transformation (acquisition of unlimited growth capacity with invasiveness potential).

Noncoding DNA sequences at the ends of chromosomes, called **telomeres**, grow shorter with each mitotic division in postnatal life owing to the absence of **telomerase**, an enzyme complex that maintains the stability of telomere length. DNA damage accompanies the loss of telomeric sequences and potentially compromises genetic information near chromosomal ends. Average telomere length decreases with cellular senescence and with increasing age of the cell donor. Thus, telomere shortening provides strong circumstantial evidence that cellular senescence occurs in vivo.

The **p53 transcription factor** blocks proliferation of damaged cells. Induction of p53 can occur in response to a variety of triggers related to putative mechanisms of aging, including unrepaired DNA damage, oxidative stress, and telomeric shortening. Interestingly, an increase in p53 activity in genetically manipulated mice confers resistance to cancer but also produces an accelerated aging phenotype. In addition, malignant cells and tumors can express telomerase. Taken together, these results suggest that aging on the cellular level may be the price an organism must pay to protect against the development of cancer.

There is limited direct evidence for actual pathophysiologic effects due to cellular senescence in the organism. An exception is evidence that vascular endothelial cells in regions of blood vessels prone to atherosclerosis may undergo more cell divisions than endothelial cells in disease-free areas of the vasculature. In addition, osteoblast senescence may play an important role in age-related osteoporosis.

In summary, replicative senescence probably plays a role in age-related processes of unregulated cell proliferation and in age-related pathology associated with the loss of proliferative capacity. The aging of cells that normally do not divide in an organism (e.g., neurons) must therefore involve other mechanisms.

11. Why are biomarkers of aging important? How can they be identified?

True biomarkers of aging, if identified, would contribute greatly to the understanding of fundamental determinants of senescence. They would help in determining the biologic age of the individual and estimate life expectancy. Furthermore, they would facilitate monitoring the impact of various interventions on the rate of aging and standardizing studies in gerontologic research.

Primary criteria for a biomarker of aging include existence of a quantitative correlation between the biomarker and the age of subjects; evidence suggesting that the parameter is not altered with a disease process; confidence that an age-related alteration in the parameter is not secondary to metabolic or nutritional changes; demonstration that factors which influence the aging rate also alter the putative biomarker; and absence of the biomarker in immortal cells. None of the previously observed changes in biological parameters satisfies all criteria.

12. Describe successful interventions in the aging process.

The only known **dietary therapy** to retard most aspects of aging in mammals is **caloric restriction**. Typically, the level of restriction required has been a 30–60% reduction of calories, which produces extensions of both mean and maximum life span. The effect has been confirmed by controlled studies in a variety of species, including rodents, fish, flies, and worms. Controlled studies are under way in nonhuman primates, but only data for surrogate outcomes, such as improvements in serum glucose and insulin levels, are currently available. Observational findings in humans suggest a reduced mortality with a low-calorie diet or low body-mass index. However, the degree of caloric restriction needed to achieve a true anti-aging effect is probably too severe to be viewed as a practical regimen in all but a very small fraction of the population. Therefore, it will become necessary to define the mechanism(s) by which caloric restriction alters age-dependent processes that cause functional decline. As mentioned above, dietary supplementation with antioxidants has not yet been shown to significantly change median or maximum life span.

Successful **cell-based therapies** have largely been restricted to clinical trials of cell transplantation to restore function lost in certain disease states. For example, reintroduction of hematopoietic stem cells to patients with aplastic anemia or after chemotherapy does restore bone marrow function. Other transplantation studies using fetal tissue in patients with neurodegenerative disease or using pancreatic islet cells in diabetic patients should be considered experimental.

Hormonal therapies such as postmenopausal estrogen replacement have been used to prevent osteoporosis; however, recent studies have suggested that the risks of such replacement in terms of breast cancer, cardiovascular disease, and thromboembolism may outweigh the potential benefit. Testosterone replacement for androgen decline in the aging male (ADAM syndrome) is gaining clinical acceptance, but there are still questions regarding the testosterone level at which men have symptoms of hypogonadism, efficacy of testosterone replacement in the elderly man, and potential side effects. Postsomatopausal growth hormone replacement in humans is still strictly investigational. Hypophysectomy (removal of the pituitary gland) and administration of dehydroepiandrosterone (DHEA) extend the life span of rodents, but this may be related to a reduction in food intake. Melatonin can also increase median life span in rats and mice by unknown mechanisms, but food intake was not carefully monitored.

Successful **genetic manipulations** have been described in both mammalian and invertebrate species. The "Ames dwarf" mutation, designated *df*, produces a developmental deficiency of the pituitary when mice receive two copies of the mutant allele. Homozygous *df/df* mice have a near-total absence of growth hormone, prolactin, and thyroid-stimulating hormone as well as a one-third reduction in normal body weight. These mice have a 49 to 68% increase in life span, depending on male or female sex, respectively. Another mouse mutation, the "Snell dwarf" mutant (*dw*), leads to low growth hormone production, a very small body size, and dramatic life span extension. Long-lived strains of fruit flies and nematodes have been obtained by selective breeding. Length of life has been increased in nematodes and yeast by specific single-gene mutations and fruit flies exhibit extended life when made to overexpress both superoxide dismutase and catalase.

Other manipulations including reduction in body temperature and voluntary exercise have also been shown to affect life span. As examples, a low body temperature increases median and maximum life span in many poikilothermic animal species (animals whose body temperatures fluctuate with the environment) and voluntary exercise in rats increases average life span. Habitual exercise does increase life expectancy in humans, but whether it also extends the maximum length of life remains an open issue.

BIBLIOGRAPHY

1. Ahmed A, Tollefsbol T: Telomeres and telomerase: Basic science implications for aging. J Am Geriatr Soc 49:1105, 2001.
2. Bohr VA: Human premature aging syndromes and genomic instability. Mechan Aging Develop 123:987, 2002.
3. Carlson JC, Riley JCM: A consideration of some notable aging theories. Exper Gerontol 33:127, 1998.
4. Cristofalo VJ, Pignolo RJ, Allen RG: Cell aging in vitro. In Maddox GL (ed): The Encyclopedia of Aging. New York, Springer Publishing Company, 2002, pp 172–175.
5. Finch CE: Longevity, Senescence, and the Genome. Chicago, University of Chicago Press, 1990.
6. Miller RA: The biology of aging and longevity. In Hazzard WR, Blass JP, Ettinger WH, et al (eds): Principles of Geriatric Medicine and Gerontology, 4th ed. New York, McGraw-Hill, 1999, pp 1–19.
7. Mooradian AD: Biomarkers of aging: Do we know what to look for? J Gerontol Biol Sci 45:B183, 1990.
8. Perls T, Kunkel L, Puca A: The genetics of aging. Curr Opin Genet Develop 12:362, 2002.
9. Sharpless NE, DePinho RA: p53: good cop/bad cop. Cell 110:9, 2002.
10. Vojta CL, Fraga PD, Forciea MA, et al: Antiaging therapy: An overview. Hosp Pract 36:43, 2001.

3. COMPREHENSIVE GERIATRIC ASSESSMENT

Mary Ann Forciea, MD

Mrs. Roosevelt is an 84-year-old retired secretary who presents for evaluation of "slowing down." She lives alone in her 2-bedroom home of 60 years. She is accompanied by her daughter, who also adds that her mother has reduced her activities outside the home, such as attendance at church, participation in bridge club, and volunteer work at the community hospital. The patient's primary care physician retired 2 years ago; the patient has not pursued medical care since that time. She takes no medications. She admits that she would like "more energy."

The initial evaluation of an older patient with a nonspecific chief complaint can be challenging for patient and practitioner. Older patients are often reluctant to seek medical care; they are often compelled by family members to participate in health evaluations. The past medical history of older patients can be extensive and retold with great relish but focused on memory rather than data. Medications are occasionally brought to the evaluation in shopping bags or suitcases! Practitioners must, in a timely manner, develop a "priority list" among complaints, ordered both by medical importance and patient preference. Comprehensive Geriatric Assessment is the approach used in health settings in which older patients are found; it allows geriatrics professionals to plan for care.

1. What does Comprehensive Geriatric Assessment imply?

Comprehensive Geriatric Assessment (CGA) is the evaluation of the older patient that is focused on

- Physical health
- Mental health
- Functional status
- Social functioning
- Environment

The goal of the evaluation is to plan care that will maximize independence and prevent future disability. CGA is usually performed by a team of professionals. The assessment is called multidisciplinary if the team members practice in different sites but are coordinated by a single practitioner (often by the primary care practitioner). Interdisciplinary evaluations are performed by teams that practice in the same site with coordination achieved through a team meeting. The resulting treatment plan must often address needs of a caregiver as well as of the patient herself.

2. Why bother with Comprehensive Geriatric Assessment?

Benefits of CGA have now been identified in a number of studies:

- Decreased nursing facility admission
- Decreased medication use
- Decreased mortality
- Decreased annual medical care costs
- Increased diagnostic accuracy
- Improved independence

At 2 years following CGA, benefits have been seen in

- Decreased permanent nursing facility stays
- Increased survival without decreased quality of life
- Increased independent functioning

Benefits found less consistently include

- Decreased use of hospital-based services
- Decreased short-term mortality rates
- Identified use of community services

Potential barriers to CGA include cost, time (CGAs require more time than routine office visits), and involvement of professionals such as social workers whose time is unreimbursed in the office setting. The availability of team members with training in geriatrics and with team practice skills can also be limiting.

3. What disciplines are represented in teams performing CGA?

The minimal team composition usually includes a physician geriatrician (internal medicine or family practice), nursing professional, and social worker (usually at the MSW level). Teams can be enriched by colleagues from geriatric psychiatry, neurology, podiatry, pharmacy, palliative care, sleep disorders, rehabilitation, dentistry, continence, and/or spiritual counselors. The composition of the team influences referrals and special expertise.

4. Which patients are candidates for CGA?

The vast majority of older patients receive excellent care from traditional primary care providers. Patients who will benefit most from CGA are considered the "frail" elderly. Frailty can be defined by

- Number of medical diagnoses
- Number of prescription medications
- Functional limitations in two or more activities of daily living (see below)

Candidates for CGA can also be selected by instruments (questionnaires) administered by mail, over the telephone, or face to face in the office. A variety of such screening instruments have been described.

5. What special features of the medical history should be emphasized during CGA?

A careful history is the foundation of any medical assessment. Thorough, careful asking and listening produce the most efficient and satisfying interaction for patient and practitioner.

The **patient profile** section of the history should include the patient's current residence (e.g., house, apartment, nursing facility) since this information is critical to either discharge planning in the hospital or care planning in the office, home, or nursing facility setting. Any caregiver who is regularly involved with the patient should also be indicated in this section. The patient's employment history is often mentioned because it can be critical to the patient's self-image.

The **history of the present illness (HPI)** is little changed from that in the traditional history. On many occasions it may have to be separated into two or even three components for the patient with several active problems.

Medication review is fundamental in CGA because errors in medication prescribing and adherence are so prevalent in older populations. Patients should be instructed to bring all medications to the visit (or have family bring them to the hospital). Pills or bottles should be shown to the patient and queries made about indication, schedules, and compliance. Over-the-counter and eye medications should always be included in the review.

The **family history** is slightly less important in patients who have already lived to old age than in children and young adults. Factors that are still important include age of parents at death and significant illnesses in parents or siblings, such as dementia, early Parkinson's disease, atherosclerotic cardiovascular disease, diabetes mellitus, hypertension, and cancer.

An extended **social history** is the most obvious difference between the medical examination of the usual primary care adult and CGA. In older patients, we must continue to ask about alcohol, tobacco, or drug use, since behaviors can still change in late life. Even frail older patients may still be sexually active; inquires about sexual activity continue to be important in late life. In addition, we need to ask about driving status and alternatives to driving available to the patient. A brief description of the home is necessary for patients still living at home. Is stair climbing required? Where are the bathrooms? Are smoke detectors in use? Who is available as a caregiver or informal supporter? Are any formal community support services, such as visiting nurses or home health aides, in place?

The **past history** should document surgery, hospitalizations, and major illnesses. Surgery involving prosthetic valves, artificial joints, and metal plates or screws is especially critical and should be documented on the problem list because of the implications for antibiotic coverage for invasive procedures and MRI scans.

The **review of systems** should pay special attention to alterations in memory, weight change, falls, sleep problems, and sensory losses. Questioning about urinary incontinence should be emphasized as well as information about bowel habits. A dietary history can be obtained as part of the systems review unless weight change is a special problem. In that case, more careful questioning should be part of the HPI.

6. What special components of the physical examination should be emphasized during CGA?

On an initial visit, the **vital signs** should include blood pressure in both arms as well as an orthostatic blood pressure determination. Since osteoporosis is so prevalent, height as well as weight should be determined.

Examination of the **skin** should involve careful searches for bruising and evidence of pressure ulceration. This aspect of the examination is especially important in the inpatient initial assessment of patients admitted from nursing facilities.

Eye examinations can be complicated by the presence of cataracts. Pupillary dilation can be performed after risk of glaucoma exacerbation is evaluated. Impacted earwax can make **auditory evaluation** difficult. This aspect of the examination may need to be postponed until wax is softened with drops or manually removed. The **oral cavity** should be inspected for dental/gingival problems in patients with teeth. Edentulous patients should still be carefully examined for irritated areas associated with dentures and for oral cancers.

Cardiovascular examinations should include information about pulse presence and bruits. Palpation for possible abdominal aortic aneurysm should be performed. Cardiac murmurs are common in older patients. Echocardiographic documentation of valvular disease and ventricular compliance may be required.

For patients with urinary incontinence, a **pelvic examination** should be performed, looking for vaginal atrophy, prolapse, or constipation. The lateral position may be more comfortable for older women, especially for those with significant hip osteoarthritis.

Examination of the **muscles and joints** should focus on tone, range of motion, and signs of inflammation.

Examination of **gait and balance** is an important aspect of CGA for any patient who is mobile. This portion of the examination should be performed with the patient in street clothes and shoes, if possible. One commonly used screening assessment of gait is the "get-up-and-go" test. The patient is timed while rising from a chair, walking 10 feet, turning, and returning to the chair. A normal time is 10 second or less.

6. Are laboratory tests a standard part of CGA?

No area of assessment is more individual than that of laboratory testing. No single laboratory test is required; many patients have periodic health determinations as part of the visit (see Chapter 19). Some require blood tests for medication monitoring. Many need a urinalysis for incontinence. Those with complaints related to the cardiovascular system require electrocardiograms. For patients in whom congregate day care or nursing facility transfer is considered, a purified protein derivative (PPD) test may be required.

Mrs. Washington is an 82-year-old retired librarian who lives alone in a 1-bedroom apartment. Her medical diagnoses include osteoarthritis of hips and knees, osteoporosis, and type II diabetes mellitus with peripheral neuropathy.

Mrs. Lincoln is an 82-year-old retired elementary school teacher who lives alone in her home. Her medical diagnoses include osteoarthritis of hips and knees, osteoporosis, and type II diabetes mellitus with peripheral neuropathy.

7. What is a functional status assessment?

If you are listening to the two patient profiles above on rounds, would you be surprised to learn that one of these women is an avid outdoorswoman who still hikes and volunteers with state park cleanups and one is housebound by immobility? Without an understanding of the consequences of disease on the activities of an individual older patient, we cannot begin to collaborate with our colleagues and with our patients themselves to maximize independence. Functional status assessment is one means to focus on the individual patient and his/her goals within the context of that patient's medical problems.

Functional status assessment is traditionally split into evaluation of:

1. **Activities of daily life** (ADLs, or skills required for basic living)
   - Mobility
   - Toilet use
   - Feeding
   - Dressing
   - Bathing
   - Transfers between bed and chair or from bed to standing
2. Instrumental activities of daily living (IADLs, or skills involving the manipulation of an instrument)
   - Shopping
   - Travel
   - Telephone use
   - Meal preparation
   - Medication administration
   - Finances
   - Laundry

Patients are often "scored" by whether they perform these tasks independently, require assistance, or are totally dependent on others to perform these tasks. Most functional status assessment is performed by patient or caregiver self-report on a questionnaire. The most thorough functional status assessments are performed by occupational therapists, and are conducted in the patient's own home. Many practices save these thorough but expensive assessments for patients who indicate serious problems on initial questionnaire-based assessments. Simple functional tests such as the "get up and go" mentioned above are often useful. Sensory assessments by hand-held audiometers and Snellen charts still have a place in screening for conditions that limit function.

8. What special areas are the domains of social work in Comprehensive Geriatric Assessment?

In no area of adult medicine does the social worker play a more essential role than in the assessment of the frail older adult. Outstanding identification of illness and cutting-edge therapy are useless for the patient who is completely isolated or cannot afford medications. The social work team member has the best training and skills to assess needs and eligibility for services such as

- Home delivered meals
- Transportation for the disabled
- Low income medication assistance programs
- Home health aides

Social workers can help patients and families with reviews of finances either for eligibility for government-supported services or for initial help in estate planning. Many social workers perform counseling for advance directive completion. Suspicions of abuse or neglect of an older patient should always be reported to the social work team member. Many social workers are able to provide bereavement support or counseling about sexuality or marital discord in late life.

9. How is the patient's home environment evaluated?

Patients undergoing CGA in the office, hospital, or nursing facility setting should be questioned about architectural features such as stairs, location of bathrooms, and front-door security. Some visiting nurse agencies are able to send a visiting nurse for a one-time assessment of the patient's home. The optimal environmental assessment is performed by a team member who makes a home visit as part of the evaluation. During this visit, access and safety features such as smoke alarms and bathroom "grab bars" can be checked. The patient can demonstrate medication adherence, and an optimal assessment of functional status performance can be done. The team member who visits the patient at home can provide critical useful information to the team meeting.

10. How is Comprehensive Geriatric Assessment concluded?

In the **multidisciplinary** model, an individual professional (usually the primary care practitioner) reviews examination findings, diagnostic studies, and consultants' reports. That professional devises an individual plan of care for the patient and meets with the patient and family to communicate results.

In the **interdisciplinary** model, the team members meet together to share findings and therapy options. Working together, the team develops a plan of care for the patient. Selected team members are designated to meet with the patient and family. At that family meeting the plan can be altered to suit the concerns of patient and family. A written report of findings and therapeutic plan is generated for patient/family and, if the patient agrees, for the referring provider.

BIBLIOGRAPHY

1. Ham RJ, Sloan PD: Primary Care Geriatrics: A Case-Based Approach, 3rd ed. St. Louis, Mosby, 1997.
2. Studenski S, Perera S, Wallace D, et al: Physical performance measures in the clinical setting. J Am Geriatr Assoc 51:314–322, 2003.
3. Wang L, van Belle G, Kukull WB, Larson EB: Predictors of functional change: A longitudinal study of nondemented people aged 65 and older. J Am Geriatr Assoc 50:1525–1534, 2002.

4. COLLABORATIVE PRACTICE

Jean Yudin, MSN, RN, CS, and Mary Ann Forciea, MD

1. Define collaborative practice.

Collaboration is the process whereby health professionals from different disciplines plan and practice together as colleagues. Each professional works within the boundaries of his or her own discipline's scope of practice but with shared values and mutual respect for all contributions. The result of this process is a coordinated plan of care focused on the patient and caregiver. The professionals organized in this manner often refer to themselves as a team.

Medicare defines collaborative practice as a joint practice of an advance practice nurse (such as a nurse practitioner) and a physician to deliver health care services. In reality, many more varieties of professional health care teams exist.

2. Why is collaborative practice important for older patients?

Functional declines in older patients can be due to a constellation of changes in physical, emotional, or environmental homeostasis. Failure to recognize the broader context of a medical complaint can limit solutions. Managing these complex syndromes requires the skills from different disciplines. Each health professional brings a different knowledge base with which to identify and solve clinical problems. Collaboration in the elucidation of problems and in the development of solutions leads to better functional outcomes.

3. What are the benefits of collaborative practices?

Studies have demonstrated that the use of an interdisciplinary team can positively affect cost by reducing hospital admissions. The team approach has also been shown to improve mental status evaluation scores, increase functional status, and improve patients' perceived well being. Much literature and many studies have shown the positive effects of interdisciplinary teams; inherent in the concept of interdisciplinary teams is collaboration among disciplines. Most often, these studies analyzed the relationship between physicians and nurses and effect on outcomes.

Effective collaboration can:
- Ensure a comprehensive analysis of the patient's problems
- Guarantee that the team will hear and understand each provider's views
- Enhance the potential for innovative solutions to problems or care plans
- Improve relations among providers
- Encourage a high level of commitment to the plan of care

4. What are the advantages and barriers to effective collaboration?

Collaboration occurs when providers work together and demonstrate shared planning, decision making, and mutual accountability for decisions and responsibility in the care of the patient. Team members show trust, mutual respect, and understanding of each discipline's skills. Other characteristics of collaboration include collegiality and cooperation among team members.

Some health care professionals may find collaborative practice threatening because of potential role ambiguity (e.g., where do the boundaries between physician and nurse fall?) Power sharing in decision making is not always easy. The initial increase in time required to collaborate with other professionals may seem burdensome.

Financial limitations may also undermine efforts at collaboration; some team members are not reimbursed appropriately. Many third-party payors do not reimburse for team meeting time.

5. What does collaborative practice look like?

The concept of collaboration can be difficult to define. Descriptive words are often used and may describe aspects of specific practices, not necessarily the actual components of collaboration.

One component of collaboration is structure, and structure refers to communication. There are three different models of communication; one is hierarchal, whereas the other two are collaborative.

–Unidirectional
  communication
–Physician driven
–Often used in
  hospitals

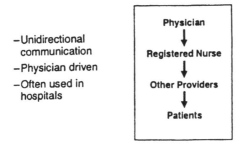

Hierarchical model.

The second model is collaborative because communication flows both ways among providers and patient. A drawback to this model is that communication is bidirectional rather than multidirectional; the physician still tends to be in the lead. There is often limited communication between physician and patient.

- Collaborative
- Physician led
- Barriers between
  physician and patient
- Often found in office
  based practice

Bidirectional communication.

The third model is also collaborative. Communication is multidirectional, and the model is patient-centered. There is the probability of equal input from all disciplines. This model allows flexibility for involvement of each discipline, and the team, including the patient, determines the plan of care.

- Patient centered
- Most ideal model
  for home care
  collaboration

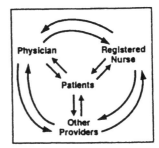

Multidirectional communication.

A second element of collaboration is process. Collaboration requires participants to be maximally assertive and cooperative rather than capitulation of one person to keep another team member satisfied. The final component of collaboration is outcomes. Most definitions of collaboration do not specify one or two outcomes that affirm one collaboration. One outcome often used is that collaboration leads to the development of a new plan of care that would not be developed by an individual provider, no matter what his or her field.

6. List important dynamics of collaboration.
- Providers are interdependent.
- Providers solve problems by dealing constructively with differences.
- Providers are responsible for reaching agreement; they "own" the decisions jointly.
- Providers are responsible for ensuring the future of the collaboration.
- A collaborative team is constantly evolving.

7. What kinds of professionals are found in collaborative practices?
Collaborative practice teams traditionally include a physician (often in primary care), an advanced practice nurse, and a social worker. Other team members can come from psychiatry, rehabilitation disciplines (physical therapy, occupational therapy, speech therapy), dentistry, pharmacy, neurology, podiatry, and community-based nursing, to name only a few. The enthusiasm of the professional for team practice and coordinated care is essential.

8. What characterizes successful collaborative practices?
- Appropriate goals are set for the patient.
- Clear role expectations are developed for team members.
- Flexible decision making is apparent.
- Shared responsibility for outcomes is evident.
- Methods of organized and regular communication are in place (a team meeting would be an example of such communication).

9. What outcomes are achieved in successful collaborative practices?
- Novel care plans are developed for each patient. The plan reflects input from all team members.
- Patient care is improved.
- Patient satisfaction is improved.
- Appropriate planning decisions are made.

BIBLIOGRAPHY

1. Arangelo V, Fitzgerald M, Carroll D, Plumb GD: Collaborative care between nurse practitioners and primary care physicians. Models Ambul Care 23(1), 1996.
2. Burchell RC, Thomas DA, Smith HL: Some considerations for implementing collaborative practice. Am J Med 74:9–13, 1983.
3. Gray B: Collaborating: Finding Common Ground for Multiparty Problems. 1999.
4. Hyer K, Fagerty E, Fairchild S, et al (eds): Geriatric Interdisciplinary Training Program Curriculum Guide. 2001.
5. Leipzig D, Hyer K, Kirsten E, et al: Attitudes toward working on interdisciplinary health care teams: A comparison by disciplines. J Am Geriatr Soc 50:1141–1148, 2002.
6. Mellor J, Hyer K, Howe J: Geriatric interdisciplinary team approach: Challenges and opportunities in educating trainees together from a variety of disciplines. Educ Gerontol 28:867–880, 2002.
7. Ruble TL, Thomas KW: Support for a two-dimensional model of conflict behavior. Organ Behav Hum Perform 16:143–155, 1976.
8. Siegler E, Whitney F: Nurse-Physician Collaboration Care of Adults and the Elderly. New York, Springer, 1994.

5. MEDICARE: A BRIEF GUIDE FOR PROVIDERS AND PATIENTS

Jennifer Tjia, MD, MSCE, and Donna Brady Raziano, MD, MBA

1. What is Medicare? How is Medicare financed?

Medicare is a federally funded health insurance program implemented in 1966 under President Lyndon Johnson's Great Society as a health insurance program for the elderly. Medicare has two parts: Part A (Hospital Insurance), which helps cover inpatient care in hospitals, skilled nursing care, some home health care, and hospice care, and Part B (Medical Insurance), which helps cover physicians' services, outpatient hospital services (including emergency room visits), ambulatory surgery, diagnostic tests, laboratory services, and durable medical equipment.

Parts A and B are financed from four different sources, including mandatory contributions by employers and employees, general tax revenues, premiums paid by beneficiaries, and deductibles and copayments. The most important of these are employer and employee contributions. Some 151 million employees make mandatory contributions to Medicare's Part A Hospital Insurance Trust Fund during their working years, with the expectation of receiving benefits at retirement. The money contributed by employees that finances Medicare's Hospital Insurance Trust Fund is not set aside to meet their own future health expenses. Rather, it is used to cover the medical bills of people who are currently covered by Medicare.

2. Who is eligible for Medicare? How do patients enroll in Medicare?

In general, people over the age of 65 (and their spouses) who have had Medicare taxes deducted from their paychecks for at least 10 years (40 calendar-year quarters) are entitled to coverage through Part A without paying a premium. Others may be able to purchase Part A coverage. In addition, people who qualified for Social Security or Railroad Retirement disability benefits for at least 24 months and people with end-stage renal disease (permanent kidney failure requiring dialysis or a kidney transplant) are eligible to receive Medicare benefits.

People sign up for Medicare at the Social Security office. All eligible Medicare beneficiaries are automatically enrolled in Part A. The enrollment period begins three months before the 65th birthday and ends three months after. After this enrollment period, people may enroll during the general enrollment period of January 1 through March 31. Medicare coverage begins on the first July 1 after enrollment. For people who delay enrollment beyond the initial enrollment period at age 65, any Part A or B charge that they subsequently pay will be higher. At age 65, people become eligible for Part B coverage if they are entitled to Part A coverage or if they are citizens or permanent residents of the United States. Enrollment in Part B is voluntary, although most beneficiaries participate. For enrollment in Part B, Medicare beneficiaries must pay a premium (currently $50 a month) that usually is taken out of their monthly Social Security checks. In addition, the enrollee is responsible for deductibles and copayments under both Parts A and B.

3. If a beneficiary is hospitalized, how much does Medicare pay? How much does the beneficiary pay?

Part A coverage pays for inpatient care for up to 90 days of a spell of illness. A spell of illness or benefit period begins the day when the patient enters the hospital and ends when the patient has been out of the hospital for 60 consecutive days. For each hospital spell of illness, the patient is required to pay a separate deductible ($812 in 2002). Medicare then pays for all covered services for the first 60 days. For days 61–90 in a spell of illness, the patient is required to pay a daily copayment. The Medicare inpatient benefit ends at 90 days for a given spell of illness. However, each Medicare recipient is entitled to 60 lifetime reserve days that can be used if a spell of illness lasts longer than 90 days. The patient decides when and how many reserve days to use. Patients and their families should choose wisely; they should budget their use of 60 days over their lifetime or consider purchasing a Medigap plan to cover additional reserve days (see question 10).

4. What is the difference between a deductible, copayment, and coinsurance?

A **deductible** is a set dollar amount that person must pay before insurance coverage for medical expenses can begin. A **copayment** is a fixed amount that a beneficiary pays to the provider for a specific service (e.g., $5 or $10 per service). **Coinsurance** is a percentage of costs of medical care that patients pay themselves. Coinsurance rates are generally in the 10–20% range.

Summary of Traditional Medicare 2002

Part A	
Benefits	**Beneficiary Pays**
Inpatient hospital	Deductible of $812 per spell of illness/benefit period
Days 1–60	No copay
Days 61–90	$203 per day
60 lifetime reserve days	$406 per day
Skilled nursing facility	
Days 1–20	No copay
Days 21–100	$101.50 per day
After 100 days	Pay 100% cost per day
	There is a limit of 100 days of Medicare Part A SNF coverage in each spell of illness/benefit period.
Home health care	No coinsurance
Hospice	Small payment for drugs and inpatient respite care
Part B	
Benefits	**Beneficiary Pays**
Deductible	$100 (once per calendar year)
Physician and other medical services	
MD accepts assignment	20% coinsurance
MD does not accept assignment	20% coinsurance plus up to 15% over Medicare-approved fee
Outpatient hospital care	20% coinsurance
Ambulatory surgical services	20% coinsurance
X-rays, durable medical equipment	20% coinsurance
Physical, speech, and occupational therapy	20% coinsurance, maximum benefit $1500.00
Clinical diagnostic laboratory services	No coinsurance
Home health care	No coinsurance
Outpatient mental health services	50% coinsurance
Preventive services	
Flu shots	No coinsurance
Pneumococcal vaccines	No coinsurance
Colorectal cancer screenings	
Fecal occult blood test	No coinsurance
Flexible sigmoidoscopy or colonoscopy	25% coinsurance
Prostate-cancer screening	
Prostate-specific antigen (PSA) test	No coinsurance
Digital rectal examination	20% coinsurance
Mammogram	20% coinsurance
Pap smear	No coinsurance
Pelvic exam	20% coinsurance
Bone mass measurement	20% coinsurance
Glaucoma screening	20% coinsurance
Diabetes monitoring	20% coinsurance

5. How do hospitals and providers get paid by Medicare Part A?

Medicare Part A uses regional insurance companies ("intermediaries") to pay hospitals, nursing homes, home-care agencies, and hospice programs for the Medicare-covered services they provide. Participating organizations that meet Medicare's conditions of participation take part in the program without regard to whether they are affiliated with health plans or aggregated medical groups. Coverage amounts and limits for inpatient hospitalizations are determined under a fixed prospective rate rather than the amount hospitals bill or spend. Prospective payments are determined in advance, based on the average cost of treating the patient's principal diagnosis (diagnosis-related groups or DRGs), adjusted for area wages, costs of medical teaching programs, and a hospital's share of low-income patients.

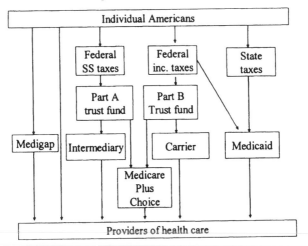

Flow of funds for the health care for older Americans. (From Boult C: Geriatric Review Syllabus, 5th ed., 2002, with permission.)

6. If a beneficiary makes an outpatient physician visit, how much does Medicare pay? How much does the beneficiary pay?

Medicare pays for services only by participating providers. Because of the regulations for reimbursement, most providers participate in Medicare. Traditional Medicare recipients are responsible for paying an annual deductible of $100. After the deductible, Medicare pays 80% of allowable charges for the rest of the calendar year and the patient is responsible for 20% of the Medicare-allowed charges for services rendered during the visit.

7. How do physicians get paid by Medicare Part B?

Providers that meet Medicare's conditions of participation can submit claims to their regional insurance companies ("carriers"). These providers accept Medicare's fee for the service (80% of the pre-established allowed amount) and bill the patient or their secondary insurer for no more than 20% coinsurance payment. For services not covered by Medicare, the physician may bill the patient, if the provider discloses the charges before the services are rendered and the patient agrees in advance in writing. Participating providers include physicians, nurse practitioners, social workers, psychologists, rehabilitation therapists, home-care agencies, ambulances, outpatient facilities, and suppliers of durable medical equipment.

8. What services are not covered by Medicare?

Neither Traditional Part A nor Part B of the Medicare program covers outpatient medications, dental care, hearing aids, eyeglasses, foot care, orthopedic shoes, cosmetic surgery, care in foreign countries, or long-term custodial care in nursing homes. Few preventive services other than mammography, Pap smear, immunization, prostate-specific antigen screening, and bone mineral density testing are covered by traditional Medicare.

9. What is Medicaid?

Medicaid, like Medicare, is a joint federal and state program that provides health insurance to people who have low incomes and limited savings. Medicaid was enacted in 1964 and is part of the federal and state welfare system. Before 1965, physicians and hospitals often gave out charity care or billed on a sliding-scale basis. States have some discretion in determining which groups their Medicaid programs will cover and the financial criteria for Medicaid eligibility. Within broad national guidelines that the federal government provides, each of the states: (1) establishes its own eligibility standards; (2) determines the type, amount, duration, and scope of services; (3) sets the rate of payment for services; and (4) administers its own program. The exact income eligibility criteria differ by state but it generally does not include private homes in asset evaluation. In several states, one can become eligible after "spending down" assets. The types of services covered include payment of Medicare deductibles and copayments, outpatient prescription drugs, and long-term custodial care in nursing homes.

10. What is Medigap?

In July 1992, the federal government approved 10 types of standardized insurance policies (A through J) designed to supplement or fill the gaps of Medicare coverage. Private insurance companies offer fee-for-service (FFS) Medigap plans according to the benefits they cover. These plans pay the deductibles, coinsurance, and some out-of-pocket expenses not covered by Medicare. Before these plans were standardized, Medicare beneficiaries had to choose among many vague Medicare supplemental policies, resulting in patients purchasing either inadequate or duplicative coverage. Both federal and state laws govern the sales of Medigap insurance and insurers may not sell a policy that duplicates the patient's present health plan or sell a policy that is not one of the ten approved standard policies.

Each plan includes a core benefit package that includes both Part A hospital coinsurance, starting from day 61, and Part B coinsurance (20% of Medicare approved charges). All ten plans cover an additional 365 days of reserve days. The core benefits do no include the Part A inpatient deductible ($812 in 2002) or the Part B $100 annual deductible. Medigap plans do not cover long-term care, dental care, eyeglasses, hearing aids, or private-duty nursing.

Ten Standard Medigap Policies by Plan Type and Number of Policies Purchased, 1999

BENEFITS	A	B	C	D	E	F	G	H	I	J
Core benefit	X	X	X	X	X	X	X	X	X	X
SNF coinsurance			X	X	X	X	X	X	X	X
Part A deductible		X	X	X	X	X	X	X	X	X
Part B deductible			X		X					X
Part B balance billing						X	X		X	X
Foreign travel emergency			X	X	X	X	X	X	X	X
Home health care				X			X		X	X
Prescription drugs								X	X	X
Preventive medical care				X						X
Percent of policies	4%	13%	26%	6%	2%	37%	2%	2%	2%	4%

From Kaiser Family Foundation: Medicare Chart Book, 2nd ed. 2001, with permission.

For a new Medicare beneficiary at age 65, the premium for A-level plans ranges from $40 to $125 per month. J-level plans cost from $175 to $400 per month. Within 6 months of initial enrollment in Medicare Part B, beneficiaries are entitled to purchase any Medigap policy on the market at advertised prices. After this open enrollment period, Medigap insurers can refuse to insure individual beneficiaries or charge them higher premiums because of their past or present health problems.

11. What is Medicare + Choice?

With the enactment of the Balanced Budget Act of 1997, Congress and the Clinton adminis-tration approved extensive reforms and new provisions to the Medicare program. The reforms were intended to expand the choices among private health plans that beneficiaries may select by creating Medicare Part C, also known as the Medicare + Choice program. These provisions ex-panded the array of insurance plan choices beyond fee-for-service indemnity coverage and health maintenance organizations to include:

- Provider-sponsored organizations (PSOs): partnerships of physician groups and hospitals that accept capitation payments and deliver Medicare-covered health services to their en-rolled patients
- Preferred provider organizations (PPOs): alliances of providers that accept capitation pay-ments and deliver Medicare-covered health services to their enrolled patients
- Private fee-for-service plans (FFS): plans that may charge beneficiaries a premium, pay providers more liberally than the original Medicare FFS plan does, and allow physicians to charge their patients copayments of up to 15%
- Medical savings accounts (MSAs): available on a limited basis, these are accounts into which Medicare beneficiaries can make tax-deductible contributions and out of which they can with-draw funds to purchase routine health-related goods and services from any Medicare provider.
- Medicare health maintenance organizations (HMOs): a type of managed care plan in which care is delivered within a network of providers. This is the most important and prevalent type of Medicare + Choice plan available to beneficiaries.

If a beneficiary chooses to enroll in Part C, Medicare pays a set amount of money per benefi-ciary every month to the participating health plan. In turn, the Medicare + Choice plan manages the Medicare coverage for its members and is responsible for paying for services that beneficiaries re-quire. At a minimum, Part C plans must provide all services that traditional Medicare covers. In order to attract enrollees, most Medicare HMOs often offer additional benefits such as prescription drugs or additional reserve days for inpatient hospitalizations at low or no premiums, deductibles, or copayments. The HMOs achieve cost savings by managing the patient's use of services, including restriction of care to contracted providers and limit care through various managed care techniques.

Each November, beneficiaries covered by Part A and Part B have their option of joining any Medicare HMO (a managed care organization or [MCO]) operating in their area and cannot be denied enrollment because of any preexisting health problem except end-stage renal disease. Enrollees continue to pay their monthly Medicare Part B premium and may also have to pay an additional monthly fee to the HMO. Availability of HMO plans depends on the beneficiary's geo-graphic area.

12. Does Medicare pay for outpatient prescription drugs?

Medicare does not pay for outpatient prescription drugs except for medications related to some types of cancer or end-stage renal disease. For qualifying low-income beneficiaries, Medicaid covers outpatient prescription drugs through individual state plans. Additionally, as of 2003, 24 states* offer prescription drugs for low-income beneficiaries who do not qualify for Medicaid. Other Medi-care beneficiaries may obtain coverage for outpatient prescription drugs through a Medigap plan type H, I, or J. However, these plans are of limited benefit because of high monthly premiums, high annual deductibles (~$1,500), and/or maximum annual prescription limits ($1500 to $3000).

A low-cost alternative to paying out of pocket for the full cost of medications is to enroll in a Medicare HMO that offers an outpatient prescription drug plan. But this managed care benefit is offset by formularies, tiered copayments, and annual coverage changes. Most pharmaceutical companies offer outpatient prescription assistance programs for eligible low-income seniors and

---

* California, Connecticut, Delaware, Florida, Illinois, Indiana, Iowa, Kansas, Maine, Maryland, Massa-chusetts, Michigan (closed except for emergency coverage as of 2003), Minnesota, Missouri, Nevada, New Hampshire, New Jersey, New York, North Carolina, Pennsylvania, Rhode Island, South Carolina, Vermont, West Virginia, Wyoming

the disabled. These programs are becoming more innovative in ways to market to the consumer and simultaneously minimize the negative publicity of rising drug costs.

13. If a beneficiary needs skilled nursing and rehabilitation after an acute hospitalization, how much does Medicare pay? How much does the beneficiary pay?

Medicare pays up to 100 days. The first 20 days are fully covered. Days 21–100 have copayment ($101.50 in 2003). In order to qualify, a beneficiary must require skilled nursing needs 7 days a week. There is no benefit that covers custodial care in a nursing home. Medicare will cover skilled care only if **all** these conditions are met:

1. You have Medicare Part A (Hospital Insurance) and have days left in your benefit period to use.

2. You have a qualifying hospital stay. This means an inpatient hospital stay of 3 consecutive days or more, not including the day you leave the hospital. You must enter the SNF within a short time (generally 30 days) of leaving the hospital. After you leave the SNF, if you re-enter the same or another SNF within 30 days, you don not need another 3-day qualifying hospital stay to get additional SNF benefits. This is also true if you stop getting skilled care while in the SNF and then start getting skilled care again within 30 days.

3. Your doctor has decided that you need daily skilled care. It must be given by, or under the direct supervision of, skilled nursing or rehabilitation staff. If you are in the SNF for skilled rehabilitation services only, your care is considered daily care even if these therapy services are offered just 5 or 6 days a week.

4. You get these skilled services in a SNF that has been certified by Medicare.

5. You need these skilled services for a medical condition that:
   • Was treated during a qualifying 3-day hospital stay, or
   • Started while you were getting Medicare-covered SNF care. For example, if you are in the SNF because you had a stroke and you fall and sprain your wrist.

14. What about hospice benefits?

Hospice care is paid by Medicare Part A. Beneficiaries must have advanced illness with a life expectancy less than 6 months. Covered services include:

• Physician services	• Social services
• Nursing care	• Physical and occupational therapy
• Medical equipment	• Speech and language pathology services
• Short-term inpatient care, including respite care	• Nutritional counseling
	• Home health aide and homemaker services

A Medicare recipient can receive up to 5 days of inpatient care at a time for respite. There is no limit to the number of times that a patient can get respite care. There are no deductibles for this coverage. Prescriptions directly related to hospice care (such as pain medicines) also are covered. However, there is a copayment of 5% of the reasonable cost of drugs, not to exceed $5 per prescription. For respite care, copayment is $5/day. If Medicare benefits are used for the treatment of an illness unrelated to the terminal illness, the patient is responsible for paying any applicable deductibles and coinsurance.

15. What is respite care?

Respite care is care given to a hospice patient by another caregiver so that the usual caregiver can rest. For example, a hospice patient may have a family member providing the care. The caregiver may require 1 to 2 weeks away from caregiving either as a "rest" or to perform other duties. The family member may thus seek respite care in a Medicare-approved facility, such as a hospice facility, hospital, or nursing home.

16. List sources of additional information.

   • Social Security Administration at 1-800-772-1213
   • Medicare Hotline at 1-800-MEDICARE (1-800-633-4227)

• Centers for Medicare and Medicaid Services (CMS) 7500 Security Blvd., Baltimore, MD 21244-1850; www.cms.gov or www.medicare.gov

BIBLIOGRAPHY

1. Boult C: Financing coverage, and costs of health care. In Cobbs EL, Duthie EH, Murphy JB (eds): Geriatric Review Syllabus: A Core Curriculum in Geriatric Medicine, 5th ed. Malden, MA, Blackwell Publishing for the American Geriatric Society, 2002, p 28.
2. Gross DJ, Branagan N: The Medicare Program. Public Policy Institute, AARP, April 1998.
3. Hsieh D, Samakur M, Lavizzo-Mourey R: The ABCs of Medicare reimbursement. In Forciea MA, Lavizzo-Mourey R, Schwab E (eds): Geriatric Secrets, 2nd ed. Philadelphia, Hanley & Belfus, 2000.
4. Inglehart JK: Health Policy Report: The American Health Care system—Medicare. N Engl J Med 340:327–332, 1999.
5. Inglehart JK: Health Policy Report: The American Health Care system—Medicaid. N Engl J Med 340:403–408, 1999.
6. McClellan M: Medicare reform: Fundamental problems, incremental steps. J Econ Perspect 14(2): 21–44, 2000.
7. Medicare Chart Book, 2nd ed. Henry J. Kaiser Family Foundation, 2001.
8. Medicare and You 2003. US Dept Health and Human Services, Centers for Medicare and Medicaid Services. 2003.
9. Powell SK: Insurance. In Case Management: A Practical Guide to Success in Managed Care, 2nd ed. Philadelphia, Lippincott, 2000, pp 140–153.
10. Talking to Your Parents about Medicare Health Coverage. Henry J. Kaiser Family Foundation, 2001.
11. Vladeck BC: The political economy of Medicare. Health Affairs 18(1):22–36, 1999.

WEBSITES

www/cmwf.org/programs/medfutur/medicare_survey97
www.medicare.gov
www.cms.gov

6. GERIATRIC PHARMACOTHERAPY

Angela C. Cafiero, PharmD, CGP

1. What age-related physiologic changes in renal function influence medication use?

Age-related physiologic changes in the renal system result in a decline in the clearance of renally excreted drugs and therefore prolong the activity of those drugs in the body. The kidney tends to lose up to 20–25% of its mass as people age from 30 to 80 years. Most of the functional loss occurs in the renal cortex. Correspondingly, glomerular filtration rate (GFR), which is measured by creatinine clearance (CrCl), decreases by about 10% per decade of life from the age of 30 as determined by cross-sectional and longitudinal studies. The causes for such a decrease have been attributed to intrarenal vascular changes, such as stenosis, and hyalinization or fibroelastic hyperplasia of the arterioles. The reduction in GFR has been reported to decline by an average rate of 1 ml/min/year in the majority of elderly patients; therefore, it is important to adjust dosage regimens accordingly.

In determining renal function in the elderly patient, a common misconception is to assess GFR solely based on serum creatinine (SCr). Elderly patients may present with normal SCr values but have severe renal dysfunction. This can be attributed to a decrease in muscle mass, resulting in a decrease in the production of creatinine. A more appropriate and common method for determining GFR is by using the Cockcroft and Gault estimation of creatinine clearance, which takes into account a person's age and weight:

$$CrCl = \frac{(140 - \text{age in years})(\text{IBW or ABW in kg})}{72 \times (\text{serum creatinine in mg/dl})} \times 0.85 \text{ (females only)}$$

where IBW = ideal body weight = 50 kg (45.5 kg/females) + 2.3(height in inches – 60 in) and ABW = adjusted body weight = IBW + 0.4(total body weight – IBW) for obese patients.

A major limitation to this equation is that it often overestimates the creatinine clearance. Alternatively, measurements of 24-hour urine samples may be useful but not always practical. In addition, therapeutic drug monitoring of drugs with narrow therapeutic indices should be done to assess drug therapy and renal function. Common medications that need to be adjusted and monitored in patients with renal dysfunction are listed below.

Renally Excreted Medications

Allopurinol	Clarithromycin	Gancyclovir	Phenobarbital
Aminoglycosides	Colchicine	Hydrochlorothiazide	Procainamide
Amoxicillin	Digoxin	Levofloxacin	Ramipril
Ampicillin	Disopyramide	Lisinopril	Ranitidine
Atenolol	Enalapril	Lithium	Spironolactone
Captopril	Famotidine	Metformin	Sulfamethoxazole
Chlorpropamide	Fluconazole	Methotrexate	Tetracycline
Cimetidine	Furosemide	Penicillin	Trimethoprim
Ciprofloxacin	Gabapentin		

2. What age-related physiologic changes in the liver influence medication selection?

The liver, which is responsible for drug metabolism, plays a vital role in normal physiology and pharmacokinetic profile as related to drug therapy. Common age-related factors that can affect drug therapy are liver mass size, hepatic blood flow, and enzyme activity. Numerous studies have shown overall reduction in mass by 25–35% with increasing age. Hepatic blood flow can significantly decrease by 35–40%. Because of a decrease in hepatic blood flow, medications that undergo extensive first pass metabolism will have a longer duration of effect. Age-related changes in the activity of the cytochrome P450 enzyme systems remain controversial due to intervariability in hepatic enzyme studies.

Two major reaction pathways, phase I and II, affect the metabolism of medications. The phase I reaction pathway involves the biotransformation of a medication to a more polar product for excretion; this process is affected by a decline in age. Typical reactions include oxidation/reduction, hydroxylation, dealkylation, and hydrolysis reactions, which are mediated through the CYP450 enzyme system. The ability of the liver to metabolize medications in the phase I pathway is reduced, therefore increasing their free concentrations, which may be potentially toxic. Examples of medications that undergo phase I metabolism are codeine, diphenhydramine, and warfarin. Phase II reactions are unaffected by age-related changes and involve the conjugation of drugs through processes such as glucuronidation or acetylation, which also make the drug more soluble and readily excreted. Examples of medications that undergo phase II metabolism are isoniazid and lorazepam. Age-related changes within the liver can significantly impact the pharmacologic activity of medications.

3. How do age-related changes in the central nervous system affect medication use?

Age-related physiologic changes in the central nervous system (CNS) include an increase in blood-brain barrier permeability and a decrease in cerebral blood flow. Consequently, the elderly have an increased sensitivity to medications that affect the CNS. In fact, studies have shown that 11–30% of hospitalized elderly patients experience drug-induced delirium. Delirium, sedation, depression, and confusion are the most common CNS effects that have been associated with anticholinergics, antidepressants, analgesics, neuroleptics, digoxin, and anticonvulsants.

The toxicity associated with anticholinergic medications is clinically associated with vivid hallucinations and agitated behavior, which vary in degree with different drugs. Long-acting benzodiazepines, such as diazepam and flurazepam, have a low hepatic clearance and a wider volume of distribution, therefore enhancing their CNS effect. Hence, shorter-acting benzodiazepines, such as lorazepam, oxazepam, and temazepam, are preferred in the elderly. Opioids can have a profound CNS effect due to a decrease in the number of receptors and an alteration of the opioid receptor affinity. Thus, the elderly are more sensitive to the effects of opioids and require lower doses. These medications should be used with caution and monitored in the elderly.

Methods to avoid adverse outcomes from CNS medications include initiating therapy at low doses and titrating the dose slowly. Narrow therapeutic drugs should be carefully monitored for drug levels and doses. Many centrally acting medications can have overlapping side effects. For instance, antihistamines (e.g., diphenhydramine) in combination with tricyclic antidepressants (e.g., amitriptyline) or antipsychotics (e.g., haloperidol) can significantly increase the anticholinergic side effects of confusion and sedation. It is important to monitor patients especially for additive CNS adverse effects.

4. How do age-related changes in protein binding affect medication sensitivity?

Two major plasma proteins, albumin and alpha-1-acid glycoprotein (AAG), are present in the serum to bind drugs. Serum albumin usually has a high affinity for acidic drugs (warfarin, phenytoin, naproxen), whereas AAG tends to bind with more basic drugs (lidocaine, propranolol, quinidine). Malnutrition associated with an increase in age can significantly decrease serum albumin. As a result, medications that are highly albumin-bound may have elevated free drug concentrations, leading to a higher incidence of drug toxicity.

Interpretation of serum drug concentrations also can be affected by changes in the serum albumin. Therapeutic ranges are normally reported as total serum drug concentration (bound drug + unbound drug), where unbound drug is therapeutically active. In elderly patients, a decreased total serum drug concentration may not necessarily indicate low therapeutic levels but rather a higher fraction of unbound drug.

Similarly, AAG can affect interpretation of serum drug concentrations. AAG levels are usually elevated under conditions of trauma, acute illness, or burns. Consequently, free drug concentrations decrease as a result of a lower fraction of unbound drug and may require close monitoring for efficacy more than side effects. Common highly protein-bound medications are listed below.

Highly Protein-bound Medications

Amiodarone	Ceftriaxone	NSAIDs	Sertraline
Amlodipine	Cilostazol	Omeprazole	Sulfonylureas
Antipsychotics	Citalopram	Pantoprazole	Tamsulosin
Atovaquone	Diltiazem	Phenytoin	Terazosin
Bepridil	Dipyridamole	Prazosin	Tiagabine
Bicalutamide	Efavirenz	Propranolol	Tolcapone
Bupropion	Felodipine	Quinine sulfate	Tolterodine
Buspirone	Lansoprazole	Rabeprazole	Valproic acid
Carbamazepine	Midazolam	Raloxifene	Verapamil
Cefazolin	Nelfinavir	Rapaglinide	Warfarin
Ceftotetan	Nifedipine	Rifabutin	

5. How do age-related changes in body composition influence medication use?

With an increase in age the body composition begins to change. Total body fat increases while total body water and lean body mass decrease. These age-related changes affect the distribution of medication. Water-soluble medications have a decreased volume of distribution, leading to a higher plasma concentration. Examples of water-soluble medications include cimetidine, digoxin, ethanol, and lithium. With an increase in total body fat, fat-soluble medications have a larger volume of distribution with a decreased plasma concentration. Fat-soluble medications are excreted from the body at a slower rate and thus have a longer half-life with extension of the pharmacologic property. Examples of fat-soluble medications include chlordiazepoxide and diazepam. In turn, body composition may affect duration of action and plasma concentration of medications.

6. Which medications have a high incidence of adverse effects in the elderly?

An adverse drug reaction (ADR) is a drug response that is noxious or unintended and occurs at prophylactic, diagnostic, or therapeutic doses. Adverse drug reactions can present atypically in the elderly. For example, in elderly patients the symptoms from constipation may present as confusion.

Certain types of medications with an increase in adverse effects vary according to patient settings (long-term care, outpatient, inpatient). Errors most commonly occur in initiating a new medication during a transition from one setting to another. The cardiovascular and psychotropic medications are commonly prescribed in this population and elicit the highest risk of medications associated with ADRs. Since older people have an increased sensitivity to CNS medications, these medications have an increased risk to cause an adverse effect of excessive sedation and delirium. Anticholinergic adverse effects or orthostasis can be more pronounced in older people due to the age-associated unsteady gait and additive effects from other medications.

It is controversial whether increased age or female gender has an impact on the development of adverse effects. However, there has been a direct association between age and medication use. There is a strong relationship between the number of medications and the incidence of adverse reactions. When a new medication is initiated, the patient should be thoroughly monitored for any changes in condition.

7. What are the mechanisms by which drug–drug interactions occur?

The elderly tend to suffer from multiple chronic diseases (e.g., coronary artery disease, benign prostatic hyperplasia, congestive heart failure, hyperlipidemia, diabetes mellitus, depression, insomnia, alzheimer's disease, parkinson's disease), which require several medications for treatment. With an extensive medication list, the potential for drug–drug interactions increases significantly and becomes difficult to manage. The incidence of drug interactions can be further confounded by the fact that many elderly patients visit different providers for care as well as obtain their medications at different pharmacies.

To recognize potentially severe interactions, it is important to understand the mechanisms by which they occur. Interactions can result from a pharmacodynamic or pharmacokinetic effect. Pharmacodynamic mechanisms usually result when medications have either an additive or opposing effect when combined. For example, additive pharmacodynamic interactions can cause postural hypotensive events in patients taking alpha-1 blockers (e.g., prazosin) with calcium channel blockers (e.g., nifedipine) or additive anticholinergic effects in a patient taking tricyclic antidepressants combined with antihistamines. Pharmacodynamic interactions that exert opposing effects are another concern. For example, the chronic use of NSAIDs (e.g., naproxen) potentially reduces the effects of antihypertensive medications such as angiotensin-converting enzyme inhibitors (e.g., lisinopril).

Pharmacokinetic mechanisms involve drugs that alter the absorption, distribution, metabolism, or excretion of other drugs. The most common types of pharmacokinetic interactions occur through the inhibition or induction of the cytochrome P450 (CYP450) enzyme system or protein binding, which includes six major isoenzymes. The table below shows examples of drugs that are substrates, inhibitors, or inducers for five of the CYP450 enzyme system.

Common Substrates, Inhibitors, or Inducers of CYP450

ISOENZYME	CYP 1A2	CYP 2C9	CYP 2C19	CYP 2D6	CYP 3A4

Substrate	Acetaminophen
	Mirtazapine
	Olanzepine
	TCAs
	Theophylline
		Carvedilol
		Celecoxib
		Diclofenac
		Fluvastatin
		Ibuprofen
		Indomethacin
		Losartan
		Phenytoin
		Piroxecam
		Tolbutamide
		Warfarin
			Diazepam
			Naproxen
			Phenobarbital
			Phenytoin
			Propranolol
			Proton pump
			  inhibitors
			TCAs
				Carvedilol
				Codeine
				Donepezil
				Fluoxetine
				Haloperidol
				Metoprolol
				Mirtazapine
				Paroxetine
				Propranolol
				Risperidone
				TCAs
				Tramadol
				Trazodone
				Venlafaxine
					Alprazolam
					Amiodarone
					Azole antifungals
					Buspirone
					Ca chan block
					Carbamazepine
					Cyclosporine
					Donepezil
					Diazepam
					Erythromycin
					Fentanyl
					HMG Co-A reductase
					  inhibitors
					Mirtazapine
					Nefazodone
					Quetiapine
					Sildenafil
					Trazodone
					Warfarin

Inhibitors	Amiodarone Cimetidine Ciprofloxacin Diltiazem Tacrine	Amiodarone Cimetidine Cotrimoxazole Fluconazole Fluoxetine Isoniazid Omeprazole	Fluoxetine Omeprazole Ticlopidine Topiramate	Amiodarone Celecoxib Cimetidine Paroxetine Quinidine Sertraline Terbinafine Thioridazine	Amiodarone Azole antifungals Cimetidine Fluoxetine Grapefruit juice Macrolides Nefazodone Verapamil
Inducers	Cigarette smoke Phenobarbital Phenytoin Rifampin	Phenobarbital Phenytoin Rifampin	Phenobarbital Rifampin		Carbamazepine Phenytoin Phenobarbital Pioglitazone Rifampin Topiramate

TCAs = Tricyclic antidepressants.

Protein binding, as discussed previously, has the potential for drug–drug interactions whereby two highly protein-bound drugs can displace one another from the binding site. For example, warfarin in combination with phenytoin may increase patients' risk for bleeding, because phenytoin has a higher affinity for the plasma proteins than warfarin. Thus, more warfarin is unbound and pharmacologically active.

Common medications that are big offenders of drug interactions in the elderly include warfarin, amiodarone, phenytoin, digoxin, carbamazepine, quinolones, and azole antifungals. However, many steps can be taken to avoid drug–drug interactions. A thorough medication history is imperative to assess a patient's complete medication list. Medications should be screened for both pharmacodynamic and pharmacokinetic mechanisms. Interactions should also be monitored to assess severity as well as signs and symptoms of drug toxicity. Minimizing the number of providers and pharmacies used by the patient helps in identifying significant drug interactions. Patient education is essential in maintaining compliance and assessing drug-related events in the elderly.

8. What is polypharmacy? How can it be avoided?

Polypharmacy is defined as the use of multiple medications. The exact number of medications that defines polypharmacy varies with the source. Some investigators report 3–5 medications/day per patient to be polypharmacy. The Health Care Financing Administration (HCFA) identified polypharmacy as taking 9 or more medications. A more complete definition of polypharmacy is the administration of more medications than clinically indicated. This definition takes into consideration that each medication should have a medical indication specific to that individual.

Risk factors that contribute to the development of polypharmacy include increased age, increased number of physicians and pharmacies, and increased number of office/hospital visits. Decline in health status and the influence of pharmaceutical industry advertising also increase the risk of polypharmacy. A contributing factor to polypharmacy is the treatment of an adverse effect of one drug with another medication. For example, a patient taking the alpha blocker, terazosin, presents to his or her provider complaining of dizziness. The provider prescribes meclizine to relieve the dizziness when, in fact, the original medication could have been changed or dosed at bedtime when the patient would not be rising.

Polypharmacy increases the risk of adverse drug reactions, drug interactions, medication noncompliance, decline in medical status, and increase in health care costs. Polypharmacy can be prevented by improving communication among health care professionals and patients and by thorough medication education. A periodic review of the medication profile helps in identifying unnecessary medications.

The Medication Appropriateness Index (MAI) is a tool developed to assess polypharmacy and medication use in the elderly. It examines the use of medications with regard to indication, effectiveness, dosage, practical directions, correct directions, drug–drug interactions, drug–disease interactions, duration, duplication, and cost. Evaluation of a patient's medication profile by the use of the MAI can help to decrease the amount of polypharmacy. Polypharmacy is a modifiable risk factor that can lead to a decrease in the amount of adverse effects, drug interactions, and medication noncompliance.

9. Which medications are considered inappropriate in the elderly?

Medications are defined as inappropriate when the risk outweighs the benefits. Although practicing geriatric clinicians have long had clinical experience in which medications to avoid in the elderly, few published data supported their experience. In 1991, Beers and colleagues published the first article to examine which medications are inappropriate to prescribe in the elderly. The investigators surveyed a group of expert geriatric clinicians about their opinion of which medications were inappropriate in the elderly. The survey included prescription medications that should be avoided entirely in the elderly, excessive dosage, and excessive duration of treatment. The findings of this study evolved into a list of inappropriate medications in the elderly, also known as the "Beer's List," which as updated in 1997. These medications are deemed inappropriate because there are safer, equally efficacious alternative medications. Whenever possible, the use of medications on the Beer's List should be avoided.

Prescribing medications on the Beer's List increases the risk of drug-related morbidity and mortality; however, not all of these medications are inappropriate in all older patients. Some healthy 80-year-olds can tolerate medications on this list while a 60-year-old with many comorbid conditions would not. It is important to take into consideration the whole patient, including comorbid conditions and medications.

Beer's List of Inappropriate Medications in the Elderly

MEDICATION CLASS	SAFER ALTERNATIVES	RATIONALE FOR INAPPROPRIATE USE
Antihistamines (first generation: diphenhydramine)	Nonsedating antihistamines (loratadine)	↑ Anticholinergic effects
Benzodiazepines (long-acting: diazepam, chlordiazepoxide, flurazepam)	Short acting benzodiazepines (lorazepam, oxazepam, temazepam)	Long-acting agents accumulate in the body ↑ Risk of sedation
Antidepressants (TCAs: amitriptyline, doxepin) Combination antidepressants	Nortriptyline, desipramine	↑ Anticholinergic effects ↑ Sedation
Narcotics (propoxyphene, meperidine)	Morphine	Active metabolites, propoxyphene: equal efficacy to APAP, CNS stimulation
Sedative/hypnotics (meprobamate)	Short acting benzodiazepines	↑ Sedation, highly addictive
Hypoglycemic agents (chlorpropamide)	Nonrenally eliminated, shorter-acting (glipizide)	Long half-life, renally excreted ↑ Risk of an hypoglycemic event
NSAIDs (indomethacin)	Acetaminophen, ibuprofen	↑ CNS activity
Skeletal muscle relaxants (methocarbamol, cyclobenzaprine, carisoprodol)		↑ Anticholinergic effects ↑ Sedation
Antipsychotics (first generation: haloperidol)	Atypicals (risperidone, olanzapine)	↑ Risk of extrapyramidal symptoms
Antiplatelet agents (dipyridamole)	Aspirin, clopidogrel	Orthostatic hypotension

BIBLIOGRAPHY

1. Aronoff GR, Berns JS, Golper TA, et al: Drugs Prescribing in Renal Failure, 4th ed. Philadelphia, American College of Physicians, 1999.
2. Beers MH: Explicit criteria for determining potentially inappropriate medication use by the elderly. Arch Intern Med 157:1531–1536, 1997.
3. Beers MH: Explicit criteria for determining inappropriate medication use in nursing home residents. Arch Intern Med 151:1825–1832, 1991.
4. Chapron DJ: Drug disposition and response. In Delafluente JC, Stewart RB (eds): Therapeutics in the Elderly, 3rd ed. Cincinnati, OH, Harvey Whitney Books, 2001, pp 257–288.
5. Cockcroft DW, Gault MH: Prediction of creatinine clearance from serum creatinine. Nephron 16:31–41, 1976.
6. Danziger RS, Tobin JD, Becker LC, et al: The age-associated decline in glomerular filtration in healthy normotensive volunteers. J Am Geriatr Soc 38:1127–1132, 1990.
7. Francis J, Martin D, Kapoor WN: A prospective study of delirium in hospitalized elderly. JAMA 263:1097–1101, 1990.
8. George J, Bleasdale S, Singleton SJ: Causes and prognosis of delirium in elderly patients admitted to a district general hospital. Age Ageing 26:423–427, 1997.

9. Hammerlein A, Derendorf H, Lowenthal DT: Pharmacokinetic and pharmacodynamic changes in the elderly. Clin Pharmacokinet 35:49–64, 1998.

10. Hanlon JT, Schmader KE, Samsa GP, et al: A method for assessing drug therapy appropriateness. J Clin Epidemiol 117:684–689, 1992.

11. Herrlinger C, Klotz U: Drug metabolism and drug interactions in the elderly. Best Pract Res Clin Gastroenterol 15:897–918, 2001.

12. Larson EB, Kukull WA, Buchner D, et al: Adverse drug reactions associated with global cognitive impairment in elderly persons. Ann Intern Med 107:169–173, 1987.

13. Le Couteur DG, McLean AJ: The aging liver. Drug clearance and an oxygen diffusion barrier hypothesis. Clin Pharmacokinet 34:359–373, 1998.

14. McLachlan M, Wasserman P: Changes in size and distensibility of the aging kidney. Br J Radiol 54:488–491, 1981.

15. Moore AR, O'Keeffe ST: Drug-induced cognitive impairment in the elderly. Drugs Aging 15:15–28, 1999.

16. Rowe JW, Andres RA, Tobin FD, et al: The effect of age on creatinine clearance in man: A cross-sectional and longitudinal study. J Gerontol 31:155–163, 1976.

17. Starr JM, Whalley LJ: Drug induced dementia: Incidence, management and prevention. Drug Saf 11:310–317, 1994.

18. Stewart RB: Drug use in the elderly. In Delafluente JC, Stewart RB (eds): Therapeutics in the Elderly, 3rd ed. Cincinnati, OH, Harvey Whitney Books, 2001, pp 235–256.

II. Symptoms

7. AGING AND NEUROCOGNITIVE FUNCTIONING

Ruben C. Gur, PhD, Paul J. Moberg, PhD, Matthew M. Kurtz, PhD, and Raquel E. Gur, MD, PhD

1. What is the pattern of cognitive decline in normal aging?

As you might suspect, most cognitive abilities decline with age after adulthood is reached, just like physical abilities. However, not all "mental muscles" "shrivel" at the same rate, and it is important to weigh the negative effects of reduced mental abilities against the positive impact of experience. Thus, even though psychological test performance may decline with age, for particular real-life tasks the relevant experience of an individual may be much more important than the score on a cognitive test. For example, a test may show decline in verbal fluency, but an experienced lawyer would perhaps be better able to select the more effective, if fewer, words compared with younger and likely more fluent counterparts.

Numerous specific changes in cognitive performance are exhibited by persons with dementia. Such changes differ both in magnitude and extent from those seen in the normal aging process. Abilities more commonly affected in dementia include verbal and nonverbal memory, perceptual-organizational abilities, communication skills, and psychomotor performance. The nature, extent, and rate of decline depend on the cause, the person's educational attainment, activity level, and general health status. It is important to remember that about 80% of people living into very old age never experience a significant memory loss or other symptoms of dementia. A slight forgetfulness is common as we age, but it is usually not enough to interfere with our functioning. Pablo Picasso, Margaret Mead, and Duke Ellington were productive well past their 75th birthdays, suggesting that successful aging is both possible and probable.

A long-standing body of research has documented differential patterns of age-related decline on different measures of intelligence. Based on these data, prior research has proposed a taxonomy of cognitive abilities in which cognitive skills can be grouped into one of two functional domains: *crystallized* versus *fluid* intelligence. In this context fluid intelligence represents cognitive abilities that handle novel problems and require flexible and rapid information processing skills. These skills are highly sensitive to the effects of age and are thought to be more closely linked to neurobiologic changes. In contrast, crystallized intelligence represents the repertoire of cognitive skills that are the result of the application of fluid intelligence to the environment. These skills include overlearned information, such as expressive vocabulary, or our general fund of information. These skills are highly influenced by our educational and social history and are relatively resistant to the impact of aging.

Most recent research suggests that cognitive changes associated with aging are most intimately related to a generalized slowing of "cognitive speed." This theoretical model has generated increasing attention to the cognitive processes that underlie performance on a variety of cognitive tasks. By this view, performance on tasks that "load" on, or are more dependent upon, overlearned verbal knowledge are preserved during aging, relative to tasks that require cognitive speed. This "slowing" of cognition, however, may be modified to some extent by general health, use of medications, and physical activity.

2. How is cognition assessed?

To understand which cognitive activities decline more than others, we need to divide cognition into components or domains. It is customary to evaluate the following clusters of cognitive abilities:

Executive functions: the ability to plan, to abstract principles from examples of a set, to shift sets, and to keep ongoing operations in "working memory."

Attention and vigilance: the ability to select relevant stimuli for further processing and response and to concentrate on specific tasks for extended periods.

Learning and memory: the ability to acquire new information and to retrieve it on demand. This ability seems to differ—and perhaps follow specific rules—for verbally encoded and spatial information.

Language and related functions: the ability to speak fluently, communicate effectively, to comprehend accurately and effectively, to name and identify things and people in the environment, to retrieve words in running speech, reading abilities, and writing skills.

Intellectual functions: analytic abilities, fund of information and vocabulary, and effectiveness of processing complex information. These abilities also seem to differ for verbal and spatial functions.

Sensorimotor functions: the acuity of the senses and the speed and accuracy of motor responses.

Of these domains of behavior, there is evidence for age-related decline in attentional processing, memory (both verbal and spatial), intellectual functions (primarily spatial), and the sensorimotor domain, particularly motor speed. On the other hand, executive functions seem relatively preserved. Declines in speed of response and processing are among the most characteristic changes seen with aging and can be observed in any of the above domains.

3. Can the effects of age on cognition be separated from the effects of illness?

A difficulty in answering the question of domain-specific cognitive decline is the need to separate normal aging effects from the effects of age-related disorders likely to influence cognitive dysfunction. As we age, we are more likely to experience accidents in which we lose consciousness, our arteries harden, and we may experience subclinical ischemic episodes that could nonetheless affect specific cognitive abilities. Other brain disorders also are more prevalent in older age. One way to address this methodologic problem is to screen research subjects carefully for any disorder that may affect cognition. In addition, it is helpful to examine the effects of aging within the younger age range, where it is less likely that age-related disorders have occurred. Obviously the effects of age will be smaller in this population, but the effects observed would point to the cognitive systems that are most vulnerable to the normal aging process. One should also bear in mind that some functions may show little if any decline initially and steeper decline after a certain age.

4. Are there sex-related differences in this decline?

This issue has been relatively less investigated, because for a long time such differences were ignored and frequently only men were studied. However, there seems to be evidence that the rate of decline with age is faster for men than for women. (See figure at top of opposite page.)

5. What causes age-related changes in cognitive functioning?

Most likely the cognitive decline associated with aging is linked to brain function, and indeed there is evidence for both anatomic and physiologic brain changes with normal aging. Brain volume is reduced with normal aging, and the reduction in the volume of brain tissue is accompanied by an increase in the volume of the cerebrospinal fluid (CSF). This was demonstrated initially by direct postmortem measurements of brains, using the old Archimedes method of measuring the volume of displaced liquid into which the brain is immersed. More recently, computed tomography (CT) and magnetic resonance imaging (MRI) have been used to measure brain volume. These methods are based on computerized "segmentation" of tissue into brain and CSF, which give different image intensities. Such studies confirm the results of postmortem measurements and also suggest sex differences in the rate at which tissue is lost with normal aging. Men show a steeper loss of tissue and increase in CSF than women. Indeed, the decline in the frontal

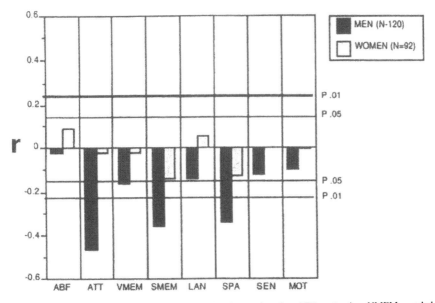

Rates of cognitive decline in men and women. ABF = abstract function; ATT = attention; VMEM = verbal memory; SMEM = spatial memory; LAN = language; SPA = spatial function; SEN = sensory perception; MOT = motor function.

and temporal regions is so pronounced in men compared with women that, whereas young men have larger volumes than young women (commensurate with their overall larger bodies), the volumes in elderly men and elderly women are identical. (See figure below.)

6. How is the pattern different in the dementias?

As noted earlier, changes in brain structure and function are inevitable with the aging process. For example, speed of response tends to slow, and mild forgetfulness is usually present as a person gets older. Some level of cognitive decline is expected with age, but at what point

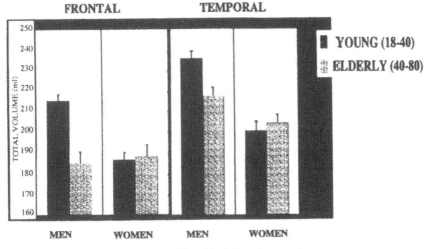

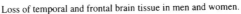

Loss of temporal and frontal brain tissue in men and women.

does it become abnormal? The basic question is whether a person exhibits cognitive changes above and beyond those expected for his or her age. Research with healthy, aged individuals provides a benchmark of mental abilities for people of various ages and educational and occupational backgrounds as well as gender. Such abnormality is typically assessed against this benchmark. For example, an elderly person with a dementing illness may remember only 50% of what is said to them, whereas a healthy person matched in age, gender, and education may remember 80% or more. In addition, the person with dementia shows other deficits of a substantial scope and magnitude in addition to "forgetfulness." Deficits in problem-solving, language, and visual-perceptual abilities are often present. The stigma attached to cognitive decline is not applied to age-associated physical ailments. Older adults suffering from heart disease are not labeled as abnormal, but this term is applied to those suffering from "dementia." Yet just as the definition of aging can include heart disease, so can it include dementia. Many names have been given to the symptoms of memory loss and loss of cognitive abilities in older adults. Terms such as *senility, hardening of the arteries,* and *organic brain syndrome* have been commonly used. *Alzheimer's disease, multi-infarct disease,* and *senile dementia* are terms often used by health care professionals. The word *dementia* means a loss or impairment of mental abilities; it does not mean "crazy": It comes from two Latin words which translate into *away* and *mind.* Dementia is a term chosen by health care professionals to describe a group of symptoms expressed by various disease states. The question is whether dementia is the inevitable end-point of the normal aging process if one lives long enough. While the evidence for either outcome is not entirely clear, the prevailing thought is that the degenerative organic brain state known as dementia is not part of normal aging. Many types of illnesses are associated with dementia, including Alzheimer's disease, multi-infarct disease, Parkinson's disease, Pick's disease, and progressive supranuclear palsy. The most common causes of dementia in elderly persons are Alzheimer's disease and multi-infarct disease.

Dementia knows no social or racial lines: rich and poor, wise and simple alike can be victims. Many brilliant and famous people have suffered from dementing illnesses, and it is likely that we all know someone with such cognitive impairment. Many elderly people live in the community with mild levels of dementia. Typically they can function if environmental supports (e.g., a caring wife, husband, family members) are available. This impairment becomes clinically meaningful when it impairs the person's level of day-to-day functioning. Although we may all be irritated by occasional forgetfulness, it does not prevent us from performing our daily duties and activities.

Although many cognitive functions (e.g., episodic memory, speed of processing, visuospatial skill, verbal fluency) decline across the adult life span, there is considerable variability among normal elderly persons with regard to the size of the age-related cognitive impairment (e.g., Hultsch, Hertzog, Dixon, and Small, 1998; Luszcz, Bryan, and Kent, 1997). A number of studies have indicated that individual differences within demographic (e.g., gender, education), life-style (e.g., activity patterns, substance use), and health-related (e.g., vascular factors, vitamin use and status) domains may impact the magnitude of cognitive deficits in old age (see Bächman, Small, Wahlin, and Larsson, 1999 for review).

7. How do the medicines that older people take affect cognitive function?

The concept that medicine can alter a person's cognitive processes is generally well-accepted by most investigators. Aging brings changes in the way that medicine is broken down and used by the body. For example, studies have shown that age-related changes in the gastrointestinal system, increases in body fat, cardiovascular alterations, reduction in blood flow in the brain, reductions in liver and kidney function, and changes in tissue response to hormones interact with medicines and their effect on the patient. In addition, age has a definite impact on the person's ability to adapt to internal or external stressors. For example, elderly people tend to recover more slowly from the adverse side effects of many medications. This issue becomes more complicated if the older adult is also taking more than one medicine. The disorders for which elderly people most commonly receive medication are depression, anxiety, and apprehension; cognitive and memory impairment; sleep disturbances; and behavior disorders. Drugs with anticholinergic properties (e.g., antidepressants, antihistamines, antimotion sickness medications) are the most likely to cause cognitive side effects. Whereas younger people may experience minimal cognitive effects, such effects are magnified in the elderly by physiologic changes. The cognitive effects of drugs used to treat most medical conditions have not, however, been studied systematically.

The greater sensitivity to drug effects in elderly persons also makes the ingestion of "social drugs" problematic and can clearly increase the frequency of negative drug reactions. It is a common practice for patients with diabetes to change their diet to help control the illness. In contrast, it is not unusual to see patients arrive at a precise combination of medicines and dosages through close consultation with their physician—and yet ingest 10–20 cups of coffee a day! Caffeine, nicotine, and other chemicals in common day-to-day beverages and foods can also interact with medicine (or act on their own) to produce adverse cognitive and physiologic effects. Coffee and cola drinks are not the only culprits in such "social drug" consumption. Tea, chocolate, cocoa, cigarettes, and alcohol also must be listed. In addition, seemingly harmless over-the-counter medications (e.g., cold capsules, sleep medicines, pain relievers) can interact with prescribed medications. Perhaps the claim of homeopathic physicians that they successfully treat patients with a minimal dosage of drugs can be explained by their close attention to diet and its direct relationship to the taking of prescribed drugs.

In general, many medicines can have an impact on cognitive processes, especially when the increased vulnerability of the brain and associated physical systems is considered. However, such concerns are often secondary to the cognitive effects of the illnesses for which such medications are prescribed. For example, untreated hypertension or diabetes has a greater adverse effect on cognitive function than the medicines used to treat either condition.

BIBLIOGRAPHY

1. Bäckman L, Small BJ, Wahlin Å, Larsson M: Cognitive functioning in very old age. In Craik FIM, Salthouse TA (eds): The Handbook of Aging and Cognition, 2nd ed. Mahwah, NJ, Erlbaum, 1999, pp 499–458.
2. Birren JE, Fisher LM: Aging and speed of behavior: Possible consequences for psychological functioning. Ann Rev Psychol 46:329–353, 1995.
3. Cowell PE, Turetsky BT, Gur RC, et al: Sex differences in aging of the human frontal and temporal lobe. J Neurosci 14:4748–4755, 1994.
4. Hultsch DF, Hertzog C, Dixon RA, Small BJ: Memory Change in the Aged. Cambridge, Cambridge University Press, 1998.
5. Luszcz MA, Bryan J, Kent P: Predicting episodic memory performance of very old men and women: Contributions from age, depression, activity, cognitive ability, and speed. Psychol Aging 12:340–351, 1997.
6. Salthouse TA: Adult Cognition: An Experimental Psychology of Human Aging. New York, Springer-Verlag, 1982.
7. Salthouse TA: Pressing issues in cognitive aging. In Schwarz N, Park DE (eds): Cognition, Aging, and Self-reports. Hove, UK, Erlbaum, 1999.
8. Salthouse TA, Hambrick DE, McGuthry KE: Shared aged-related influences on cognitive and noncognitive variables. Psychol Aging 13:486–500, 1998.
9. Salzman C, Shader RI, Van Der Kolk BA: Clinical psychopharmacology and the elderly patient. N Y State J Med 76:71–77, 1976.
10. Stuart-Hamilton I: Intellectual changes in late-life. In Woods RT (ed): Clinical Psychology of Ageing. New York, Wiley, 1996.
11. Wilson RS, Bennett DA, Schwartzendruber A: Age-related change in cognitive function. In Nussbaum PD (ed): Handbook of Neuropsychology and Aging. New York, Plenum, 1997.

8. CONFUSION AND AMNESIA

Joel E. Streim, MD

1. Are confusion and memory loss part of the normal aging process?

Aging is normally associated with some decline in specific areas of cognitive performance, especially information acquisition, processing, and retrieval, and some language functions. Mild forgetfulness may also be apparent.

Despite this decline in the *speed* of several cognitive functions, older adults normally retain full or nearly-full *capacity* to learn and remember new information, perform problem-solving, and communicate. Confusion and disorientation, or a pattern of memory loss that interferes with the person's ability to function in everyday activities, are *not* normal aging phenomena. They are almost always manifestations of pathologic processes, and some may represent medical emergencies. (See also Chapter 26.)

2. Which conditions are associated with confusion in elderly patients?

Delirium and **dementia** are the two syndromes most often associated with confusional states in older adults. These syndromes, in turn, may each be caused by a wide variety of underlying illnesses and may be exacerbated by environmental factors. Delirium and dementia may also be concurrent.

3. How is delirium distinguished from dementia?

Delirium involves a disturbance of consciousness associated with impaired attention. This may be manifest clinically as waxing and waning lethargy or diminished arousability, with or without intercurrent periods of agitation. By contrast, patients with **dementia** are consistently arousable and able to remain alert without alterations in their level of consciousness, even though they too may have difficulty concentrating on a task or may become agitated at times.

The onset and clinical course of confusion also help to distinguish delirium from dementia. Confusional states with acute onset should always suggest **delirium**. Typically, the syndrome of delirium develops over a short time, becoming clinically apparent over a few minutes, hours, or days—with the level of consciousness and cognitive and perceptual disturbances tending to fluctuate. By contrast, when confusion is due to **dementia**, it usually begins insidiously and becomes apparent over weeks, months, and years. While patients with dementia may exhibit some day-to-day variability in level of confusion, their cognitive and perceptual capacities do not change dramatically over a period of hours or days, and for most patients, the clinical course tends to be stable or gradually progressive, depending on the underlying cause of the dementia syndrome.

4. What causes acute confusional states or delirium?

Almost any medical illness and many medications. The differential diagnosis includes any condition associated with:

- Cerebral hypoperfusion (e.g., hypotension, myocardial infarction, low cardiac output states, arrhythmias)
- Cerebral hypoxia (e.g., pneumonia, COPD, congestive heart failure, pulmonary emboli) or hypercarbia
- Dehydration (mild dehydration as well as intravascular volume depletion)
- Electrolyte disturbances (e.g., hypo- and hypernatremia, hypo- and hypercalcemia, hypo- and hypermagnesemia)
- Hypo- and hyperglycemia and hyperosmolar states
- Infection (e.g., cystitis, urosepsis, pneumonia, peritonitis, and less common CNS infections such as meningitis and encephalitis)

• Fever or hypothermia
• Pain or discomfort (including urinary retention or severe constipation/fecal impaction)
• Intracranial processes (e.g., stroke, subdural hematoma, neoplasm, infection)
• Intoxication or withdrawal states (e.g., alcohol and other drugs)
• Other adverse drug effects (e.g. central anticholinergic, antihistaminic effects)

While this list of potential causes includes conditions that occur commonly in older patients, it is not exhaustive. In many cases of acute confusion or delirium, it is impossible to identify or confirm a single cause. More often, one identifies multiple factors that are suspected to cause, contribute to, or aggravate confusion.

5. Which classes of drugs commonly cause confusion in older adults?

Virtually all drugs that affect CNS function have the potential to cause confusion.

Sedative/hypnotic drugs (e.g., benzodiazepines, barbiturates)
Analgesics (e.g., opiates, NSAIDs?)
Histamine blockers (used for GI disorders, insomnia, pruritus, allergy)
Antisecretory agents (atropinic-like drugs)
Antidiarrheals
Incontinence agents
Tricyclic antidepressants
Antipsychotics (esp. chlorpromazine, thioridazine, mesoridazine)
Antiarrhythmic drugs (e.g., lidocaine, procainamide)
Some antineoplastic agents

6. Who is at risk for developing delirium?

Persons most likely to develop delirium are the very old, those with preexisting brain damage (e.g., from degenerative dementia, cerebrovascular insults, traumatic brain injury), and those with sensory loss (e.g., hearing and visual impairment). Acute confusional states are also more likely to occur in unfamiliar surroundings and environments that cause sensory overload or sensory deprivation.

7. Is sensory deprivation the cause of "sundowning"?

The term "sundowning" usually refers to acute confusional episodes that begin late in the day or at night. The temporal association with the sun's going down has suggested that sensory deprivation may be a cause. However, patients often exhibit a pattern of confusion that has its onset late in the day but before the sun sets. Also, nocturnal confusion has frequently been observed to persist even when adequate lighting and sensory stimulation are maintained after nightfall. Thus "sundowning" may be a misnomer, and some diurnal factor other than altered sensory input may explain the time of onset of confusion.

8. Why is it always important to recognize and evaluate acute confusion or delirium?

Delirium often is the only apparent clinical manifestation of a serious medical illness. For example, myocardial infarction or pulmonary embolus in older adults may present initially with confusion in the absence of chest pain or dyspnea. Urosepsis and pneumonia often occur in older adults without somatic complaints, fever, or leukocytosis, and delirium may be the sole initial clue to these and other infectious diseases. Similarly, abdominal catastrophes (e.g., bowel infarction, perforation, peritonitis) may be heralded by confusion in the very old. Thus, delirium can be an important clinical sign that leads to early recognition, diagnosis, and treatment of serious illness.

Even when delirium is caused by less serious conditions (mild dehydration, constipation, use of low-dose antihistamines), it can lead to significant, potentially reversible comorbidity and excess disability, especially in frail, older adults. When the underlying conditions are identified and are properly managed, the confusion and other cognitive disturbances associated with delirium are usually reversible. Treatment interventions can also alleviate comorbidity, reduce distress and disability, increase function, and improve quality of life. Recognition and evaluation of acute confusion or delirium is therefore essential for the identification and treatment of reversible conditions. The Confusion Assessment Method (CAM) is a validated and widely used approach for the detection of delirium that can be used for screening and case identification.

9. How should acute confusion be evaluated?

The workup for acute confusion or delirium should include:
Complete history
Chart review (with close attention to medications administered, including PRNs)
Physical and mental status examinations
Laboratory evaluation including:
    Urinalysis
    Complete blood count
    Chemistry profile (with electrolytes including calcium and magnesium)
    Electrocardiogram

The use of further tests, such as chest x-ray, CSF examination, electroencephalogram, or brain imaging, should be directed by the specific findings from the history, record review, and patient examination.

10. How is acute confusion or delirium treated?

Appropriate treatment of delirium begins with ensuring the patient's safety, attending to medical emergencies, and managing any other underlying medical conditions, medication effects, or environmental factors that are thought to be contributing to the delirium. Thus, the treatment of delirium and amelioration of the acute confusional state will depend on the specific etiologic factors identified.

11. When should psychotropic medications be used in the management of elders with acute confusion or delirium?

Psychotropic medications are often used in acute and long-term care settings when acute confusional states are associated with agitated or combative behaviors, psychotic symptoms (e.g., hallucinations and delusions), or severe disruption of the normal sleep-wake cycle. The medications usually used for calming these agitated patients are the high-potency neuroleptic/antipsychotics and the short half-life benzodiazepines. One study found haloperidol to be more effective than lorazepam in reducing symptoms. Unfortunately, placebo-controlled clinical trials have not been conducted to determine the efficacy or safety of these drugs in elderly patients with delirium. In particular, it is not known whether such drugs diminish or exacerbate agitation, combativeness, psychosis, insomnia, or confusion; whether they shorten or prolong the course of the delirium; or whether they reduce the excess disability and mortality associated with delirium.

Although clinical experience suggests that some patients' agitation and psychosis may be effectively quieted with these medications, these agents can also complicate the course of delirium. They can cause sedation and worsen lethargy. The benzodiazepines can also cause increased confusion, anterograde amnesia, disinhibition, and paradoxical excitation. The neuroleptic/antipsychotics can induce akathisia, a syndrome of motor restlessness that may worsen the agitation. When this occurs, it is usually difficult to distinguish the effects of the drugs from the symptoms and signs of delirium.

For this reason, it is usually preferable to manage agitation, sleep disruption, and psychosis by first addressing medical conditions, medication effects, and environmental factors that may be causing these symptoms, with an emphasis on proper nursing care. Pharmacologic strategies should be used for those patients who are refractory to these measures and who remain highly distressed or physically unsafe without medication to calm them down. Otherwise, benzodiazepines and neuroleptics should not be used as a treatment for acute confusion when it is uncomplicated by agitation, insomnia, or psychosis. Benzodiazepines are considered first-line treatment for delirium due to alcohol or benzodiazepine withdrawal.

12. What safety precautions should be observed for acutely confused patients?

For many patients with delirium, acute confusion will be accompanied by lethargy or agitation. Patients whose level of responsiveness is diminished may require airway protection or aspiration precautions. For those who are agitated, there may be a need for safeguards against injury: prevention of falls; restriction of access to arterial lines, urinary catheters, tracheostomy cannulae, and ventilator hoses; enforcement of precautions for new joint prostheses; avoidance of trauma from motor restlessness; and surveillance to avert wandering into unsafe situations.

13. What other nursing interventions are indicated to manage delirium?

Beyond immediate safety measures, nursing staff can be instrumental in reducing confusion by setting a calendar and clock in the patient's field of vision, providing frequent verbal reorientation cues, surrounding the patient with familiar personal possessions, pictures, and objects from home, and enlisting the help of family and friends in providing comfort and reassurance. Adjustment of the level of sensory stimulation may also be helpful, increasing the amount of stimulation for patients who have sensory impairment or deprivation and reducing the level for those who are overwhelmed by external stimuli. Nursing staff can also employ sleep hygiene measures to manage the disruption of sleep-wake cycles that typically occurs in patients with delirium.

14. Describe the follow-up care that should be provided after delirium has resolved.

Delirium is a traumatic experience for most patients. Although some are amnestic for events that occur during the course of delirium, many have distressing memories of their confusional state. Even after their acute confusion has resolved, their recollections of illusions, hallucinations, and delusions may be confusing and upsetting, and they may harbor misunderstandings about events and treatment, sometimes attributing malicious intentions to caregivers and family members. For those patients who are not persistently confused due to underlying dementia, it is usually helpful to conduct a debriefing session. This gives the patient an opportunity to express residual concerns, fears, and anger; and it gives the health care provider a chance to provide a medical explanation for the confusional state and to counsel the patient and family. It is especially important to reassure patients about the resolution of their confusion and to discuss prognosis, emphasizing that they are not expected "to go crazy" or "lose their mind," though they may be at risk for recurrence of confusion if exposed to similar circumstances in the future. Therefore, patients and families should be advised to inform future health care providers about their history of confusion and any known causal or precipitating factors. This history can be extremely valuable for prevention.

15. Which conditions are most commonly associated with complaints of amnesia or memory impairment in older adults?

Depressive disorders, dementing illnesses, and effects of drugs and alcohol account for most of older adults' complaints about memory problems. When neuropsychological testing provides objective evidence of memory deficits, dementia is often the cause. However, depression can also impair performance on formal tests of cognitive function, and it accounts for a substantial proportion of subjective memory complaints among elders, with and without dementia (see also Chapter 24).

Alcohol can affect memory in several ways. Acute alcohol intoxication can cause "blackouts," with amnesia for the period of intoxication. Chronic alcohol abuse can lead to alcohol amnestic syndrome, though these patients seldom have insight into their memory impairment and rarely complain about it. Although this condition is also known as "Korsakoff's psychosis," it is actually a disorder of memory function and not a psychotic illness. It is also distinct from dementia in that cognitive functions other than memory are relatively spared.

Drugs other than alcohol can interfere with memory function. Elderly patients commonly receive anesthetic agents, narcotic analgesics, and benzodiazepines, all of which can cause amnesia.

Of note, the syndrome of **delirium** usually includes memory impairment, but memory difficulty is usually not a specific presenting complaint of patients suffering from delirium.

16. When does a patient with memory impairment qualify for a diagnosis of dementia?

Memory impairment, by itself, is not sufficient to diagnose dementia. At least three other criteria must be met:

- Mental status examination must demonstrate that other aspects of cognitive function are impaired. Evidence for this may include agnosia, aphasia, apraxia, or deficits in executive functions.
- The cognitive deficits must be clinically significant in that they interfere with social or occupational functioning or ability to care for oneself.
- The cognitive deficits must not be attributable to depression or delirium or other nondementing neuropsychiatric syndromes.

17. When is memory impairment reversible?

Numerous conditions associated with memory impairment are treatable and reversible. The memory deficits in **nondemented patients** with delirium almost always resolve when the condition causing the delirium is successfully treated. Memory complaints in nondemented patients with depression improve with effective treatment for the depression. Various drugs may impede memory without causing the full syndrome of delirium, dementia, or depression, and in these cases, memory often improves after reduction or discontinuation of the drug.

Approximately 10% of older adults with dementia may have a reversible component to their cognitive dysfunction. In **demented patients** with comorbid depression or delirium or adverse drug effects involving memory, treatment of the comorbid condition usually leads to some improvement in memory function. When the dementing process is due to such conditions as hypo- or hyperthyroidism, vitamin B12 or folic acid deficiency, neurosyphilis, Lyme disease, subdural hematoma, normal pressure hydrocephalus, or autoimmune disease, prompt treatment may help reverse memory impairment. However, when these conditions remain untreated for > 6 months to 1 year, clinical experience suggests that the prognosis for recovery of memory function becomes poor.

18. What is pseudodementia?

Pseudodementia is a term used to describe the reversible cognitive impairment commonly associated with major depressive disorder in older adults. However, this term is misleading, as there are several ways that memory problems appear to be related to depression. Some depressed patients have memory *complaints* despite intact cognitive *performance*, and others have poor memory *performance* due to apathy or lack of motivation despite intact cognitive *capacity*. However, there is evidence that some patients with onset of major depression in late life have measurable changes in cerebral function associated with diminished cognitive capacity. When depression is treated, many patients experience improvement in cognitive function, but a significant proportion have persistence of cognitive impairment consistent with a diagnosis of dementia, or they go on to develop dementia within 2 years of their episode of depression. For these patients, the dementia associated with their depression is clearly not simply "pseudo" dementia.

19. How are memory complaints evaluated?

If memory problems are evident, the evaluation should focus on identifying potentially reversible causes. A comprehensive evaluation includes a careful history, physical and mental status examination, and screening laboratory tests. It is often helpful to use standardized instruments for assessment of both cognitive function (e.g., Mini-Mental State Exam or Blessed Information-Memory-Concentration Test) and affective status (e.g., Geriatric Depression Scale). Laboratory evaluation usually includes a urinalysis, complete blood count, chemistry profile including indices of hepatic and renal function, thyroid function tests, serum B12 and folic acid levels, and serologic test for syphilis. The need for borrelia titers, erythrocyte sedimentation rate, or other laboratory tests depends on the findings from the history, physical, and mental status examinations. Although brain imaging (e.g., CT or MRI scan) is often done routinely, the need for this depends on the duration of memory problems as well as other findings from the history, physical, and mental status examination.

20. How should memory problems be managed?

As with confusion, appropriate management of memory loss begins with ensuring the safety of the patient and treating causal factors and comorbid conditions. Patients with mild memory loss may benefit from mnemonic aids (e.g., making lists and using signs or reminders) and cognitive strategies (self-cueing). Those with moderate and severe memory impairment usually require assistance of a caregiver who can provide cues, prompts, and supervision. Home safety includes measures to ensure that kitchen, plumbing, and electrical appliances are properly turned off. When memory problems are severe, patients usually require supervision or assistance with most activities of daily living.

Effective pharmacologic treatment of memory problems has been limited. Cholinesterase inhibitors have been shown to delay cognitive decline and produce modest improvement in memory performance for some patients with mild-to-moderate dementia due to Alzheimer's disease, but controlled clinical trials in patients with memory impairment associated with delirium are lacking.

BIBLIOGRAPHY

1. American Psychiatric Association: Practical guideline for the treatment of patients with delirium. Am J Psychiatry 156(Suppl):1–20, 1999.
2. Delirium, dementia, and amnestic and other cognitive disorders. Diagnostic and Statistical Manual of Mental Disorders, 4th ed. Washington, DC, Amercian Psychiatric Press, 1994, pp 123–163.
3. Eisdorfer C, Sevush S, Barry PP, et al: Evaluation of the demented patient. Med Clin North Am 78:773–793, 1994.
4. Inouye SK, Charpentier PA: Precipitating factors for delirium in hospitalized elderly persons: Predictive model and interrelationships with baseline vulnerability. JAMA 275:852–857, 1996.
5. Inouye SK, Van Dyck CH, Alessi CA, et al: Clarifying confusion: The Confusion Assessment Method. A new method for the detection of delirium. Ann Intern Med 113:941–948, 1990.
6. Jones BN, Reifler BV: Depression coexisting with dementia: Evaluation and treatment. Med Clin North Am 78:823–840, 1994.
7. McNicoll L, Pisani MA, Zhang Y, et al: Delirium in the intensive care unit: Occurrence and clinical course in older patients. J Am Geriatrics Soc 51:591–598, 2003.
8. Rabins PV: Psychosocial and management aspects of delirium. Int J Psychogeriatr 3:319–324, 1991.

Website
http://www.psych.org/psych-pract/treatg/pg/pg-delirium.cfu.

9. DEMENTIA

*Valerie T. Cotter, MSN, CRNP, Jason H. T. Karlawish, MD,
and Christopher M. Clark, MD*

1. What is dementia?

The term *dementia* describes a clinical syndrome of at least 6 months of chronic and progressive impairments in two or more domains of cognitive function in the absence of delirium or a psychiatric or medical illness that can cause cognitive dysfunction. In addition, the impairments must interfere with usual and everyday activities. A key point in this definition is the need for symptoms of dysfunction in two or more domains of cognitive function such as memory and language. A "preclinical" diagnosis of dementia is not logically possible, and memory loss alone is not dementia.

2. Is dementia primarily defined by progressive memory loss?

Dementia is not just memory loss. Alzheimer's disease (AD), the most common cause of dementia, does present with prominent impairments in short-term memory that correspond with the early pathologic changes of neurofibrillary tangles in the hippocampus where short-term memory is processed. But even in its early stages, patients with AD have deficits in other domains of cognition, especially language and visuospatial skills. The appropriate descriptor for a patient who has a single cognitive deficit, such as memory loss, and is not demented, is *mild cognitive impairment*, not dementia.

3. What is mild cognitive impairment and how is it different from dementia?

The concept of mild cognitive impairment is in transition, but the current consensus is that it is a "diagnosis" reached when a nondemented patient has an impairment in only one domain of cognition. In this case, *impairment* is defined as performance that is greater than two standard deviations below the performance of age-matched persons. One significant controversy is whether mild cognitive impairment is a state of "preclinical dementia." Cohort studies suggest that persons with mild cognitive impairment are at higher risk to progress to dementia compared to persons without it.

4. Is *any* degree of memory loss "normal"?

Memory loss that may be annoying but not severe enough to interfere with daily function can occur as part of the normal aging process. In addition, intellectual response time slows with aging. It takes nondemented elderly people longer than younger people to complete memory tasks and solve problems. However, accuracy is unaffected. See Chapter 3 for a discussion of cognition and aging.

5. Can a patient who is aware of his or her memory loss have AD?

Many patients with early-stage AD are aware of their cognitive deficits, especially the memory loss. However, patients often minimize the deficit's severity and clinical significance. As the disease progresses (sometimes even in the earliest stages), the patient's and caregiver's reports of disease severity begin to diverge. The patient usually rates his or her disease severity far lower than the caregiver does. It is likely similar disparities will occur with quality-of-life ratings.

6. How is dementia clinically different from delirium and affective disorders such as schizophrenia and depression?

A patient's history is the key to sort out the different clinical presentations of these disorders that can affect cognitive function. Of course, a patient can have two diagnoses, especially dementia and depression or dementia and delirium. A patient with delirium may appear to have dementia. The cognitive impairment seen in delirium starts abruptly (especially during a hospitalization) and is marked by periods of waxing and waning alertness. In contrast, patients with dementia generally retain their level of alertness.

Patients with depression also can seem like a patient with dementia, but again, the patient's history may show that the depressed patient may have an antecedent event, such as the death of a spouse or a new diagnosis of a significant disease. In addition, the depressed patient characteristically exaggerates the degree of cognitive impairment compared to his performance on cognitive testing.

Patients with schizophrenia have predominant thought disorders, the hallmark of which is beliefs that do not adhere to reality testing (e.g., "I am Napoleon!"). A patient with dementia also can have delusions, but these usually occur in the middle to late stages of the syndrome. Also, the demented patient will have prominent signs of cognitive dysfunction, such as errors in calculation, language, and memory. The schizophrenic will have relatively preserved cognitive function. Finally, schizophrenia typically presents between the ages of 20 and 35. Dementia typically presents after age 60.

7. How common is dementia in America?

Currently there are more than 4 million Americans diagnosed with AD, and it is projected that the prevalence will quadruple in the next 40 years, when approximately 14 million or 1 in 45 Americans will be affected by the disease. Prevalence increases with age from less than 5% in 60 year olds to over 20% in 80 year olds.

8. Are there risk factors for dementia?

Case-control and cohort studies suggest that the following may place a person at an increased lifetime risk of developing dementia (specifically AD):

- Lower education (less than 12 years of school)
- Advanced age
- Family history of dementia
- Previous head injury
- Genes: two copies of the ApoE ε4 allele (not well established in nonwhite races) and mutations on chromosome 1, 14, and 21

9. What diseases can cause dementia?

After a thorough assessment for medical illnesses and medications that can cause or contribute to cognitive impairment, the clinician should consider four common causes of dementia:

DISEASE	PREVALENCE	DESCRIPTION
Alzheimer's disease (AD)	~60–80%	**Onset:** ages 70–80, range 50–90. **History:** initial changes in memory, language, and judgment followed by changes in personality, behavior, and function. Early-stage patients typically preserve social conduct and well-learned roles despite cognitive impairments. **Neurologic exam:** typically normal during mild and moderate stages of dementia.
Frontotemporal dementia	~10%	**Onset:** ages 50–70. **History:** initial changes in personality, behavior, or language *followed* by changes in memory. **Neurologic exam:** signs of frontal reflexes (e.g., palmomental reflex) may be present.

(Cont'd.)

DISEASE	PREVALENCE	DESCRIPTION
Dementia with Lewy bodies	~10%	**Onset:** ages 60–80 **History:** cognitive dysfunction much like AD except for delusions and visual hallucinations seen early in the course. **Neurologic exam:** parkinsonian signs such as a slow gait, masked face, and cogwheeling.
Ischemic vascular dementia	5%	**History:** stroke closely antecedent to onset of cognitive dysfunction and in a neuroanatomic location that may explain cognitive dysfunction. Most patients with small-vessel disease and periventricular white matter changes on MRI actually have AD.

Although it is best to select the fewest diagnoses to explain the most symptoms, a skilled clinician should recognize that a patient may have more than one cause of dementia or that a patient may have a blend of criteria for different diseases. For instance, "Alzheimer's disease or "vascular dementia" are potential coexistent diagnoses.

Other causes of dementia are Huntington's disease, Jakob-Creutzfeldt disease, progressive supranuclear palsy, Parkinson's disease, and corticobasilar degeneration. Key features of these diseases include rapid progression, focal weakness, impaired eye movements, dysarthria and dysphagia, myoclonus, tremor, and movement disorders. With the exception of Parkinson's disease, all are uncommon. The dementia of Parkinson's disease typically occurs later in the course of the illness, a key feature that distinguishes it from dementia with Lewy bodies.

10. What is a caregiver?

Dementia is a disease that impacts the patient's entire family and social network. At the center of this family are at least one caregiver and the patient. The standard of care for the *patient* with dementia must include care for the *caregiver* of that patient. A caregiver occupies at least four roles:

Caregiver Roles

ROLE	FEATURES OF ROLE
Knowledgeable informant about disease progression and response to therapies	Day-to-day experience of the patient provides valuable knowledge of the patient's cognitive and physical function. Clinicians should teach caregiver how to observe and record these functions.
Decision-maker for the patient	Cognitive impairment can cause a patient to be incapable of making a decision. Caregiver acts as a surrogate decision-maker. Clinicians should teach caregiver how to serve the patient's best interests.
Caretaker for the patient	Cognitive impairment can cause a patient to be incapable of performing IADLs and BADLs. Caregiver will assume these tasks. Clinicians should teach caregiver when to expect functional losses and ways to cope with them.
Second patient	Caregivers are likely to experience emotional, social, and financial burden. Clinicians should assess caregiver for depression and related illnesses.

IADLs = instrumental activities of daily living (e.g., using the telephone, cooking, cleaning, managing money, using transportation, shopping). BADLs = basic activities of daily living (e.g., feeding, transferring, toileting, dressing, bathing/grooming).

Although one person can fulfill all four of these roles, it is highly likely that multiple persons will share one or more of these roles. Dementia is a disease that requires a biopsychosocial approach that challenges the traditional ethic that autonomous patients self-determine their care. Proper care of the patient requires careful attention to family dynamics. If caregivers are to properly fulfill these roles, they need core knowledge and skills, including information about diagnosis, prognosis, and treatment, and support for emotional and financial burden. Randomized trials demonstrate providing information and support to caregivers may postpone the need for 24-hour nursing care.

The clinician should develop skills to respect the balance between the provision of a standard of care and the individuality of each family. This is particularly important for managing issues such as discussing the patient in his or her presence and disclosing the diagnosis to the patient.

11. What is caregiver burden and why should we care about it?

The term *caregiver burden* describes the emotional, social, medical, and financial impact of caregiving on a person. Manifestations include depression, isolation, stress-related illnesses, and poverty. Caregiver burden is significant for at least three reasons. First, research shows that a caregiver's ability to accurately assess a patient is influenced by the caregiver's mood and burden. Second, research shows that patients and caregivers benefit when caregivers receive interventions to relieve burden. Third, the caregiver is a person, not an instrument, who deserves the dignity and respect accorded to all persons.

12. Discuss the work-up of a patient who has signs and symptoms of cognitive impairment.

A thorough history is the cornerstone of a work-up. The clinician should interview both the patient and the caregiver; and some portion of each person's interview should be separate from the others. A skilled clinician should prompt the caregiver to narrate the patient's history of cognitive dysfunction in as much detail as possible. The clinician should assess for evidence of impairment in several categories:

Categories and Features of Impairment

CATEGORY OF IMPAIRMENT	TYPICAL FEATURES
Memory	Difficulty retaining new information and recalling information acquired in the past
Function: Advanced activities of daily living (AADLs): Work, hobbies, and leisure activities, such as going to church, reading, and golf	Inability or partial ability to complete a function that patient was fully capable of doing before. AADLs and IADLs are characteristically lost before BADLs in AD.
Instrumental activities of daily living (IADLs): Using the telephone, cooking, cleaning, managing money, and medications, using transportation, shopping	
Basic activities of daily living (BADLs): Feeding, toileting, dressing, grooming, and bathing, and walking	BADLs are characteristically lost in the reverse order that they are acquired in infancy*
Language	Substitution of words; agrammatical speech; changes conversation topics without proper cuing; paucity of speech output
Behavior and personality	*Changes commonly seen in frontal lobe dysfunction:* Disinhibited behavior, such as hypersexuality, public nudity, and cursing Repetition of tasks *Changes commonly seen other than frontal lobe dysfunction:* Blunting of affect; blunting of social engagement

* A pattern that does not fit these criteria is highly suggestive of an illness other than dementia.

13. Which tests of cognitive function are most useful for evaluating cognitive impairment?

The clinician should be able to administer and interpret a standardized set of cognitive tests that cover the range of cognitive and emotional functions described above. The Mini-Mental Status exam (MMSE) is a common test, it combines tests of multiple cognitive functions to determine whether the patient is cognitively impaired. The following table lists standard tests and their normal values:

Standard Tests and Their Normal Values

FUNCTION	MEASURES	SCORING
Affect	Geriatric depression scale (GDS)—short form; evaluate answers to simple questions "Are you depressed?" and "Are you anxious?"	GDS < 5(+) out of 15
Memory	Five-minute recall of 3 words; recite full date, home address, and telephone number	Recall 2 or 3 out of 3
Language	Naming parts of objects; generating from a category a list of words in one-minute (e.g., "Tell me all the animals you can think of."); following a multi-step command	10 or more words in 60 seconds
Visuospatial	Draw the face of a clock to show that it is 8:20 (the instructions can be repeated if necessary; this is not a test of memory); draw two interlocking pentagons	10 angles and 4 interlocking sides
Judgment	Ask what they would do in a real-life situation (e.g., "What would you do if you arrived in a strange city and wanted to find a friend that lived there?")	Judgment of examiner
Attention and calculation	Spell *world* backwards; count down from 100 to 85 by 3's	No errors for individuals with ≥ 12 years schooling

14. What laboratory and imaging tests are most useful for evaluating dementia?

After medical illnesses have been excluded as the cause of a patient's cognitive impairment, few (if any) clinically useful laboratory tests can diagnose the cause of a dementia. One goal of clinical research is to develop tests that measure biologic markers of disease. At present, candidate biomarkers for AD are cerebrospinal fluid tau protein (a component of the neurofibrillary tangles) and beta-amyloid (a component of the neuritic plaques). Clinicians should carefully follow the literature that reports the operating characteristics of these diagnostic tests.

Neuroimaging tests can be useful to confirm a diagnosis of the cause of dementia. Functional neuroimaging studies such as positron emission tomography (PET) and single photon emission computed tomography (SPECT) scans demonstrate cerebral metabolism (directly with PET, indirectly with SPECT). These studies are not recommended in the diagnostic evaluation of dementia at this time. Structural neuroimaging tests such as computed axial tomography (CAT) and MRI scans demonstrate neuroanatomy. MRI is the preferred study for assessing focal or global cortical atrophy, mass lesions, and cerebral infarcts. Two key issues should temper the clinician's ordering hand: the administration and interpretation of these tests is operator-dependent (decreasing reliability and validity), and many insurance companies will not reimburse the charges when used for the diagnosis of dementia.

15. What treatments are available for dementia?

There are two classes of treatments for dementia: disease-slowing and symptomatic. At present, few disease-slowing therapies are available. Vitamin E (at doses of 1,000 international units twice a day) has been shown to slow the progression of Alzheimer's disease. Selegiline may do the same. The ability of cholinesterase inhibitors to slow progression is debatable. Clinicians should keep close attention to the literature for developments. The multiple symptomatic treatments may be categorized in categories of behavioral and pharmacologic treatments. They can affect cognition, function, mood, and behavior.

Multiple Symptomatic Treatments

TREATMENT CATEGORY	COGNITION AND FUNCTION	MOOD	BEHAVIOR
Pharmacological	Cholinesterase inhibitors (e.g., donepezil, rivastigmine, galantamine)	Serotonergic reuptake inhibitors (e.g., sertraline) Tricyclic antidepressants	Antipsychotics Benzodiazepines Mood stabilizers
Behavioral	Remove hazards from environment Emphasize assistance over dependence in early-stage patients	Nonstressful activities during the day (e.g., adult day care) Supportive counseling	Identify and then re-direct patient from sources of stress Identify calming activities such as aroma or music therapy

16. How do we know that treatment for a dementia is working?

Patients with dementia lack the insight and judgment to assess their own symptoms. The general goal of all treatment is to maximize the patient's quality of life and function, but how to assess these is unclear. The caregiver is a key person here. The caregiver not only acts as a knowledgeable informant, but also can help to assess the degree of patient response. The clinician's role is to help the caregiver assess the areas of function, cognition, mood, and behavior. The goal of the caregiver and clinician is to arrive at a consensus concerning the direction and degree of a patient's global change, including agitation and psychosis, whether it is improved, unaltered, or worse.

17. A patient with severe-stage dementia develops aspiration. How can this be managed?

If aspiration occurs in a patient with severe-stage dementia, it is reasonable to approach the problem with exclusive attention to maintaining the patient's dignity and quality of life. The clinician should carefully assess the patient's ability to swallow food and liquid safely and comfortably. A speech therapist may be useful here. In general, careful oral feeding with attention to the pace of feeding and the portion and consistency of foods can significantly decrease complicated episodes of aspiration. The data describing the inability of enteral feeding to reduce aspiration risk and the 6-month and 1-year mortality rates suggest that this intervention should follow only after considerable discussion of its risks and potential benefits in the context of the patient's dignity and quality of life. Time-limited trials of interventions also help to settle uncertainty. Decision-makers must be comfortable with withdrawing an ineffective treatment.

18. How do patients die of dementia?

Most of the research on prognosis comes from patients with AD. Survival after diagnosis ranges from 2–10 years. Death follows complications of functional impairments in swallowing, movement, and nonstarvation-related loss of lean body mass. Typical causes are pneumonia, urinary tract infection, and infected stage 4 pressure ulcers.

19. How is dementia staged?

Valid instruments that stage the progression of AD include the Clinical Dementia Rating (CDR) and Dementia Severity Rating Scales (DSRS). The DSRS is completed by the caregiver.

In general, the five broad categories of disease severity are mild, moderate, severe, profound, and terminal. The following table describes the typical patient who fits in each category. Note that for a patient with frontotemporal dementia, behavior symptoms are frequntly more prominent in the "mild stage." A patient also may fit in between stages, such as "moderate to severe."

Stages of Dementia

	MILD	MODERATE	SEVERE	PROFOUND	TERMINAL
Function	IADL-independent or decreased ability with complex tasks ADL-independent	IADL-dependent or assistance needed ADL-independent or reminders, assistance needed	IADL-dependent ADL-dependent (incontinent, able to feed self, still ambulatory)	IADL-dependent ADL-dependent (loss of ambulation, feeds with assistance)	Inability to walk or sit up without assistance Inability to smile or hold head up > 10% body weight loss, pressure ulcers > stage 2 urinary tract infection, aspiration pneumonia
Cognition	Difficulty in learning new information, memory loss interferes with everyday functions Difficulty with time relationships Mild word finding difficulty Able to carry on social conversation Mild judgment impairment	Substantial memory loss, disoriented in time, often to place Conversation disorganized, rambling Judgment impaired Decreased attention span	Oriented to person only Only fragments of memory remain Severe language impairment Inconsistent recognition of familiar people Very short attention span	Speaks < 6 words Consistent difficulty in recognizing familiar people	Few words spoken
Behavior	Mild personality changes Less engaged in relationships Appears normal	May have psychotic, wandering, elopement, agitated verbal or physical symptoms Sleep disturbance Appears well enough to be taken to functions outside of home	Emotional lability Restlessness Inability to focus on tasks Appears too ill to be taken to functions outside the home	Repetitive vocalizations, calling out More passive	Passive
Cognitive scores	MMSE ≥ 19	MMSE 12–19	MMSE 0–11	MMSE < 11	Not testable

From Cotter VT: Forgetfulness. In Goolsby MJ (ed): Nurse Practitioner Secrets. Philadelphia, Hanley & Belfus, 2002, pp 64–70, with permission.

20. How do you know if a patient with dementia is competent to make medical decisions?

A diagnosis of dementia *does not* mean that the patient is incompetent, but it does raise clinical suspicion that the patient *may* be incompetent. A clinician should be skilled in competency assessment, which relies on assessing the patient's specific abilities to understand, appreciate, and rationally manipulate the information needed to make a decision. A patient's decision-making abilities should be weighed against the balance of the risks and potential benefits of the decision. Because competency is specific to each decision the patient must make, the context of each decision is very important. For instance, a patient with AD may not be competent to decide to take a nonsteroidal anti-inflammatory drug (which has unproven benefits in AD and real risks such as gastrointestinal bleeding). However, the same patient may be competent to decide whether to take vitamin E to slow the progression of AD (which has proven benefits and few if any risks).

ACKNOWLEDGMENTS

The authors thank the participants of the Washington University in St. Louis e-mail discussion group on Alzheimer's disease for their thoughtful suggestions (www.biostat.wustl.edu/alzheimer/).

BIBLIOGRAPHY

1. Clark CM, Ewbank D: Performance of the dementia severity rating scale: A caregiver questionnaire for rating severity in Alzheimer's disease. Alzheimer Dis Assoc Disord 10:31–39, 1996.
2. Cotter VT: Forgetfulness. IN Goolsby MJ (ed): Nurse Practitioner Secrets. Philadelphia, Hanley & Belfus, 2002, pp 64–70.
3. Doody RS, Stevens JC, Beck C, et al: Practice parameter: Management of dementia (an evidence-based review). Neurology 56:1154–1166, 2001.
4. Finucane TE, Bynum JPW: Use of tube feeding to prevent aspiration pneumonia. Lancet 348: 1421–1424, 1996.
5. Grisso T, Appelbaum PS: Assessing Competence to Consent to Treatment. A Guide for Physicians and Other Health Care Professionals. New York, Oxford University Press, 1998.
6. Haley WE: The family caregiver's role in Alzheimer's disease. Neurology 48:S25–S29, 1997.
7. Knopman DS, DeKosky ST, Cummings JL, et al: Practice parameter: Diagnosis of dementia (an evidence-based review). Neurology 56:1143–1153, 2001.
8. McKhann GM, Albert MS, Grossman M, et al: Clinical and pathological diagnosis of frontotemporal dementia: Report of the work group on frontotemporal dementia and Pick's disease. Arch Neurol 58:1803–1809, 2001.
9. Mittelman M, Ferris S, Shulman E, et al: A family intervention to delay nursing home placement of patients with Alzheimer's disease: A randomized controlled trial. JAMA 276:1725–1731, 1996.
10. Office of Technology Assessment: Losing a Million Minds: Confronting the Tragedy of Alzheimer's Disease and Other Dementias. Washington, D.C., U.S. Government Printing Office, 1987.
11. Rogers S, Farlow M, Doody R, et al: A 24-week, double-blind, placebo-controlled trial of donepezil in patients with Alzheimer's disease. Donepezil study group. Neurology 50:136–145, 1998.
12. Sano M, Ernesto C, Thomas RG, et al: A controlled trial of selegiline, alpha-tocopherol, or both as treatment for Alzheimer's disease. N Engl J Med 336:1216–1222, 1997.
13. United States General Accounting Office: Alzheimer's disease: Estimates of prevalence in the United States. Washington DC, GAO/HEHS-98-16. Report of the Secretary of Health and Human Services, 1998.

WEBSITE

www 1/9/03 http://ww.alz.org/About AD/statistics.htm

10. DEPRESSION

David S. Miller, MD

1. What is the difference between depression and normal sadness?

Depressive illnesses in older people, like those in younger adults, can occur without obvious causes or precipitants. More often, however, late-life depression occurs in the context of medical illness, psychosocial stress, and loss, and so most depressions make sense empathetically and intuitively. Unfortunately, this often leads to the view that depression is a "natural" state of aging rather than a medical symptom requiring evaluation.

Despite these misconceptions, the distinction between depressive illness and normal sadness is straightforward. Depressive illnesses are persistent, lasting for several weeks or longer. Depressive illnesses can be disabling, interfering with social, instrumental, or self-care activities either by themselves or by amplifying the disability associated with medical illness. Although the relationships between depression and disability can be complex and bidirectional, patients who have persistent depression coexisting with functional impairments require medical evaluation.

2. What subtypes of depression are relevant in late life?

Major depressive disorder is characterized by episodes in which the following symptoms persist:

Persistent depressed mood	Hypersomnia
Markedly decreased interest or pleasure in usual activities	Psychomotor agitation or retardation
Decreased appetite and weight loss	Fatigue or loss of energy
Increased appetite and weight gain (more rarely)	Feelings of worthlessness or excessive guilt
	Decreased ability to think or concentrate
Insomnia	Suicidal thoughts, wishes, plan, or intent

According to the *Diagnostic and Statistical Manual for Mental Disorders* (DSM-IV), the diagnosis of a **major depressive episode** can be made when patients have depressed mood and/or loss of interests or pleasure and a total of five of the above symptoms to a significant degree for a period of at least 2 weeks.

Major depression can occur as a *single* episode or as part of a *recurring* pattern of episodes. Depressions occurring in the elderly can be of *early onset*, in which the late-life depression occurs as a recurrence of an illness that began in younger adulthood, or *late onset*, in which illness began initially at an older age. Recurrent depression can be *bipolar*, where both depressive and manic or hypomanic episodes occur, or *unipolar*, in which only depressions occur. This distinction between unipolar and bipolar is important because antidepressant treatment of bipolar patients may precipitate manic or hypomanic episodes. Depressions can also be associated with *psychotic* features (hallucinations or delusions). Psychotic depressions do not, as a rule, respond to antidepressants alone and instead require both antidepressants and antipsychotic medications or electroconvulsive therapy.

Although less severe, other types of depressions are also clinically significant. **Dysthymic disorder** is a condition in which lower levels of depressive symptoms exist chronically for a period of 2 years or more. **Minor depressions** include those in which symptoms of depression and anxiety coexist and those in which more severe depressive symptoms occur briefly but recurrently.

3. How is depression related to other medical illness?

The NIH consensus conference on the diagnosis and treatment of late-life depression noted that the hallmark of depression in the elderly was its association with medical illness. Late-onset depressions, in general, emerged in the context of chronic medical or neurologic illness, and a growing body of epidemiologic research demonstrates an increased prevalence of major depression in medical care settings. Major depression occurs in approximately 2–4% of healthy elderly in the community, 10–12% of elderly medical inpatients, and 20–25% of cognitively intact nursing home residents. In addition, as many as 30–50% of patients in medical care settings have clinically significant minor depressions. Clinicians should systematically determine whether comorbid depression is present in all elderly patients with significant medical illness whom they see. Conversely, all elderly individuals who present to mental health care settings for evaluation of depression should be evaluated for significant medical illnesses. Major depression is now thought likely to increase the risk of developing a number of different medical conditions. Among them are dementia, osteoporosis, myocardial infarction, diabetes, breast cancer, and Alzheimer's disease.

4. How do you treat depression that occurs as part of a medical illness?

When depression complicates significant **acute medical illnesses**, patients require support. Specific treatment is necessary when depression is severe or when it interferes with medical management. For more moderate depressions, continued monitoring of affective symptoms during the course of recovery from the medical illness is necessary. Treatment for depression should be instituted when the depression persists despite improvement in medical status.

When depression occurs in medically stable patients with **chronic illness**, systems should be reviewed to identify possible medical causes of the affective symptoms. Common causes include unrecognized acute illnesses (e.g., heart failure, urinary tract infections), side effects of medications (e.g., beta blockers), electrolyte abnormalities (e.g., hyponatremia, hypercalcemia), thyroid dysfunction, and vitamin B_{12} or folate deficiency. A review of systems is also necessary to identify medical conditions that could complicate treatment; for example, before use of tricyclic antidepressants, patients must be evaluated for disorders of cardiac conduction, prostate hypertrophy, and glaucoma.

5. How can you tell if a particular symptom is due to medical illness or to depression?

Extensive literature in the field of consultation-liaison psychiatry has focused on the possibility that medical symptoms can obscure the diagnosis of major depression. Some symptoms, such as fatigue, can be due to medical illnesses (e.g., heart failure) or to depression. Experienced clinicians can evaluate the etiology of symptoms and "factor" them into their medical and depressive components. Even with truly ambiguous symptoms, utilizing an inclusive approach to diagnosis based on all observed symptoms, regardless of their apparent etiology, can still be helpful. Despite the theoretical difficulties, current approaches to diagnosis have, in fact, been validated in patients suffering from many of the comorbid medical disorders that are common in late life. Controlled clinical trials have demonstrated that depressions diagnosed in patients with medical illnesses as diverse as stroke, parkinsonism, cancer, ischemic heart disease, chronic obstructive pulmonary disease, and arthritis still respond to treatment.

6. What is depressive pseudodementia?

Classically, most textbooks in geriatric psychiatry emphasized the difficulties in identifying patients in whom major depression caused significant cognitive impairment and in distinguishing between these potentially treatable cases of "pseudodementia" and irreversible dementias such as Alzheimer's disease. The use of the term *pseudodementia* has been criticized by some investigators who note that severe depression can cause real cognitive impairment. The name **dementia syndrome of depression** has been proposed to emphasize that although these conditions are treatable, there is nothing "pseudo" about the disability resulting from severe depression.

More significantly, Reifler and colleagues noted that patients with coexisting depression and cognitive impairment could have either one disease or two. Patients could have a pure depressive disorder associated with cognitive impairment (pseudodementia), in which case, treatment of depression could restore normal levels of functioning. Alternatively, they could have an irreversible dementia with a superimposed depressive disorder. In these cases, treatment of depression could reverse only a component of the patient's disability. In either case, recognition, diagnosis, and treatment of depression could be of benefit to the patient.

7. What is the long-term prognosis for patients having dementia syndrome with depression?

Recent research has been reevaluating the long-term prognosis of patients with depression associated with cognitive impairment that is alleviated through treatment. Two generations ago, there were concerns that all depressions with onset in late-life were prodromes of dementia. A generation ago, systematic follow-up studies on patients hospitalized for depression demonstrated that depression and dementia were, in fact, separable disorders and that the long-term outcome of most patients with late-life depression did not include cognitive deterioration. New research in this area, however, suggests that patients with depression associated with reversible cognitive impairment are at increased risk for developing dementia over the subsequent few years. At present, these findings should not be taken to reflect nihilism about outcomes for these patients but rather should underscore the importance of long-term follow-up and treatment.

8. What are the problems associated with untreated depression?

Untreated or undertreated depression is associated with both psychiatric and general medical consequences. Psychiatric morbidity includes chronicity with its associated psychosocial disability, risks of alcohol or substance abuse in attempts at self-treatment, and suicide. The most compelling case for the importance of the recognition of depression by primary care physicians comes from the finding that 75% of older people who kill themselves saw their physicians within 30 days of their deaths.

Suicide can occur not only when depression is missed but at any time during the treatment course of a depressive episode. Closer surveillance is indicated if the patient expresses suicidal thoughts, intent, and/or describes a plan. There is a transient increased suicide risk in the early stages of treatment, as patients gain the energy and capacity to act on their earlier plans.

Medical morbidity associated with depression includes increased disability, protein-calorie undernutrition, increased pain complaints, and greater sensitivity to subjective side effects of medications. There are also increases in utilization of general medical care services (inpatient and outpatient) and in caregiver burden. Finally, there is an increase in mortality, even after controlling for the increased severity of medical illnesses in patients with depression.

9. When should patients receive antidepressant medications?

The efficacy of antidepressant medications has been established for the treatment of patients with major depression. Thus, clinicians should inquire about the presence of the DSM-IV diagnostic symptoms. Significantly (and counterintuitively), evaluating a patient's need for antidepressant medication requires knowledge about symptoms but not about the presence or absence of reasons for the depression.

In addition to their well-established use in the treatment of major depression, antidepressants may be of value in patients who have dysthymia or minor depression with more severe functional impairment as well as in patients who do not respond to psychosocial treatment.

10. When should older patients receive psychotherapy?

Structured psychotherapies, such as cognitive-behavioral therapy, interpersonal therapy, or brief dynamic therapies, may be the treatments of choice for dysthymia or minor depression. They may also be a first-line treatment for milder major depression; however, if these patients do not experience a significant amelioration of their symptoms within several weeks, use of antidepressants should be reconsidered.

In general, depression in the elderly frequently has associated functional and social difficulties. Among these are loss of or changed roles, lack of social support, chronic medical illnesses, hopelessness, disability, and bereavement. Therefore, psychotherapy can be extremely useful as an adjuvant to pharmacotherapy in patients with major depression of moderate severity.

11. What are first- and second-line agents used in the pharmacotherapy of depression?

Selective serotonin reuptake inhibitors (SSRIs—e.g., fluoxetine, sertraline, paroxetine, citalopram): Given their tolerable side effect profile and safety in overdose, these agents are appropriate first-line treatments for depression in ambulatory elderly, especially those seen by primary care providers. They have fewer anticholinergic and cardiac side effects but may cause nausea, diarrhea, somnolence, and headache. Their once-daily dosing and tolerability may enhance compliance. However, although SSRIs are somewhat less effective in people over 75-years-old, their efficacy and safety in frail or medically ill elderly patients have not been established. In such patients, SSRIs may cause lethargy, anorexia, and syndrome of inappropriate antidiuretic hormone secretion. In the elderly, who frequently take multiple medications, particular attention must be paid to the effect of SSRIs on hepatic metabolism of other medications via the cytochrome P450 system. Additional problems may include drug interactions, extrapyramidal symptoms, bradycardia, and sexual dysfunction.

Tricyclic antidepressants (TCAs): The secondary amine TCAs nortriptyline and desipramine are preferred for use in the elderly. Their efficacy in the elderly, including patients with significant medical comorbidity, has been well-established. Moreover, these agents are less likely to produce orthostasis (which can lead to falls and fractures), excessive sedation, anticholinergic symptoms, or cardiac toxicity than the tertiary amine TCAs (e.g., amitriptyline or imipramine). The secondary amine TCAs can be used safely in patients who do not have cardiac conduction problems, acute narrow-angle glaucoma, and prostatic hypertrophy with urinary retention. With these agents, plasma level–response correlations have been established, and therapeutic blood levels (80–120 ng/ml for nortriptyline and > 125 ng/ml for desipramine) can be utilized to individualize doses for the individual patient.

	SEDATION	HYPOTENSION	ANTICHOLINERGIC SIDE EFFECTS	CHANGES IN CARDIAC RATE AND RHYTHM
Desipramine	+	+/++	+	+
Nortriptyline	+	+	++	+

Other agents: Among the newer antidepressants, mirtazapine, bupropion, and venlafaxine may be of value in treating older patients. Some of these agents target more than one neurotransmitter system to enhance effectiveness.

12. How do you select an appropriate medication?

Before an antidepressant is chosen one must consider the risks and benefits for that particular patient. Factors to be mindful of are concurrent medical conditions and medications, substance abuse problems (e.g., alcohol abuse), and the likelihood of overdose, either by suicide attempt or secondary to cognitive problems. Several basic principles can be outlined:

- For ambulatory outpatients with major depression that is mild to moderate in severity, the first-line use of SSRIs or other well-tolerated agents is reasonable.
- For patients with more severe depression, early use of the better-established TCAs should be considered.
- In patients who are frail or with specific medical conditions that could complicate use of these agents, hospitalization may be necessary to optimize safety during the institution of treatment. Frequently, an extensive list of medications can and should be pared down (generally in consultation with the geriatric medicine team). This affords the treatment team an opportunity to determine to what degree the patient's presenting symptoms are iatrogenic. Concurrently, as the patient's medical conditions are treated, the depression may lessen or remit. When it does not, antidepressants are indicated.
- Regardless of which medications are used initially, it is necessary to monitor patients to evaluate both therapeutic responses and to identify side effects.
- If patients do not show early signs of response within 4–6 weeks, it is important to consider modifying the treatment plan.

13. Should St. John's wort be used?

St. John's wort has been shown to be better than placebo and as effective as tricyclic antidepressants and selective serotonin reuptake inhibitors for mild-to-moderate but not for severe depression. It should be noted, however, that this herbal preparation induces various drug-metabolizing enzymes. Therefore, caution must be used in patients taking oral contraceptives, warfarin (Coumadin), and HIV protease inhibitors, among others.

14. How long should treatment be continued?

Treatment of depression can be divided into three phases:

Acute phase (goal: to achieve symptom remission)—The median time to recover from the acute phase of an index episode of depression is 12 weeks (longer than for younger patients). Discerning whether a patient is responding can only reliably be done after 4–6 weeks.

Continuation phase (goal: to stabilize patients during a period when they are highly vulnerable to relapse)—All patients recovering from an episode of depression are vulnerable to relapse during the first 6–9 months after symptom remission. All patients should remain in continuation-phase treatment for this period of time.

Maintenance phase (goal: to prevent recurrence)—At the completion of the continuation phase, patients and their physicians must decide whether treatment should be discontinued (by slowly tapering antidepressant doses) or whether the patient should remain on long-term maintenance treatment to decrease the probability of recurrences. If treatment is discontinued, the patient and family should be educated and informed about the need for continued monitoring to facilitate the early identification of recurrences. If the patient has had > 2 episodes of depression, or if the initial episodes were particularly severe or lengthy, long-term (possibly lifetime) maintenance therapy should be considered.

15. When should electroconvulsive therapy (ECT) be considered?

The indications for ECT in both younger and older patients include severe major depression and mania. Older patients with severe depression often present with psychotic symptoms and suicidality (occasionally taking the form of food refusal). They may respond to SSRIs less consistently and may be less able to tolerate the anticholinergic and cardiac side effects of the TCAs. Therefore, the elderly are more likely to require ECT. They actually account for a disproportionate percentage of those who get ECT (receiving > 30% of all ECTs despite representing < 10% of all hospitalized psychiatric patients).

ECT is safe and effective, even when there are physical comorbidities or dementia. It should be considered the treatment of choice when a rapid response is needed for severely depressed patients. It should also be considered in patients who have previously not responded to adequate trials of antidepressant treatment.

16. What can be done when patients don't respond to treatment?

Between 20 and 30% of patients fail to respond satisfactorily to initial treatment with an antidepressant medication. Possible explanations include improper diagnosis, inadequate treatment, and failure to identify and treat concurrent general medical and psychiatric disorders.

Obstacles to administering adequate treatment include:

- Poor compliance by both patient and family (who may fail to understand the illness, its course, and/or the importance of compliance)
- Side effects
- Hidden self-medication (e.g., alcohol)
- Adverse psychosocial factors (which may diminish the desire to comply)
- Medical comorbidities (which can interfere with antidepressant response or attainment of adequate dosages)

Steps the clinician can take to enhance compliance include creating an alliance with and providing education about depression to the patient and family, being mindful of side effects so as to decrease them when they occur, and maintaining a supportive attitude.

Once satisfied on all counts that the initial trial was adequate, one can either augment the present medication or switch to another agent (from another class of antidepressant). Adjuvant treatments include:

- Lithium (a response should be seen within a few days to a few weeks; blood levels indicating therapeutic levels are not clear)
- Thyroid hormone
- Psychostimulants

The anticonvulsants carbamazepine and valproic acid have been used both as primary and adjuvant agents for treatment-resistant depression. Occasionally the clinician will choose an antidepressant that targets more than one neutrotransmitter system. Sometimes, multiple antidepressants are used simultaneously. Combined treatment, however, carries the risk of adverse interactions and may require dose adjustment (e.g., SSRIs can increase TCA blood levels, and thus TCA doses may need to be reduced to avoid toxicity). If a patient fails two separate trials of antidepressant medication, ECT should be considered.

17. Under what circumstances are psychostimulants indicated?

In the elderly, psychostimulants such as methylphenidate (Ritalin) are generally used for two purposes. The first is to treat patients who, although not severely depressed, become apathetic or discouraged, frequently in the context of chronic disease or rehabilitation from illness or surgery. Although not effective in treating major depression, psychostimulants have been found to be helpful in medically ill patients and apathetic nursing home residents. The second use is to augment an ongoing antidepressant trial in which the response has been suboptimal.

Ritalin is well tolerated and works quickly. It should be given in the morning to avoid insomnia. Dosing should begin at 2.5–5.0 mg/day and titrated to a maximum of 20 mg/day (generally divided between 8:00 AM and noon). The most common side effects are tachycardia and mild elevation in blood pressure.

18. What are the most important points about late-life depression for primary care doctors?

1. The diagnosis of late-life depression is as valid as that of other significant medical disorders.
2. Major depression in the elderly is a significant disorder associated with both psychiatric and medical morbidity, increased utilization of general health care services, and increased mortality.
3. Late-life depression is a treatable disorder.

BIBLIOGRAPHY

1. Alexopoulos GS, Meyers GS, Young RC, et al: The course of geriatric depression with "reversible dementia": A controlled study. Am J Psychiatry 150:1693–1699, 1993.
2. Conwell Y: Suicide in elderly patients. In Schneider LS, Reynolds CF, Lebowitz BD, Friedhoff AJ (eds): Diagnosis and Treatment of Depression in Late Life. Washington D.C., American Psychiatric Press, 1994, pp 397–418.
3. Jones BN, Reifler BV: Depression coexisting with dementia: Evaluation and treatment. Med Clin North Am 78:823–840, 1994.
4. Katz IR: Drug treatment of depression in the frail elderly: Discussion of the NIH consensus development conference on the diagnosis and treatment of depression in late life. Psychopharmacol Bull 29(1):101–108, 1993.
5. Katz IR: Diagnosis and treatment of depression in patients with Alzheimer's disease and other dementias. J Clin Psychiatry 59(Suppl 9):38–44, 1998.
6. Katz IR, Miller D, Oslin D: Diagnosis of late-life depression. In Salzman C (ed): Clinical Geriatric Psychopharmacology, 3rd ed. Philadelphia, Lippincott Williams & Wilkins, 1998, pp 153–183.
7. Katz IR, Streim J, Parmelee P: Prevention of depression, recurrences, and complications in late life. Prev Med 23:743–750, 1994.
8. Reynolds CF, Alexopoulos G, Katz IR, et al: Treatment of geriatric mood disorders. Curr Rev Mood Disord 1:189–202, 1997.
9. Schneider LS, Reynolds CF, Lebowitz BD, Friedhoff AJ (eds): Diagnosis and Treatment of Depression in Late Life: Results of the NIH Consensus Development Conference. Washington, D.C., American Psychiatric Press, 1994.
10. Wallace AE, Kofoed LL, West AN: Double-blind placebo-controlled trial of methylphenidate in older, depressed medically ill patients. Am J Psychiatry 152:929–931, 1995.

11. INSOMNIA

Nalaka Gooneratne, MD

1. What changes occur in the typical sleep patterns of adults as they age?

Sleep is divided into five stages. Each stage is characterized by unique electroencephalogram (EEG) findings. The sleep of older adults is characterized by a decrease in stage III/IV sleep (slow-wave sleep), possibly the most restful phase of sleep. However, this may be due in part to a technicality: due to age-related changes such as atrophy, elderly subjects may continue to have stage III/IV sleep yet do not meet the technical definitions of stage III/IV sleep. In addition, the elderly have more frequent nocturnal arousals (awakenings) and their sleep efficiency (total time asleep ÷ total time in bed) is decreased.

Sleep Stages and Their Characteristics

SLEEP STAGE	CHARACTERISTICS	LENGTH (MIN)	CHANGE WITH AGING
I	Decreased muscle tone, slow eye movements	30	Increased
II	EEG with spindles and K-complexes	200	Stable
III/IV	Delta waves present on EEG	30	Decreased
REM	Rapid eye movements, decreased muscle tone, low amplitude EEG	150	Shortened time to first REM episode

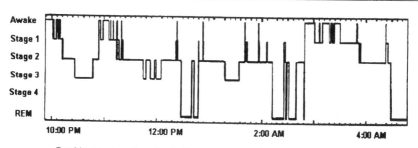

Graphic overview of a patient's sleep stages during the course of a sleep study.

Patients with Alzheimer's disease (even those with mild disease) have a generalized slowing of background EEG activity, a decrease in rapid eye movement (REM) sleep, a significant increase in nocturnal awakenings, reduction in slow-wave sleep, and altered stage I and II morphology. The decline in REM sleep often parallels the patient's intellectual decline. Patients with severe Alzheimer's disease may spend as much as 40% of their bedtime hours awake and up to 14% of their daytime hours asleep.

2. How is insomnia defined?

The term *insomnia* often is used loosely to describe the symptom of difficulty initiating or maintaining sleep. **Transient insomnia** refers to self-limiting cases that last < 1 month and usually do not require treatment. **Chronic insomnia** is defined as lasting > 1 month and is the focus of this chapter. The prevalence of the complaint of chronic insomnia in the elderly varies from study to study, with a range of 10% to 35%. There are many classification systems for insomnia, but most broadly distinguish between **primary insomnia** and **secondary insomnia** (insomnia due to other causes). The *Diagnostic and Statistical Manual of Mental Disorders, 4th ed. (DSM-IV)* is primarily used in this discussion because it is straightforward and widely recognized. To satisfy the *DSM-IV* criteria for primary insomnia, a patient must have the following:

A. A predominant complaint of insomnia for ≥ 1 month
B. The sleep disturbance (or associated daytime fatigue) causes clinically significant distress
C. Insomnia does not occur during other sleep disorders (e.g., sleep apnea)
D. An absence of coexisting mental disorders (e.g., major depressive disorder)
E. The disturbance is not due to substance abuse or a general medical condition.

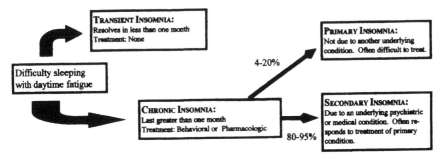

Types of insomnia and their relationship to one another.

Prevalences of primary insomnia may vary: in the elderly, it may constitute 4.1% of cases of insomnia (with a 1.2% population prevalence), but it may be as high as 20.2% of the total cases of insomnia. Secondary insomnia differs from primary insomnia in that criteria C, D, or E above may not be met. It accounts for the remaining 80–95% of insomnia cases. Women tend to have more complaints of insomnia than men.

A large discrepancy exists between the number of individuals who state they have difficulty sleeping and the clinical diagnosis of insomnia using the *DSM-IV* because of its more rigorous criteria in the classification paradigms. The elderly in particular are a diagnostic challenge and often report a lack of daytime repercussions of their insomnia complaint, thus failing to satisfy criterion B of the *DSM-IV* system; often they remain without a specific diagnosis to a greater degree than younger subjects. Fortunately, many of these patients will respond to the behavioral treatments outlined in question 8.

3. What are the different types of secondary insomnia?

Secondary insomnia may be due to psychiatric diseases or comorbid medical problems. The following is a list of their specific subtypes and incidences based on the *DSM-IV*:

- **Psychiatric diagnosis associated with an insomnia complaint.** In these cases, the patient has a primary psychiatric diagnosis, most commonly generalized anxiety disorder or major depressive disorder, and the insomnia is but one of many aspects of the disease. The insomnia often does not warrant specific attention and improves as the underlying problem is treated. Some studies suggest that more than one-half of all individuals who complain of insomnia fall into this category.
- **Insomnia due to an underlying mental disorder.** In certain situations the insomnia is the *main complaint* of a patient who actually suffers from a mood disorder; this insomnia is severe enough to warrant specific attention. Such patients often "focus on their sleep disturbance to the exclusion of the symptoms characteristic of the mental disorder, whose presence may become apparent only after specific and persistent questioning." Thus, this type of secondary insomnia is distinguished from psychiatric diagnosis associated with an insomnia complaint, in which case the insomnia is a minor (not the major) part of the symptom complex of another primary psychiatric diagnosis. Insomnia

due to an underlying mental disorder affects 2.0% of people older than 65. It may account for up to 44% of cases of insomnia.

- **Sleep disorder due to a general medical condition, insomnia type.** In this case, the insomnia is severe enough to warrant attention and is due to a general medical condition such as arthritis, congestive heart failure, hyperthyroidism, or gastroesophageal reflux. Typically, sleep apnea, narcolepsy, and periodic leg movements are not included in this category. The specific prevalence is estimated to be 1.8% of the elderly.
- **Substance-induced sleep disorder, insomnia type.** (See table below.)

Substances That May Cause Insomnia

Alcohol	Diuretics (furosemide)	Caffeine (teas, soda, chocolate)
Beta-blockers	Levodopa/carbidopa	Withdrawal from sedatives
Bronchodilators (albuterol)	Methyldopa	Illegal drug use
Cimetidine	Nifedipine	
Corticosteroids	SSRIs	
Decongestants (pseudoephedrine)	Theophylline	

SSRIs = serotonin reuptake inhibitors.
Adapted from Ancoli-Israel S: Sleep problems in older adults. Putting myths to bed. Geriatrics 52:20, 1997.

- **Circadian phase disorders, such as delayed sleep phase type or jet lag type.** These disorders result from a mismatch between the subject's endogenous sleep-wake regulation system and fundamental demands. Currently, it rarely is diagnosed in the elderly; however, new research suggests that it may play a greater role than initially suspected.
- **Dyssomnia not otherwise specified.** This broad category includes:
  - **Sleep hygiene and sleep deprivation.** These refer to the environment in which sleep occurs. They may be impaired by elevated noise levels, frequent disruptions from family members, and uncomfortable sleeping conditions. Institutionalization often is accompanied by the development of insomnia.
  - **Periodic limb movements** (PLMs). PLMs are characterized by repetitive leg movements that occur every 20–40 seconds and cause an arousal that can lead to a perception of disrupted sleep; a patient must have > 40 per night to meet diagnostic criteria. PLMs may be associated with peripheral neuropathies, chronic renal failure, dementia, anemia, and tricyclic antidepressants and occur in up to 44% of elderly patients.

4. How is insomnia diagnosed?

The diagnosis of insomnia is primarily a clinical one and does not require lab testing for confirmation. As long as the patient's condition satisfies the criteria outlined in question 1, he or she meets the definition of primary insomnia. Note that patients who complain of insomnia have a tendency to over-report their problem; often a discrepancy is found between the objective sleep latency and sleep efficiency on objective sleep testing and the patient's subjective complaints.

5. When should a patient with insomnia have a formal sleep study (polysomnography)?

In a position paper on the role of nocturnal polysomnography in insomnia, the American Sleep Disorder Association (ASDA) recommends that a patient should have a polysomnogram when:

- The insomnia remains persistent despite behavioral or pharmacologic therapy.
- The insomnia may be due to precipitous arousals or violent behavior during sleep.
- The insomnia may be caused by circadian rhythm disorders.
- Other diagnoses (e.g., sleep apnea or PLMs) are highly suspected or the actual clinical diagnosis is unclear.

6. What are important aspects of the history and physical examination in an elderly patient with insomnia?

- **Clarify sleep habits.** In addition to standard questions, also ask about what he or she does before falling asleep (e.g., reading in bed or watching TV) and his or her coffee and/or nicotine consumption.
- **Check for any symptoms of sleep-disordered breathing**, such as snoring, witnessed apneas (although these patients usually do not complain of insomnia), or nocturnal leg movements.
- **Perform a review of psychiatric symptoms to screen for depression or anxiety.** Also determine if the patient has any prior experiences or expectations that may increase anxiety about sleep (e.g., "I always sleep poorly; I have grown to expect it").
- **Assess the severity of any comorbid medical problems** (e.g., dyspnea, pain, orthopnea, cough, nocturia).
- **Inquire about medications**, which may include prescription and over-the-counter drugs as well as alternative preparations (e.g., herbal).

The physical exam should screen for the severity of the patient's comorbid medical conditions (especially arthritis) and also evidence of hyperthyroidism, a rare but curable cause of insomnia.

7. Describe the etiology of insomnia in older adults.

Although insomnia is often due to underlying psychiatric or medical problems, there is a growing appreciation of the role of circadian rhythm abnormalities in promoting disrupted sleep in the elderly. The human body has an internal clock, which is located in the suprachiasmatic nucleus and relies on extrinsic stimuli such as light exposure and social cues to regulate the body's sleep-wake cycle. In elderly subjects, evidence shows that this clock is phase-advanced relative to younger subjects and may possibly have a weaker amplitude. The elderly may be inclined to go to bed sooner but wake up earlier, thus creating a sense of insomnia. The decrease in amplitude, as seen by a drop in melatonin levels up to one-tenth that of younger subjects, or ablation of their melatonin rhythm altogether may lead to a greater tendency to awaken from sleep. In patients with Alzheimer's disease, neuronal degeneration in the sleep-wake regulatory pathways may lead to impaired sleep as demonstrated by histologic studies of brainstem sections from patients with Alzheimer's disease.

Furthermore, many elderly are exposed to < 30 minutes of bright light per day, which may contribute to their altered circadian physiology. Long-term institutionalization also contributes to disturbed sleep because of the frequent nocturnal interruptions, noisy environment, increased nap time, limited bright light exposure, and the multiple psychosocial issues associated with institutionalization. Nocturnal light exposure in particular may serve to blunt melatonin rhythms that may contribute to fragmented sleep. The combination of weakened circadian rhythm and comorbid medical and psychiatric conditions possibly may interact to decrease the threshold of awakening in the elderly and thereby promote insomnia.

8. What is the treatment of insomnia in the elderly?

Successful treatment should begin with amelioration of the underlying condition in secondary insomnias, such as improved nocturnal pain control and treatment of underlying psychiatric disorders. If the insomnia persists, behavioral therapy should be initiated and then incorporated with pharmacologic therapy if the response to behavioral changes alone is suboptimal.

Behavioral Therapy

- **Sleep hygiene modification** involves educating the patient about the most effective sleep habits:
  - Avoid caffeinated products, alcohol, and tobacco after 6 PM.
  - Limit naps to 30 minutes or ideally stop daytime napping altogether.

- Limit liquid intake near bedtime to reduce nocturia.
- Strive to have a sleeping environment that is quiet and free from disruptions.
- Establish a consistent bedtime.
- Avoid watching TV or reading in bed.

In patients with Alzheimer's disease, limiting daytime napping can help improve nocturnal sleep.

- **Sleep-restriction therapy** limits time spent in bed. It begins with asking the patient to estimate the amount of time he or she sleeps each night and then spend only 15 minutes more than that in bed for the first few nights. Fifteen minutes is then gradually added every few nights until a comfortable level of nocturnal sleep is reached. For example, if a patient states that he or she sleeps only 4 hours a night, instruct the patient to go to bed at 1:45 AM and awaken at 6:00 am. After the patient is able to sleep during this entire period (usually after a few days because of fatigue), instruct him to go to bed at 1:30 AM (15 minutes earlier than before), and so on.
- **Stimulus control therapy** attempts to strengthen the association between the bed and sleeping. The patient is instructed to use the bed only for sleeping and to leave the bed if she is awake for more than 15–30 minutes, which helps remove any negative conditioning that might prompt a patient to paradoxically feel more awake when lying in bed.

Pharmacologic Therapy

The pharmacologic treatment of insomnia is complicated by the decreased rate of metabolism in the elderly, increased total body fat (increased volume of distribution for lipid soluble agents), the high rate of polypharmacy in the elderly, and their increased sensitivity to the central nervous system–depressant effect of some medications. In general, starting doses should be one-half that of the standard starting doses:

- **Sedative/hypnotics** are recommended for short-term use only (< 3–4 weeks) and should not be prescribed if sleep apnea is suspected. For chronic insomniacs, sedative/hypnotics can be used intermittently (every 2–4 days) as needed, although little data verify this regimen. A short half-life is needed to minimize daytime sedation. If a patient complains of difficulty initiating sleep, then an agent with a very short half-life is appropriate (zolpidem tartrate [Ambien] with a 2.5 hr half-life, 2.5 mg starting dose); however, if the tendency is to wake up frequently or too early, an agent with a longer half-life may help (temazepam [Restoril] with a half-life of 10–17 hr, 7.5 mg starting dose).
- **Tricyclic antidepressants** also can be used to treat insomnia because of the frequent association between depression and insomnia, and they have a role in patients in whom depression is a major component. Their use is limited by their anticholinergic effects; nortriptyline and desipramine are most useful for this reason.
- **Over-the-counter medications** that are often used include analgesics such as Tylenol PM or sedating antihistamines. However, little data are available regarding efficacy of these agents.
- **Melatonin** may help certain patients with insomnia who have abnormal melatonin rhythms. However, little data presently support its routine use. Also, melatonin is not FDA-regulated, and potencies and quality vary. Doses of 0.3–1 mg most closely mimic physiologic levels. Given concern about unregulated manufacturing and the equivocal efficacy data to date, routine use of melatonin is not recommended.
- **Bright light therapy** has been shown to improve sleep quality in insomniacs in small studies and has a more well-established role in cases of seasonal affective disorder and early morning awakening insomnia. In Alzheimer's disease, some studies have shown a benefit, whereas others showed no improvement. Regimens include 2,000–10,000 lux for 2 hours usually administered in the early evening.
- **Selective serotonin reuptake inhibitors (SSRIs)** primarily are used to treat depression, but interest is growing in the use of agents such as paroxetine (Paxil), 20 mg, for insomnia.

Research is ongoing in the field and complicated by the fact that some SSRIs may actually cause insomnia.

• **Periodic limb movements** can be treated with levidopa-carbidopa (100–600 mg of the L-dopa as needed), pergolide (Permax; start at 0.05 mg 2 hr before bedtime), or clonazepam (0.5 mg–3.0 mg).

9. What are the side effects of treatment with sedatives?

Sedative use notably increases in the elderly with insomnia: 37% of elderly insomniacs used sedatives regularly versus 10.3% of elderly noninsomniacs in one Australian study. The immediate side effects of sedatives are increased risk of daytime fatigue with an associated risk of falls and cognitive dysfunction. In addition, dependence occurs in 15–30% of long-term benzodiazepine users. Patients with respiratory disease may develop carbon dioxide retention and narcosis when using sedatives. When sedatives are withdrawn, patients are at risk of rebound insomnia (i.e., worsening of their insomnia), especially with short- and intermediate-acting benzodiazepines.

10. What are the sequelae of insomnia?

Insomnia has been associated with a significantly increased risk of developing major depression, alcoholism, and anxiety disorder. In addition, there is an associated increase in daytime fatigue and sleepiness which, along with the nocturnal disruptions, impairs quality of life. The caregiver stress associated with frequent nocturnal disruptions also is a factor that may contribute to the institutionalization of a demented relative.

BIBLIOGRAPHY

1. American Psychiatric Association: Diagnostic and Statistical Manual of Mental Disorders. 4th ed. Washington, DC, American Psychiatric Association, 1994.
2. Ancoli-Israel S: Sleep problems in older adults: Putting myths to bed. Geriatrics 52:20–30, 1997.
3. ASDA–Standards of Practice Committee of the American Sleep Disorders Association: Practice parameters for the use of polysomnography in the evaluation of insomnia. Sleep 18:55, 1995.
4. Buysse D, Reynolds CI, Kupfer D, et al: Clinical diagnosis in 216 insomnia patients using the International Classification of Sleep Disorders (ICSD), DSM-IV, and ICD-10 categories: A report from the APA/NIMH DSM-IV field trials. Sleep 17:630–637, 1994.
5. Feinsilver S, Hertz G: Sleep in the elderly patient. Clin Chest Med 14:405–411, 1993.
6. Henderson S, Jorm A, Scott L, et al: The morbidity of insomnia uncomplicated by psychiatric disorders. Gen Hosp Psychiatry 19:245–250, 1997.
7. Monane M: Insomnia in the elderly. J Clin Psychiatry 53:23–28, 1992.
8. Monk TH: Sleep disorders in the elderly. Ciracadian rhythm. Clin Geriatr Med 5:331–346, 1989.
9. Morin CM, Colecchi C, Stone J, et al: Behavioral and pharmacological therapies for late-life insomnia: A randomized, controlled trial [see comments]. JAMA 281:991–999, 1999.
10. Ohayon MM: Prevalence of DSM-IV diagnostic criteria of insomnia: Distinguishing insomnia related to mental disorders from sleep disorders. J Psychiatr Res 31:333–346, 1997.
11. van Someren E, Mirmiran M, Swaab D: Nonpharmacological treatment of sleep and wake disturbances in aging and Alzheimer's disease: Chronobiological perspectives. Behav Brain Res 57:235–253, 1993.
12. Vitiello M, Prinz P: Alzheimer's disease. Sleep and sleep/wake patterns. Clin Geriatr Med 5:289–299, 1989.
13. Wooten V: Sleep disorders in geriatric patients. Clin Geriatr Med 8:427–439, 1992.

12. FALLS AND GAIT DISORDERS

Roberta A. Newton, PT, PhD, and William F. Edwards, MSN, APRN, BC, CRNP

1. What is considered a fall?

Any incident that involves unintentionally coming to the ground or some lower level is considered a fall. Older adults frequently have incidents that meet the definition of a fall, but they use other words such as "trip," "stumble," or "tumble" and may not report such incidents in their fall history. Slips and trips, although generally not considered a fall, need to be assessed and receive appropriate management, particularly in frail older adults.

2. Is falling a normal part of aging? How do falls affect the morbidity and mortality rates of older adults?

Falls in older adults are *common* but should not be viewed as *normal*. Each year, 33% of community-dwelling older adults between the ages of 65 and 69 years and 50% of adults over the age of 80 years experience a fall. The majority (50–66%) of these falls occur in the home.

Falls are the leading cause of injury-related deaths. More than 60% of people who die from a fall are over the age of 75 years. Caucasian women have the highest rate of fall-related deaths.

Of 1.6 million older adults treated in the emergency department due to falls and fall-related injuries, 22% are admitted to the hospital and 14% fall within the first month after discharge from the acute care setting.

From 30% to 56% of older adults in long-term care settings fall, with the highest incident rates occurring during the first 6 weeks after admission.

LOCATION	% FALLS/PERSON/ANNUALLY
Community	0.2–0.8
Hospital	0.6–2.9
Long-term care	0.6–3.6

Women, vigorous older adults who are risk takers, and frail older adults tend to have higher rates of falls with more serious injury. Three to 5% of the falls result in hip fractures. Other common fracture sites are wrist, forearm, ankle, vertebrae, and leg. Falls are a leading cause of head trauma. Approximately 10% of the soft tissue injury and lacerations associated with falling require medical assistance.

"Long-lie" (i.e., remaining on the floor or ground for longer than 1 hour) is a consequence of falls. A long-lie can result in increased weakness and is associated with secondary consequences such as pneumonia, rhabdomyolysis, hospitalization, and prolonged recovery.

3. What are the psychological consequences of falling?

Fear of falling occurs in nonfallers as well as fallers. Fear of falling and decreased activity are significant consequences leading to loss of confidence, self-imposed restriction of activity, muscle weakness, increased functional deficits, frailty, and increased risk for future falls. A fear of falling and/or self-imposed or family-imposed restriction of mobility can lead to nursing home admission.

4. What are the costs of falls?

Excluding physician services, the average cost for a fall and/or a fall-related injury reported in 1998 was approximately $19,500. In a 1994 report, the cost of fall injury nationwide was $20.2 billion, and this figure will increase as the population of baby boomers ages.

5. Are hip fractures more costly than other injuries?

Older adults over the age of 85 years, regardless of gender, are 10 to 15 times more likely to sustain a hip fracture. Medicare costs for hip fractures are approximately $2.9 billion with a projected increase to $35–$77 billion by 2040.

Hip fractures are the most costly injuries in terms of mortality, health problems, reduced quality of life and admission to nursing home. Older adults recover more slowly from hip fractures and have more adverse consequences postoperatively. Fewer than 50% of fracture survivors return home, and most demonstrate a decrease in routine activities of daily living and require assistance from others or a mobility device. One-third of older adults hospitalized for hip fracture die within 1 year.

6. What causes falls?

Generally falls are caused by multiple contributing factors and an interaction between the individual (**intrinsic factors** related to age or pathology) and the environment (**extrinsic factors**). The following lists include relative risk (RR) for falls when data are available.

Intrinsic Factors

1. **Central processing**
   Attentional demands
   Executive functioning, particularly judgment
   Cognitive impairment (RR = 1.8)
   Depression (RR = 2.2)
   Dementia
   Alzheimer's disease
2. **Neuromotor**
   Muscle strength/weakness (RR = 4.4)
   Decreased proprioception and somatosensation (feet and neck)
   Balance disorders (RR = 2.9)
   Gait disorders (RR = 2.9)
   Walking speed
   Parkinson's disease
   Stroke
   Peripheral neuropathy
3. **Musculoskeletal**
   Decreased range of motion (ROM)
   Osteoporosis
   Arthritis (RR = 2.4)
   Foot disorders
4. **Vestibular and auditory**
   Vertigo
   Benign paroxysmal positional vertigo
   Meniere's disease
   Decreased hearing

5. **Cardiovascular**
   Carotid sinus hypersensitivity
   Vertebrobasilar insufficiency
   Orthostatic hypotension
   Syncope
   Cardiac disease
6. **Vision**
   Visual deficit (RR = 2.5)
   Decreased contrast sensitivity
   Decreased depth perception
   Acuity < 20/60
   Cataracts
   Glaucoma
   Macular degeneration
7. **Other medical disorders**
   Acute illness
   Vitamin B12 deficiency
   Dehydration
   Diabetes
8. **Other intrinsic considerations**
   History of falls (RR = 3.0)
   Age > 80 yr (RR = 1.7)
   Impaired activities of daily living (RR = 2.3)
   Use of an assistive device (RR = 2.6)

Extrinsic Factors

1. **Support surface**
   Uneven surfaces (e.g., thresholds, stairs, sidewalks, gutters)
   Texture (compliant or patterned)
   Slippery or wet
2. **Obstacles/objects in environment**
   Pets
   Clutter in walkway
   Cords in path

5. **Lighting**
   Glare on floor or unshielded lamps
   Dim
   No night lights
6. **Weather conditions**
   Ice on curb cuts
7. **Bathroom**
   Low toilet seats
   Throw rugs

3. **Furniture**
Clear glass coffee tables
Furniture with protruding legs
Chairs without arms or with low seats
Beds too high or low

4. **Clothing**
Long skirts, coats
Shoes: high-heels, worn, too large, too
slippery (e.g., bedroom slippers) or
grippy soles

Lack of nonskid surfaces
Lack of grab bars in shower/tub

8. **Other extrinsic factors**
No handrails on stairs

7. Discuss common gait characteristics in older adults. What common gait disorders in older adults may contribute to falls?

Gait speed is a useful assessment, rehabilitation outcome measure, and marker for disease progression. Gait velocity is usually maintained until the seventh decade. Comfortable speed in women in their 70s is 1.32–1.74 m/sec with active elders having a mean gait speed of 1.42 m/sec. Inactive community-dwelling older adults are generally 15% slower than active elders. Gait speeds of nursing home residents tend to be 0.37 m/sec for fallers and 0.64 m/sec for nonfallers. A slower speed is associated with shortened stride length.

Factors that alter gait efficiency include decreases in lower extremity range of motion, muscle strength, and endurance. Alterations in speed, symmetry, and smoothness are among the indicators for gait disorders; however, the practitioner is cautioned that typical age-related gait patterns have not been described. The following table indicates the level of dysfunction (e.g., sensory impairments, muscle weakness) and indicators of a typical gait pattern.

LEVEL OF DYSFUNCTION	TYPICAL GAIT PATTERNS
Visual, somatosensory, vestibular impairments	Unsteady Uncoordinated Tentative
Arthritis, osteoporosis, painful musculo-skeletal changes	Decreased weight bearing on painful side, causing decreased time in single-leg support phase on painful side Shortened stride length Stooped posture Buckling of lower extremity joints with weight bearing
Muscle weakness	Pelvic girdle weakness: Trendelenberg (pelvic drop on the side of the elevated leg during single leg stance or gait) Distal motor weakness: foot drop or foot slap, steppage gait (increased hip flexion)
Hemiparesis (stroke)	Circumduction at the hip Genu recurvatum (hyperextension of knee joint during stance or weight-bearing phase of gait) Ankle plantarflexion and inversion Decreased or absent arm swing
Parkinson's disease	Small and shuffling steps, hesitation, festinating Decreased or absent arm swing
Cerebellar ataxia	Wide-based support Asymmetry of stepping
Cautious gait	Associated with fear of falling Wide-based support, decreased velocity Shortened stride

8. What medications are associated with a strong risk for falls?

Polypharmacy and its side effects are associated with falling. Medications associated with relative risk for falls include the following:

- Psychotropics (RR = 1.7)
- Class IA antiarrhythmic medications (RR = 1.6)
- Digoxin (RR = 1.2)
- Diuretics (RR = 1.1)

Older adults should be asked to bring in all current, previously prescribed medications, over-the-counter medications, and herbal supplements. They should be encouraged to comply with medication schedules and discouraged from sharing medicines with others.

Drugs that May Affect Fall Risk

HYPNOTICS-ANXIOLYTICS (INCLUDING BENZODIAZEPINES)	TRICYCLIC ANTIDEPRESSANTS	SSRI ANTIDEPRESSANTS	ANTIPSYCHOTICS
Chlordiazepoxide (HCL)	Amitriptyline	Fluoxetine	Haloperidol
Chloral hydrate	Amoxapine	Paroxetine	Resperidone
Diazepam	Doxepin	Sertraline	Trifluoperazine
Ethchlorvynol	Imipramine (HCl)		
Flurazepam	Nortriptline (HCl)		
Quazepam	Protriptyline (HCl)		
Temazepam			

SSRI = selective serotonin reuptake inhibitor.

9. What elements should be included in the evaluation of fall risk?

On an annual basis, practitioners should inquire whether an older adult has fallen and, if so, attempt to delineate the predicating causes. The following elements should be included:

1. History of falls in the past 6 weeks and 6 months. Is the person a recurrent faller (> 2 falls in 6 months)? Patients use a variety of terms to describe a fall. The clinician should clarify what the patient means when describing the incident.

2. Determine activity level.

3. A review of the musculoskeletal and neurologic systems will reveal most intrinsic factors and can be assessed by balance and gait testing:
   - Single-leg stance, tandem stance (normal: > 10 sec)
   - Timed up and go (normal: < 15 sec)
   - Multidirectional reach test (normal: > 8 in forward; 4 in backward lean, and 6 in right and left directions)
   - Gait can be assessed while the person is performing the timed up and go test or as a separate test, observing symmetry, speed, and ability to walk in a straight line.
   - Complaints of shortness of breath or dizziness with positional changes can also be observed as the older adult performs these tasks. Monitoring of heart rate and blood pressure provides an objective measure for orthostatic hypotension.

4. If vertigo or dizziness is present, conduct a review of the cardiovascular, vestibular, visual, and proprioceptive systems as well as neurologic status to determine mild head trauma. Review changes in current health status, medications, and vision.

10. What other aspects of the physical examination are most important in assessment of fall risk?

- Brief screen for cognitive functioning and mood (depression)
- General strength assessment to identify areas of dysfunction and weakness
- Assessment of activity level and fear of falling. For example, Do you have a fear of falling? If "yes," does the fear decrease your activity level?
- Recent changes in health/medical status, vision, medications, residency status, and level of care.

11. When is a referral for further evaluation recommended?

Assessment and intervention for falls are generally interdisciplinary concerns. Referrals may include specific services as well as rehabilitation services such as physical and occupational therapy and low vision rehabilitation. Additional referrals to cardiology, neurology, and otorhinology may be recommended for the patient with complaints of dizziness or unknown cause of falls. Referral is recommended in the following situations:

- Falls of unknown etiology and recurrent falls
- Cardiac, neurologic, vestibular/auditory, visual cause
- Postural hypotension not related to medications or dehydration
- Musculoskeletal condition, including foot pathology
- > 4 medications or high-risk medications
- Single-leg stance < 10 seconds; timed up and go > 20 seconds, limited bending of the ankles or trunk during the multidirectional reach test.
- Unstable gait and need for an assistive device

12. How is an environmental assessment done?

An environmental assessment starts with an interview of the older adult in the office. If the results of the interview raise questions about safety in the home environment, nurses, physical therapists, or occupational therapists from home-care agencies can provide an in-home evaluation for potential hazards and offer suggestions, such as installation of grab bars for the tub and toilet.

13. Can exercise or other physical activities improve function and reduce fall risk?

Several studies have demonstrated that exercise can improve functional status and reduce the risk for falls. These programs may assist with elderly persons who have not fallen (primary prevention) as well as with those who have fallen. More effective fall prevention programs include patient education as well as activity programs such as walking or tai chi. The exercise/activity program should be tailored to the needs of the older person by a knowledgeable exercise professional, such as a physical therapist, occupational therapist, or rehabilitation specialist.

The patient needs to have a work-up before participating in such programs and to follow graded exercise/activity intensity. Patients with exercise-induced angina, intermittent claudication, chronic obstructive lung disease, degenerative joint disease, orthopedic and foot problems, and neurologic abnormalities require both professional evaluation and supervised exercise programs.

Cardiac rehabilitation programs and health clubs with a physical therapy department can provide gait and balance evaluations as well as prescribe exercise/activity programs. Evaluation of cardiac risk, including exercise stress testing, depends on significant findings in the history, such as cardiac dysrhythmia, severe congestive heart failure, angina, exercise-related chest pain or myocardial infarct, diabetes mellitus, hypertension, elevated cholesterol levels, and current cigarette smoking.

The ideal program for fall prevention should include an interdisciplinary and collaborative effort with exercise physiologists, physical therapists, occupational therapists, rehabilitation nurses, cardiac specialists, and geriatrician/primary care provider.

14. Can exercise/activity programs be instituted with institutionalized older adults?

Frail older adults and adults in long-term care settings can benefit from an exercise/activity program. Studies in these frail older adults have demonstrated an increase in muscle strength after an exercise program. An interdisciplinary approach to preventing falls and improving functional status is recommended. In addition, these programs may include a continence program because many falls in the nursing home occur when the patient is getting out of bed or going to the bathroom. A cognitive rehabilitation program incorporating fall prevention strategies is also recommended.

15. What can be recommended for a nonambulatory older adult at risk of falling?

Falls in nonambulatory persons usually occur as a result of sliding or slipping out of chairs or transferring without assistance from a chair or bed. Replacing side rails with a low-height bed coupled with floor mats may reduce or prevent fall-related injuries from bed.

If the person falls because he or she is attempting to get out of an uncomfortable chair, individualized seating alternatives are currently available. Recliner chairs and wedge or other support cushions may prevent such unassisted ambulation while ensuring comfort.

Older adults who wish to be mobile despite their inability to ambulate can be given a program to improve wheelchair skills along with more user-friendly wheelchairs. Physical therapists and occupational therapists can provide guidance in prescribing these interventions.

16. Discuss the role of physical restraints in institutionalized older adults.

Despite the assumed safety of nursing home environments, falls remain an important clinical problem. Until the late 1980s, physical restraints were the primary intervention to prevent falls, although their efficacy in fall prevention has never been demonstrated. More recent work has demonstrated not only the lack of efficacy of fixed restraints in preventing falls but also significant increases in restraint-related injury and death.

Interventions such as regular ambulation and other exercises that increase strength, balance, and coordination and continence programs have been shown to be the most effective measures in preventing falls. Hip protectors have been noted to decrease the seriousness of injury related to falls. However, the compliance rate for wearing the hip protectors is low due to cosmesis and the time to don and doff the hip protector.

17. Are physical restraints useful in preventing falls in the hospitalized elder?

Fall prevention programming is essential if injuries leading to increased morbidity, length of hospital stay, institutionalization, and even death are to be prevented. The Joint Commission for Accreditation of Health Care Facilities (JCAHO) guidelines restrict physical restraint use to limited situations.

New fall prevention interventions individualized to specific patient needs are beginning to be seen in hospitals. Examples include beds equipped with transfer enablers (one-fourth or one-half length side rails with narrow bars to prevent head entrapment) and motion-activated lights. Open monitors at the nursing station, placement of high-risk patients close to the nursing station, bedside commodes, bed alarms, and video monitoring are useful interventions for patients who require assistance with transferring but are cognitively or physically unable to seek assistance or choose to not to do so. Hip protectors are another alternative; however barriers to their success include patient compliance and the difficulty of donning and doffing.

Encouraging families to stay overnight with the hospitalized older adult and the use of companions can also be helpful.

18. How can the risk of legal liability be reduced?

American physicians and nurses continue to believe that failure to restrain elder persons places clinicians and facilities at risk for legal liability. In the past, many cases favored plaintiffs against hospitals when fall-related injuries occurred in the absence of physical restraints. However, the current standard of care (as demonstrated in clinical and research literature and government regulations) reflects elimination or at least minimal usage of restraint. Settlement and court decisions in fall-related injury cases have begun to shift.

Although a number of reported cases assert the so-called failure to restrain, a careful reading of these cases demonstrates that the real basis of liability is a lack of care addressing fall risk. Only falls that are the proximate result of a deviation from the current standard of care are a liability risk. In fact, suits are being won against nursing homes and hospitals for physical restraint use that led to adverse consequences of enforced immobility or restraint-related deaths. Therefore, a well-designed and well-applied fall prevention plan is imperative.

BIBLIOGRAPHY

1. AGS Guidelines for the prevention of falls in older persons. J Am Geriatr Soc 49:664–672, 2001.
2. Capezuti E, Strumpf N, Evans L, et al: The relationship between physical restraint removal and falls and injuries among nursing home residents. J Geontol Biol Sci Med Sci 53A:M47–M53, 1998.

3. Centers for Disease Control and Prevention: Web-based Injury Statistics Query and Reporting System (WISQARS, data base online). National Center for Injury Prevention and Control, Centers for Disease Control and Preventio. Available at www.cdc.gov/ncipc/wisquars, 2001.
4. Cummings RG: Epidemiology of medication-related falls and fractures in the elderly. Drugs Aging 12:43–53, 1998.
5. Lord SR, Dayhew J: Visual risk factors for falls in older people. J Am Geriatr Soc 49:508–515, 2001.
6. Province MA, Hadley EC, Nornbrook MC, et al: The effects of exercise on falls in elderly patients: A pre-planned meta-analysis of the FICSIT trails. JAMA 273:1341–1347, 1995.
7. Tinetti ME, Baker D, McAvy G, et al: A multifactorial intervention to reduce the risk of falling among elderly people living in the community. N Engl J Med 331:821–827, 1994.
8. Tinetti ME, Williams SC: Falls, injuries due to falls, and the risk of admission to a nursing home. N Engl J Med 337:1279–1284, 1997.
9. Wolinsky FD, Fitzgerald JF, Stump TE: The effect of hip fracture on mortality, hospitalization, and functional status: A prospective study. Am J Public Health 87:398–403, 1997.

13. DIZZINESS AND VERTIGO

*Lesley Carson, MD, Dana L. Suskind-Liu, MD,
and Glenn W. Knox, MD*

1. What is the clinical difference between dizziness and vertigo?

Dizziness is a common and often complicated complaint in geriatric patients. It is one of the most common reasons for physician visits in patients over 75 years of age and the third most common reason in patients over 65 years. Dizziness can be subtyped into vertigo, presyncopal lightheadedness, and dysequilibrium; it is often multifactorial and difficult to describe. It also may have psychogenic features. **Vertigo,** which refers to a sense of rotational movement and spinning, suggests vestibular pathology. **Presyncopal lightheadedness** describes an impending faint and is due to cerebral hypoperfusion. **Dysequilibrium** describes a feeling of imbalance and unsteadiness of body, not of head, which may result from pathology in the motor control system (visual, vestibulospinal, proprioceptive, somatosensory, cerebellar, motor) and vestibular system (inner ear, middle ear, brainstem, cerebellum). Of note, apart from the above subtypes, a vague or floating feeling much of the time is highly correlated with psychologic reasons or change in vision as with cataract removal.

2. Can dizziness be a normal part of aging?

Presbystasis is the term used to describe the dysequilibrium of aging. It is thought to result from an overall decline in vestibular, visual, proprioceptive, and neuromuscular function. Although functional decrease in vestibular activity in elderly people is slight, the overall decline in compensatory mechanisms (i.e., proprioception, vision, and neuromuscular) leaves them vulnerable to unstable conditions to which a younger person could easily adapt. Presbystasis is a diagnosis of exclusion. Nearly all causes of dizziness are pathologic. Given the multifactorial etiology of "dizziness" in many an older person, it has been suggested that dizziness should be considered a geriatric syndrome. Miltipronged evaluation and intervention are more effective than identification of one cause and treatment. The elderly patient with symptoms of vertigo or dizziness often has a definable etiology. Patients diagnosed with presbystasis are prime candidates for vestibular rehabilitation, during which they learn methods of compensation.

3. What major etiologies should be considered in vertigo or dizziness in the elderly?

Vertigo—acute	Vertigo—recurrent *(cont'd.)*	Vertigo—positional *(cont'd.)*
Vertebrobasilar event	Hypothyroidism	Cervical vertigo
Toxic (drugs/illness)	Multiple sclerosis	Central causes
Infectious	Presbylabyrinth	Imbalance
Trauma	Syphilis	Medication toxicity
Tumor	Diabetes mellitus	Sensory impairment
Seizure	Small vessel	Cervical spine dizziness
Transient ischemic attack	Peripheral neuropathy	Presbystasis
Cerebrovascular accident	Vertigo—positional	Presyncope
Cardiac arrhythmia	Benign paroxysmal	Orthostasis
Vertigo—recurrent	positional vertigo	Hyperventilation
Meniere's disease	Infection	Muscle weakness
Migraine	Trauma	

Adapted from Mader SL: Dizziness and syncope. In Yoshikawa T (ed): Ambulatory Geriatric Care. St. Louis, Mosby, 1993, pp 305–315.

4. How do you differentiate among vertigo, lightheadedness, and dysequilibrium?

	COMMON EXAMPLES	TIME FRAME	CHARACTERISTIC FEATURES
Vertigo	Benign positional vertigo	Short and episodic, < 1 minute	Rapid head movements, precipitate, recurrent
	Vertebrobasilar insufficiency • Transient ischemic attack • Medullary dysfunction • Cerebellar infarcts	Longer and episodic, 20 min–2 hr or continuous	Associated neurologic symptoms, such as diplopia, hallucinations, and dysarthria, as well as nausea and vomiting
	Meniere's disease	Even longer episodes, 2 hr–2 days	Fluctuating hearing loss, tinnitus, pressure in ear
	Neurolabyrinthitis	Episodic for days	Associated with nausea, vomiting and acute onset with recent upper respiratory infection
Lightheadedness	Vasovagal episodes	Episodic	Induced by strong emotion; fall in heart rate and blood pressure
	Orthostatic hypotension	Continuous (may occur daily)	Precipitated by rapid change to standing position; medications, volume loss, autonomic dysfunction implicated
	Cardiac arrhythmia	Episodic or continuous	Syncope of sudden onset
	Valvular heart disease	Continuous or episodic	Murmur of aortic stenosis
Dysequilibrium	Multiple neurosensory deficits	Continuous	Worse with standing or walking; multiple deficits, including degenerative joint disease, medication, decreased vision
	Physical deconditioning	Continuous	Decreased activity, after recent fall, <1 wk bedrest
	Peripheral neuropathy	Continuous	Associated with acoustic neuroma, diabetes mellitus, renal failure Worse in dark
	Cerebellar disease	Continuous	Accompanied by intention tremor, incoordination, dysarthria

5. Which aspects of the physical exam need to be evaluated during the work-up for dizziness in the elderly?

Initial evaluation should include traditional orthostatics, full cardiovascular exam, and a complete neurotologic work-up. Blood pressure and pulse should be measured in the lying, sitting, and standing positions, because orthostatic hypotension is a common cause of dizziness in the elderly. Orthostatic hypotension is defined as a drop in systolic blood pressure of > 20 mmHg from lying to standing position. However, in the elderly orthostatic symptoms may occur without the 20-mmHg drop in systolic pressure even 10–30 minutes after the assumption of erect posture. Cardiovascular exams are performed to identify possible cardiac arrhythmias, significant valvular heart disease, and carotid bruits.

A complete neurotologic exam should be performed, beginning with an otologic exam and including a cranial nerve exam, evaluation of the external and middle ear, and a fistula test. The fistula test is performed by applying pressure to the ear and evaluating for vertigo and nystagmus. A positive result indicates the presence of a fistula of the labyrinth due to cholesteatoma or infection. Evaluation for nystagmus, an objective finding that accompanies vertigo, is also important. Spontaneously induced nystagmus may indicate central or peripheral vestibular dysfunction. Nystagmus is named according to the direction of the rapid component. Fixation inhibits peripheral spontaneous nystagmus with the slow phase toward the abnormal side and the fast phase toward the normal side. The Dix-Hallpike or Nylen-Barany maneuver evaluates positional nystagmus. Nystagmus with latency time of 3–10 seconds until onset, less than 1-minute duration, fatigability on repeat testing, and a rotatory nature with a vertical or horizontal component can be found in peripheral nervous system disorders. A Weber-Rinne test is performed to assess for sensorineural or conductive hearing loss. The Romberg test and tandem gait tests evaluate vestibular, proprioceptive, and cerebellar components.

6. Which basic and adjunctive tests should be ordered to evaluate the dizzy or vertiginous patient?

Routine lab tests include an electrocardiogram (EKG), blood sugar, and complete blood count. An EKG suggests the presence or absence of an arrhythmia. Anemia and hypoglycemia can be detected by a complete blood count and blood sugar.

Adjunctive tests may greatly facilitate a diagnostic work-up. They should be obtained, however, with a systematic rather than a "shotgun" approach. A complete audiogram should be obtained in all patients complaining of hearing loss and vertigo and in all patients with abnormal neurotologic exams. Electronystagmography (ENG), which evaluates the vestibular system by recording nystagmus, aids in differentiating central from peripheral vestibular dysfunction. It should be obtained in patients complaining of vertigo or patients with neurotologic findings such as nystagmus. Patients should avoid all vestibular suppressants for at least 48 hours before testing. Auditory brainstem-evoked responses should be obtained in patients with asymmetric sensorineural hearing loss to rule out acoustic neuroma. Magnetic resonance imaging (MRI) may be considered in selected patients. MRI examination of the temporal bone is often ordered in patients suspected of having acoustic neuromas or other cerebellopontine angle masses. Computed tomography (CT) of the temporal bones also may be obtained when cholesteatomas or other middle ear lesions are suspected.

Cervical spine radiographs should be obtained if cervical dizziness is suspected, whereas an echocardiogram, carotid and vertebral artery Doppler scans, tilt-table testing, and a 24-hour Holter monitor are obtained if presyncope is diagnosed.

7. What is vestibular rehabilitation? Who is a candidate?

Vestibular rehabilitation is a form of physical therapy designed specifically to help dizzy patients to cope in their environment through vestibular compensation. It is a multidisciplinary treatment program that uses vestibular provocation as well as conditioning and control exercises. It teaches the patient to use existing visual or proprioceptive cues. Vestibular exercises range from ocular fixation in all gaze positions to combined head and eye movements jumping between two targets or head movements in all directions while walking. Although vestibular suppressants may be used as adjunctive therapy, preferably patients should avoid such medication during vestibular rehabilitation. As soon as the acute nausea and vomiting have passed, vestibular exercises should be started.

Vestibular rehabilitation is used most often in patients with benign paroxysmal positional vertigo (BPPV) and dizziness secondary to presbystasis, vestibular surgery, or traumatic head injury. Although elderly patients make slower progress in vestibular rehabilitation than younger patients, they often derive significant benefit. Vestibular rehabilitation is inappropriate for patients in whom the cause of dizziness has not been identified. In addition, long-term benefits have not been found in patients with Meniere's disease.

8. What is Meniere's syndrome?

Meniere's syndrome is characterized by episodic vertigo, aural fullness, tinnitus, and fluctuating hearing loss. The pathophysiology is thought to be secondary to endolymphatic hydrops, possibly due to bacterial, viral, or syphilitic causes. The hearing loss is unilateral and involves the low-frequency range. The episodes of vertigo typically last minutes to hours, at times with nausea and vomiting. A sensation of unsteadiness may persist for days thereafter. Diagnosis is made on the basis of the typical clinical history and documentation of fluctuating hearing loss as well as episodic vertigo. Medical management includes acute management with antivertiginous medication, prophylactic salt restriction, and diuretics in an effort to reduce the hydrops. Surgical treatments, such as labyrinthectomies, vestibular nerve sections, and endolymphatic shunts, are not recommended in elderly patients, who tend to have more difficulty adapting after such procedures. Vestibular rehabilitation results in minimal improvement.

9. Define BPPV. How is it diagnosed?

BPPV is one of the most common causes of vertigo in elderly patients. It occurs usually after trauma or an episode of viral labyrinthitis. The pathophysiology is thought to be due to the release of otoconia (small calcium carbonate crystals in the saccule) into the posterior semicircular canal. With head movement the crystals are displaced, resulting in vertigo and nystagmus. Patients develop vertigo that occurs with positional changes and lasts less than 1 minute. BPPV is diagnosed by a suggestive history and a positive Hallpike maneuver on physical examination. Extensive diagnostic testing is not required. Although 90% of cases resolve spontaneously within a few months, exacerbations may last for years.

The Hallpike maneuver is used to evaluate for BPPV. Nystagmus and vertigo are assessed after the head is turned to the left and the patient is quickly lowered from a sitting to a supine position. The head is held in the supine position for 1 minute. The procedure is repeated with the head turned to the right. The test should be repeated several times on the side that is most symptomatic to check for fatigability. A positive Hallpike test classically provokes the patient's symptoms and elicits nystagmus on the affected side.

Treatment is directed toward active provocation of the vestibular system with the goal of vestibular habituation and resolution of symptoms. The Epley maneuver repositions free-floating endolymphatic particles in the posterior semicircular canal. The patient is placed in the provocative head-hanging position and remains there for several minutes. The patient is then rotated to the opposite side, with the head turned 45° downward. The patient should be aware that dizziness is exacerbated initially during the exercises but will subside with time. Theoretically this maneuver allows the floating particles to continue their course through the common crus into the utricle by rotating the posterior semicircular canal 180° in the plane of gravity. Meclizine may be useful in the short term for control of symptoms.

10. What is the role for vestibular suppressants such as lorazepam and meclizine in elderly vertiginous patients?

The use of vestibular suppressants is not contraindicated in the elderly. An antiemetic may also aid patients with severe nausea and vomiting. Elderly patients, however, may be extremely sensitive to vestibular suppressants. In addition, they may be taking other medications that interact with or affect the metabolism of such medications. Promethazine is an effective first-line suppressant of vertigo and vomiting, and prochloperazine is used for persistent vomiting. Meclizine and dimenhydrinate are effective oral agents. Lorazepam is less effective as a suppressant.

11. Which medications are possible causes of dysequilibrium?

Geriatric patients are often on polypharmacy that may either cause or exacerbate baseline dizziness or vertigo. It is extremely important to obtain a thorough medication list, including as-needed prescriptions.

CLASS OF DRUG	TYPE OF DIZZINESS	MECHANISM
Alcohol	Positional	Cerebellar dysfunction
Sedatives	Disorientation	Depression of central processing
Antihypertensives	Lightheadedness	Orthostatic hypotension
Anticonvulsants	Dysequilibrium	Cerebellar dysfunction
Aminoglycosides	Dysequilibrium, oscillopsia/vertigo	Damage to labyrinthine hair cells
Diuretics	Positional	Orthostatic hypotension

12. How does the time frame of the symptoms relate to the diagnostic etiology?

The time frame of the patient's symptoms may give an indication of the etiology. BPPV usually resolves within 30 seconds to a minute after the provoking positional change. In patients with vascular etiologies, such as transient ischemic attack, symptoms last for 20 minutes to several hours. Episodes of vertigo in Meniere's disease usually last from minutes to hours. The episodes of vertigo with neuronitis and labyrinthitis continue for days. The more continuous the symptoms, the more carefully one should consider psychological states, medications, or diseases that cause permanent structural damage, such as stroke and peripheral neuropathy.

13. Describe a general approach to the diagnosis of dizziness.

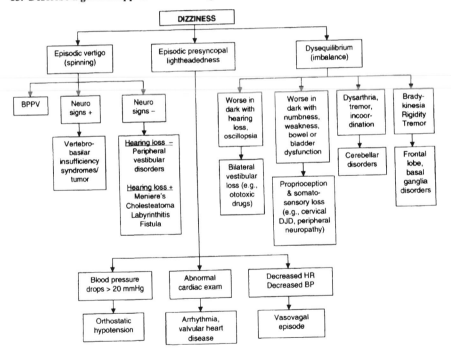

BIBLIOGRAPHY

1. Aronow WS: Dizziness and syncope. In Hazzard WR, Blass JP, Ettinger WH, et al (eds): Principles of Geriatric Medicine and Gerontology, 4th ed. New York, McGraw-Hill, 1999, pp 1519–1524.
2. Baloh RW: Dizziness in older people. J Am Geriatr Soc 40:713–721, 1992.
3. Baloh RW: Approach to the evaluation of of the dizzy patient. Otolaryngol Head Neck Surg 112:3–7, 1995.

4. Baloh R: Vestibular neuritis. N Engl J Med 348:1027–1032, 2003.
5. Cohen H, Rubin AM, Gombash L: The team approach to treatment of the dizzy patient. Arch Phys Med Rehabil 73:703–708, 1992.
6. Cohen H: Vestibular rehabilitation reduces functional disability. Otolaryngol Head Neck Surg 107:638–643, 1992.
7. Drachman DA: Occam's razor, geriatric syndromes, and the dizzy patient. Ann Intern Med 132:403–404, 2000.
8. Frohman E: Evaluation of the dizzy patient. Am Med 11:1–11, 2002.
9. Gomez CR, et al: Isolated vertigo as a manifestation of vertebrobasilar ischemia. Am Acad Neurol 47:94–97, 1996.
10. Katsarkas A: Dizziness in aging: A retrospective study of 1194 Cases. Otolaryngol Head Neck Surg 110:296–301, 1994.
11. Lempert T, Gresty MA, Bronstein AM: Benign positional vertigo: Recognition and treatment. BMJ 311:489–491, 1995.
12. Mader SL: Dizziness and syncope. In Yoshikawa T (ed): Ambulatory Geriatric Care. St. Louis, Mosby, 1993, pp 305–315.
13. Sloan PD: Evaluation and management of dizziness in the older patient. Clin Geriatr Med 12:785–801, 1996.
14. Sloane P, Coeytaux R, Beck R, Dallora J: Dizziness: State of the science. Ann Intern Med 134:823–832, 2001.
15. Tinetti ME, Williams CS, Gill TM: Dizziness among older adults: A possible geriatric syndrome. Ann Intern Med 132:337–344, 2000.

14. OSTEOPOROSIS

Robert J. Pignolo, MD, PhD, Edna P. Schwab, MD,
and Michael Pazianas, MD

1. What is osteoporosis?

Osteoporosis is a systemic disease characterized by low bone mass and microarchitectural deterioration of bone tissue, with a consequent increase in bone fragility and susceptibility to fracture.

2. Discuss the economic and functional impact of osteoporosis.

According to a prevalence report update by the National Osteoporosis Foundation (NOF), low bone mass and osteoporosis are currently estimated to affect 44 million U.S. women and men aged 50 and older. By 2010, it is estimated that this number will exceed 52 million and by 2020, over 61 million. In 2002, it was estimated that over 10 million people had osteoporosis, women accounting for about 80% of cases. One in two women and one in four men over age 50 will have an osteoporosis-related fracture in their lifetime, accounting for more than 1.5 million fractures annually, including 300,000 hip fractures, approximately 700,000 vertebral fractures, 250,000 wrist fractures, and 300,000 fractures at other sites. National direct expenditures for osteoporotic and associated fractures, including hospital and nursing home costs, was estimated to be $17 billion in 2001 ($47 million each day).

Osteoporosis is associated with a great deal of functional loss as well as skeletal deformities, pain, dependence, and depression. Vertebral fractures occur more frequently than hip fractures. Compared with women without fractures, women with a history of vertebral or hip fractures have more difficulty with bending, lifting, reaching, walking, and ascending and descending stairs and experience impairment in dressing, cooking, shopping, and housework. Approximately 40% of hip fracture survivors are able to return to their prior level of performance for activities of daily living (ADLs), whereas only 25% return to their prefracture level for instrumental activities of daily living (IADLs). The ability to perform ADLs and IADLs, along with the presence of social supports, often determines whether a person can return to independent living. Approximately 15–25% of patients with hip fractures require institutionalization.

3. What is the mechanism of bone loss in osteoporosis?

Bone is composed of two types of tissue: trabecular bone, which is metabolically more active, and cortical bone, which is less active. Bone remodeling is a tightly organized process consisting of bone formation closely coupled to bone resorption. Systemic humoral factors, such as parathyroid hormone, growth hormone, estrogens, and testosterone, and local humoral factors (e.g., IGF-1, TNF, IL-1, and IL-6) contribute to proper functioning. The majority of adult bone mass is laid down during adolescence; however, peak bone mass is not obtained until the fourth decade. Peak mass is determined by numerous genetic and environmental factors, including sex, family history, body type, and activity level. By age 40 years there is a slow decline in bone mass in both men and women. Aging alters the tight coupling between bone resorption and formation, resulting in augmented osteoclastic resorption and diminished osteoblastic activity. Estrogen deficiency accelerates the rate of bone loss. Total lifetime bone loss in men may be 20–30% of peak bone mass, whereas in women it may amount to 40–50%.

4. List the risk factors associated with osteoporosis.

- Family history of osteoporosis or fracture
- Personal history of fracture as an adult
- Increasing age
- Lifelong low calorie intake
- Poor health/frailty
- Immobilization

- Early menopause (< 45 years old)
- Late menarche (> 16 years old)
- Amenorrhea or irregular menstrual periods
- Female sex
- White or Asian ancestry
- Sedentary lifestyle
- Thin body frame or low body weight
- Calcium/vitamin D-deficient diet
- Heavy alcohol use
- Cigarette smoking

5. Which medical conditions can cause secondary osteoporosis?

Osteoporosis is a diagnosis of exclusion. Secondary causes of low bone density must be ruled out before a diagnosis of osteoporosis is made.

Secondary Causes of Low Bone Density

Endocrine	Hyperthyroidism, hyperparathyroidism, Cushing's syndrome, diabetes mellitus, prolactinoma, estrogen deficiency, hypogonadism (men)
Rheumatologic	Rheumatoid arthritis, ankylosing spondylitis, idiopathic scoliosis, sarcoidosis
Gastrointestinal/ nutritional	Malabsorption, hepatobiliary dysfunction, vitamin D deficiency, parenteral nutrition
Hematologic/ oncologic	Mastocytosis, hemolytic anemia, malignancy (general), multiple myeloma, hemophilia, thalassemia
Renal	Idiopathic hypercalciuria (on low calcium diet), renal osteodystrophy
Psychiatric	Eating disorders (anorexia, bulimia), depression
Genetic	Congenital porphyria, osteogenesis imperfecta, osteoporosis-pseudoglioma
Other	Paget's disease, amyloidosis, epidermolysis bullosa, hemochromatosis, hypophosphatasia, multiple sclerosis

6. List pharmacologic agents that are associated with low bone density.

- Glucocorticoids
- Lithium
- Antacids (chronic use)
- Heparin
- Gonadotropin-releasing hormone agonist or antagonist
- Phenothiazines
- Cytotoxic drugs
- Anticonvulsants
- Tamoxifen (premenopausal)
- Vitamin A
- Methotrexate
- Warfarin
- Excessive thyroid supplementation
- Aluminum-containing medications
- Organ transplant therapy

7. Name the various methods used to measure bone density.

- Skeletal radiographs: not a sensitive test because osteopenia becomes evident on radiographs only after more than one-third of bone mass has been lost.
- Quantitative computed tomography (QCT): estimates the amount of minerals in the bone. Although it can analyze the bone in three dimensions and even distinguish trabecular from compact bone tissue, it has a number of practical disadvantages: it is available at a small number of centers; it is expensive; the radiation dose is not negligible; the error around re-peated measurements may be high; and it evaluates only small volumes of bone.
- Peripheral quantitative computed tomography (pQCT): offers some advantages over QCT. It is portable and can measure at the forearm, which is a relatively large bone area.
- Central bone densitometry (dual energy x-ray absorptiometry [DXA]): Bone mineral density (BMD) measurement of the spine and hip has become the standard test for assessing the risk of osteoporosis. The lower the result, the higher the risk of fracture. The test is highly accurate and reproducible (less than 2% error, depending on the site measured). The scan time is short (less than 5 minutes; with the latest technology, less than 1 minute) at each site (i.e., spine and

hip), and the radiation dose to which the patient is exposed is extremely low (one-twentieth that of a chest radiograph). DXA requires lying on a table (fully clothed) while the arm of the machine swings over the torso.

• Peripheral bone densitometry
   a) Single- or dual-energy x-ray absorptiometry performed at the radius or calcaneus;
   b) Ultrasound: performed at the calcaneus or tibia;
   c) Radiographic absorptiometry: compares the density of the proximal phalanges to that of a wedge of aluminum (with known densities) placed alongside the hand.

BMD measurement at peripheral skeletal sites is most applicable to postmenopausal Caucasian women and should not be used to monitor the effects of antiresorptive agents. Also, World Health Organization (WHO) T-score criteria should not be used with peripheral devices.

8. What does the DXA report reveal?

Before you read the report, remember that the terms *osteopenia* and *osteoporosis* were introduced to label different levels of bone density and may not mean that the patient has osteoporosis for the following reasons:

   • Low BMD may be due to a number of metabolic bone diseases other than osteoporosis; osteomalacia and hyperparathyroidism are the most common examples.
   • Osteoporosis is a diagnosis of exclusion.

BMD is estimated in gm/cm^2 and then compared with prestored data from two groups of normal individuals of the same gender and race. One group consists of the same age and the other of young adults. Comparison with the same age produces a Z-score, which is the number of standard deviations (SDs) above or below the normal BMD for the same age. Comparison with the young adults produces a T-score, which is the number of SDs above or below the normal BMD of young adults. The T-score is the more important result because it shows how much bone is left compared with the peak bone mass of a normal young adult. According to WHO, a BMD of 1 to 2.5 SD below that of a normal young adult classifies the patient as osteopenic and below 2.5 SD as osteoporotic. Generally, a drop of 1 SD doubles the risk of fracture.

9. What are the indications for bone density studies?

Postmenopausal women under the age of 65 with identifiable risk factors should be screened for osteoporosis as should all women over 65. BMD can confirm the diagnosis of osteoporosis, evaluate a woman's risk for osteoporosis, and assess efficacy of treatment.

Indications for bone density screening

• Age > 65 years
• Patients with history of fractures
• Estrogen-deficient women
• Hypogonadal men
• Persons taking long-term corticosteroids
• Persons with endocrinopathy (hyperthyroidism, hyperparathyroidism, Cushing's disease/syndrome)
• Patients with significant risk factors, regardless of age
• Assessment of treatment efficacy
• Postmenopausal women considering therapy for osteoporosis when BMD will facilitate treatment decisions

10. How does one diagnose primary or secondary osteoporosis?

Osteoporosis is a diagnosis of exclusion. It is made by an assessment of bone mass or evidence of minimally traumatic fracture in the absence of secondary causes of bone loss. A skeletal history and risk factor assessment are used to determine an individual's likelihood of bone loss and fracture risk. Increasing age and an increased number of additional risk factors suggest those with the greatest predisposition for osteoporosis.

Physical examination is directed at detecting sequelae and secondary causes of osteoporosis. Previously unsuspected fractures often occur along the spine and can be detected by a combination of signs including a dowager's hump, loss of height, protuberant abdomen, paravertebral muscle spasm, and vertebral tenderness. A dowager's hump is a hunchback-looking protrusion in the upper back resulting from an anterior vertebral collapse that also causes the head to be pushed forward, shortening the chest and reducing lung capacity. Evidence for secondary causes of osteoporosis might include bony deformities in rheumatoid arthritis, stigmata of chronic alcoholism or cholestatic liver disease, scars on the neck suggesting parathyroid or thyroid surgery, and skin changes consistent with other endocrine disorders.

Screening laboratory studies should be normal in patients with osteoporosis. Serum electrolytes, liver and kidney function tests, albumin, total protein, calcium, phosphorus, thyroid-stimulating hormone, serum testosterone (in men), and a complete blood count comprise initial screening laboratory studies in patients with low bone density. These studies rule out most secondary causes of bone loss or suggest further tests. If these screening tests are within normal limits and there are no obvious predisposing factors or conditions by history or exam, a 24-hour collection for urinary calcium, sodium, and creatinine can be helpful. For example, low 24-hour urinary calcium may suggest vitamin D deficiency, osteomalacia, or malnutrition. High urinary calcium may suggest a renal tubular calcium leak, high sodium diet, absorptive hypercalciuria, or excessive bone resorption secondary to malignancy, hyperparathyroidism, hyperthyroidism, or Paget's disease. In specific cases, more specialized tests should be considered, including serum and urine protein electrophoresis, 24-hour urinary free cortisol or overnight dexamethasone suppression test, and markers of bone turnover (see below).

11. What effective medical interventions are currently available for the treatment of osteoporosis?

The best treatment is not the same in all individuals and should be determined by the physician. Adequate calcium and vitamin D intake from diet and supplements have been shown to reduce both vertebral and nonvertebral fractures. Optimal treatment of bone loss with any pharmacologic intervention also requires calcium and vitamin D intake at recommended levels, at least 1200 mg/day of elemental calcium and 400–800 IU/day of vitamin D. In addition, adequate intake of vitamin D ameliorates secondary hyperparathyroidism, a common age-related cause of increased bone resorption.

Pharmacologic agents approved by the Food and Drug Administration (FDA) can be divided into **antiresorptive agents** and **bone-forming agents**. The antiresorptive agents (bisphosphonates, estrogen and estrogen-like drugs, calcitonin) have inhibition of osteoclast function as their common mechanism of action. Bone-stimulating agents work by promoting osteoblast activity.

TREATMENT	MECHANISM OF ACTION	INDICATIONS	OTHER BENEFITS	ADVERSE EFFECTS
Bisphosphonates (alendronate and risedronate)	Inhibition of osteoclast function	Treatment and prevention of osteoporosis; increase BMD at spine and hip; reduce risk of vertebral fractures; decrease subsequent non-vertebral fractures in women with osteoporosis; glucocorticoid-induced osteoporosis		Abdominal pain, nausea, dyspepsia; esophagitis, gastritis; absolute contraindications of achalasia and esophageal stricture; relative contraindication of gastroesophageal reflux

(Cont'd.)

TREATMENT	MECHANISM OF ACTION	INDICATIONS	OTHER BENEFITS	ADVERSE EFFECTS
Estrogen replacement therapy (estrogen and estrogen with progestin products)	Inhibition of osteoclast function	New FDA labels recommend that when products are considered solely for prevention of postmenopausal osteoporosis, they should be used only after nonestrogen treatments are carefully reviewed	Decrease in colorectal cancers	Women's Health Initiative Study showed overall health risks, including invasive breast cancer, cardiovascular disease, stroke and pulmonary embolism
Selective estrogen-receptor modulators (SERMS) (e.g., raloxifene)	Antiestrogen with estrogenic effect on bone	Treatment and prevention of osteoporosis; reduce risk of vertebral fracture	Positive effect on lipids; no effect on breast or endometrium	Increased risk of "hot flashes" and venous thromboembolism
Calcitonin, as injection or as nasal spray used daily in alternating nostrils	Inhibits bone resorption by directly inhibiting osteoclast function	Prevention and treatment of osteoporosis, but not a first-line agent; reduces risk of vertebral fracture	Analgesic properties in patients with vertebral fractures	Injection is inconvenient with local reaction and pain at injection site; nasal spray may cause nasal irritation
Teriparatide, once daily injection	Stimulates new bone formation	Treatment of postmenopausal women or hypogonadal men with osteoporosis who are at high risk for fracture; increases BMD at the spine and hip; reduces the risk of vertebral and nonvertebral fractures		Nausea, dizziness, leg cramps, osteosarcoma in animals; therapy for more than 2 years is not recommended
Vitamin D	Increases calcium absorption ameliorates secondary hyperparathyroidism		May reduce fracture risk in those > age 65; useful in institutionalized patients, in whom deficiency is common	
Calcium, as carbonate or gluconate (40% or 9% elemental calcium, respectively)		Calcium with or without vitamin D can reduce bone loss and fractures in older adults		Constipation

The bisphosphonates **alendronate** and **risedronate** increase BMD at the spine and hip, reduce the risk of vertebral fractures, and decrease subsequent nonvertebral fractures in women with osteoporosis and adults with glucocorticoid-induced osteoporosis. Because these agents are poorly absorbed, they must be taken in the morning before the first meal. The most common adverse effects are abdominal pain, nausea, and dyspepsia; esophagitis and gastritis are potential complications. People receiving these medications should take them at the prescribed time with a full glass of water and then remain upright for at least 30 minutes. Absolute contraindications include achalasia and esophageal stricture. Both alendronate and risedronate are available as daily and weekly formulations for treatment of osteoporosis and in lower dosages for prevention of osteoporosis.

Estrogen replacement therapy has been a popular approach for prevention (and treatment) of osteoporosis. However, its relative benefit has been called into question by The Women's Health Initiative Study in light of overall health risks, including invasive breast cancer, cardiovascular disease, stroke and pulmonary embolism. The Food and Drug Administration (FDA) has approved new labels for all estrogen and estrogen with progestin products and recommends that when these products are considered solely for prevention of postmenopausal osteoporosis, they should be used after nonestrogen treatments are carefully reviewed. **Selective estrogen-receptor modulators (SERMs)** confer the beneficial effect of estrogen on bone and minimize or antagonize deleterious effects on breast and other end-organs. Raloxifene, a SERM approved for the treatment and prevention of osteoporosis, reduces the risk of vertebral fracture. There may be an increased risk of "hot flashes" and venous thromboembolism with raloxifene.

Calcitonin, either as an injection or more commonly as a nasal spray used daily in alternating nostrils, may reduce the risk of fracture by mechanisms not well understood. Calcitonin could also have analgesic properties in patients with vertebral fractures. It is not a first-line agent for the treatment of osteoporosis but may be reserved for patients with contraindications to other drugs and, in women, those who are at least five years postmenopausal.

In contrast to all of the aforementioned drugs that are predominantly antiresorptive agents which directly or indirectly inhibit osteoclast function, **teriparatide** is the first FDA-approved agent that *stimulates* new bone formation. Teriparatide is a recombinant portion of the parathyroid hormone molecule that is administered by injection once daily in the thigh or abdomen. It increases BMD at the spine and hip and reduces the risk of vertebral and non-vertebral fractures. It is indicated for the treatment of postmenopausal women or hypogonadal men with osteoporosis who are at high risk for fracture. Common side effects include nausea, dizziness, and leg cramps. Based on findings in animal studies, a theoretical safety issue is the development of osteosarcoma; therefore, although no osteosarcomas have been reported in human trials, therapy for more than 2 years is not recommended.

12. How is a person with osteoporosis monitored for treatment response?

Treatment response is usually monitored by BMD testing or by biochemical markers of bone turnover. The interval for monitoring using bone densitometry is usually every 1–2 years. No increases in BMD are common during the first monitoring period, but values usually rebound by the next period. Also, BMD losses should not prompt change or discontinuation of treatment as they may actually be *less* than the decreases that would have occurred in the absence of treatment.

Markers of bone formation include bone-specific alkaline phosphatase, osteocalcin, and procollagen peptides; those for bone resorption are various collagen breakdown products (pyridinoline, deoxypyridinoline, N-telopeptides, and C-telopeptides). Unlike BMD measurements, these markers detect more acute changes in bone turnover that occur after weeks or months. Treatments that decrease bone resorption cause a decrease in markers for bone resorption and formation, whereas the converse is true for treatments that increase bone formation. Although the routine use of markers in the clinical setting is limited due to high inter- and intra-assay variability, there may be a specialized use for these markers in assessing high bone turnover and response to treatment. Earlier evidence that a treatment regimen is working may also serve to reinforce a patient's desire to continue therapy.

13. Discuss the differences with osteoporosis in men.

Osteoporosis is less common in men due to larger skeletons, bone loss starting later in life with slower progression, and the absence of going through a phase of rapid bone loss as women do during menopause. However, men can be at high risk for the disease; a Caucasian man at age 60 has an approximate 25% chance of osteoporotic fracture sometime during the remainder of his life. Osteoporosis in men accounts for one-fifth to one-third of all hip fractures, and men have much higher mortality rates and chronic disability after a hip fracture compared to women. Symptomatic vertebral fractures occur about one-half as often in men. More than half of all men with osteoporosis have secondary causes that produce bone loss, including declines in testosterone levels or hypogonadism, history of steroid therapy, alcohol abuse, significant smoking history, hyperparathyroidism, intestinal disorders, malignancies, and immobilization. Evaluation, treatment, and prevention are similar to those in women, although in many cases there is a paucity of information about the success of these approaches in men.

14. Describe factors that contribute to skeletal health maintenance and osteoporosis prevention throughout life.

Bone loss of a degree that causes hip or vertebral fractures is largely irreversible. Therefore, prevention should start early—in teenage years, when bone mass attained is one of the most important determinants of prolonged skeletal health. Modifiable factors that influence peak bone mass include adequate nutrition and body weight, undisrupted sex hormones at puberty, physical activity, and avoidance of cigarette smoking. A diet that is optimal for bone health includes a balanced, adequate calorie diet containing age-appropriate amounts of calcium and vitamin D. Although a diet high in protein, caffeine, phosphorus, or sodium can adversely affect calcium balance, it can be minimized by adequate calcium intake. Regular physical activity, especially resistance and high-impact exercise, slows the decline in BMD seen with age and reduces the risk of falling. Gonadal sex hormones influence bone fidelity throughout life.

BIBLIOGRAPHY

1. Chan GK, Duque G: Age-related bone loss: Old bone, new facts. Gerontology 48:62, 2002.
2. Crandall C: Parathyroid hormone for treatment of osteoporosis. Arch Intern Med 162:2297, 2002.
3. Cummings SR, Bates D, Black DM: Clinical use of bone densitometry. JAMA 288:1889, 2002.
4. Dawson-Hughes B: Bone loss accompanying medical therapies. N Engl J Med 345:989, 2001.
5. Fitzpatrick LA: Secondary causes of osteoporosis. Mayo Clin Proc 77:453, 2002.
6. Kleerekoper M: Evaluation of the patient with osteoporosis or at risk for osteoporosis. In Marcus R, Feldman D, Kelsey J (eds): Osteoporosis, 2nd ed. New York, Academic Press, 2002.
7. Miller PD, Njeh CF, Jankowski LG, et al: International Society for Clinical Densitometry Position Development Panel and Scientific Advisory Committee. What are the standards by which bone mass measurement at peripheral skeletal sites should be used in the diagnosis of osteoporosis? J Clin Densitom 5:S39, 2002.
8. National Institutes of Health Consensus Development Panel: Osteoporosis prevention, diagnosis, and therapy. JAMA 285:785, 2001.
9. National Osteoporosis Foundation: Physician's Guide to Prevention and Treatment of Osteoporosis. Washington, DC, National Osteoporosis Foundation, 1999.
10. Nelson HD, Helfand M, Woolf SH, et al: Screening for postmenopausal osteoporosis: A review of the evidence for the U.S. Preventive Services Task Force. Ann Intern Med 137:529, 2002.
11. Teitelbaum SL: Bone resorption by osteoclasts. Science 289:1504, 2000.

15. PAIN MANAGEMENT

Jennifer M. Kapo, MD, and Janet Abrahm, MD

1. What are the major types of pain? How do they present?

There are three main types of pain: somatic, visceral, and neuropathic. **Somatic pain**, such as postoperative pain or pain from bony metastases, arises from cutaneous or deep tissues. The pain is usually very well-localized and is dull or aching in character.

Visceral pain, arising from organ infiltration, compression, or stretching, is poorly localized, deep, squeezing, and pressure-like. It may be referred to cutaneous sites, such as the diaphragmatic pain that is felt in the shoulder region. When it is acute, there is often associated nausea, vomiting, or sweating. Patients with an acute myocardial infarction, cholecystitis, bowel obstruction, or liver enlargement due to tumor infiltration present with visceral pain.

Neuropathic pain arises from traumatic or ischemic injury to the peripheral or central nervous systems or from nerve infiltration, compression, or other damage. The pain is usually severe, burning, or vise-like, but is occasionally shooting, like an electric shock. Patients with diabetic or alcoholic neuropathy or herpes zoster have neuropathic pain, as do patients with spinal cord compression.

Pain complaints also may arise in people who have no anatomic lesions. The pain complaint may be the only manner in which the patient is able to express nonspecific feelings of distress caused by anxiety, financial problems, anger, loneliness, depression, or grief over poor health or lost relatives. Because these concerns may exacerbate any concomitant painful sensations, alleviating them can treat the cause of the distress and thereby significantly decrease the need for pain medications.

2. What are the components of an adequate pain assessment?

Effective pain management requires repeated, comprehensive assessment of the patient's pain(s). Although the elderly experience pain to the same degree as younger patients, they often under-report their pain, ascribing it to normal changes expected with aging. Scales that quantify patient reports of pain are valid, reliable, and reproducible. They should be used, much as a blood sugar determination is used in diabetes, to monitor the efficacy of therapy. Cognitively impaired patients may not be able to recall and compare pain levels before and after therapy has been introduced, but they can reliably report their pain at any given time. Repeated assessments, therefore, will accurately reflect the adequacy of the pain control.

If, for example, you are using a scale of 0 (no pain) to 10 (the worst pain imaginable), the change in the rating 1 hour after pain medication is given will indicate how to adjust the medication. The physician must determine both the intensity of the pain and the functional distress caused by the pain (e.g., is it interfering with the patient's ability to eat, sleep, interact with others, move, walk, or talk or with the patient's emotions or concentration). The goal is to lower the pain to a level acceptable to the patient.

3. How does chronic pain differ in its manifestations from acute pain?

Patients in chronic pain do not present the common autonomic manifestations of acute pain (i.e., tachycardia, elevated blood pressure, sweating, or facial grimacing). Such patients will often be quiet and withdrawn, manifesting little spontaneous movement; they can be depressed or irritable and will complain of discomfort if moved. When their pain is relieved, however, they often become mobile and engaged and involved with other people.

4. What common nonpharmacologic methods are effective for pain control?

Hypnosis: Simple hypnotic techniques to minimize patient anxiety and pain include rehearsing the planned test or procedure, distraction techniques (e.g., listening to music), and dissociation (e.g., daydreaming or imagining to be somewhere else). Even without formal hypnotic induction, the words used by the practitioner to describe procedures are very important. Using the phrase "You will feel something; everyone feels this a little differently" in place of "This is going to hurt a lot!" gives the patient permission to alter the sensation and also may diminish the experience of pain. Other cognitive therapies, such as relaxation training or psychological or spiritual counseling, are also helpful.

Hyperstimulation analgesia: Ice massage, using a paper cup filled with ice, is a form of hyperstimulation analgesia that is particularly well-accepted by elderly patients with cancer pain. **Acupuncture** can be helpful for patients with osteoarthritis or neuropathic pain. It is the intensity, not the precise site, of the mechanical stimulation that induces the anesthesia. This anesthesia is not simply due to placebo effect. **Transcutaneous electrical nerve stimulation** (TENS) devices using electrical hyperstimulation are indicated for patients with dermatomal pain, such as postherpetic neuralgia or radiculopathy from spinal cord compression. For optimal effect, a physiatrist or physical therapist familiar with the device should train the patient in its use.

Other: For arthritis pain, **dry heat** or **hydrotherapy** often is used, as is **physical therapy**, which maximizes function and minimizes disability. **Orthotic devices** or prostheses to reduce joint loading and minimize abnormal stresses can limit pain as well as progression of joint damage. Removing fluid from the joint also can provide relief. In certain patients with extensive deformities, synovectomy, joint replacement, or **other surgeries** are indicated for pain relief. **Trigger point injection** can provide relief for many patients with myofascial or certain neuropathic pain syndromes (e.g., post-thoracotomy pain).

5. How are the nonpharmacologic and pharmacologic therapies used for different types of pain?

Pain Regimens for Geriatric Patients

SEVERITY	FREQUENCY	TYPE	AGENTS
Mild	Intermittent	Somatic, visceral	Acetaminophen, COX-2 "selective" NSAID
			Nonacetylating salicylates
			Trigger point injection
			Nonpharmacologic means (hypnosis, ice massage, wet or dry heat)
			Orthotic devices
Moderate	Intermittent	Somatic, visceral	Combination agent (ASA, acetaminophen/NSAID with codeine, oxycodone, hydrocodone)
			Acupuncture
			Hypnosis
	Intermittent or continuous	Neuropathic	Combination agent
			Tramadol
			Tricyclic antidepressant or anticonvulsant
			Steroids, capsaicin
			TENS, hypnosis
			Peripheral nerve, ganglion block, lysis
Severe	Intermittent	Somatic, visceral, neuropathic	Strong, short-acting opioids
			Tricyclic antidepressants
			Nonacetylating salicylates or acetaminophen
	Continuous	Somatic, visceral, neuropathic	Substitute a sustained-release or long-acting opioid for the short-acting opioid[†] in the regimen for severe, intermittent
			Steroids
			Peripheral, central nerve ablation

* Significant toxicities at therapeutic doses in geriatric patients. ASA = acetylsalicylic acid; NSAIDs = nonsteroidal anti-inflammatory drugs.
† Short-acting: oxycodone (alone), Dilaudid (hydromorphone), immediate-release morphine, transmucosal fentanyl.

6. Which patients would benefit from nonopioid analgesics?

Nonopioid analgesics (aspirin, acetaminophen, NSAIDs, nonacetylating salicylates) should be given to patients with **mild pain**, especially of somatic or visceral type. Acetaminophen or nonacetylating salicylates, such as salicylic acid and choline magnesium salicylate, cause less toxicity and therefore should be the first-line agents for elderly patients. Selective inhibitors of COX-2 (e.g., celecoxib, rofecoxib) also may cause less gastrointestinal toxicity and inhibition of platelet function than the nonselective agents that inhibit both COX-1 and COX-2. They may be preferred for patients who have developed serious side effects from a nonselective NSAID or who have other contraindications. It is important to prescribe an adequate dose of the drug at regular intervals, switching to another nonopioid analgesic only when maximal doses of the first are ineffective. The limited metabolism of salicylates can, however, lead to salicylate toxicity if the patient takes the pills more often than recommended. The nonopioid analgesics should be continued in patients with moderate pain when opioid analgesics are added, as they will potentiate the pain-relieving effect of the opioid.

Tramadol is a nonopioid that binds opiate receptors and is effective for mild to moderate pain. Starting dose is 50 mg 4 times/day; patients > 75 with normal renal/hepatic function should not exceed 300 mg/day.

7. What drugs are particularly helpful for patients with bone pain?

The nonopioid analgesics are especially useful in patients with bone pain. For patients with bone pain caused by cancer the bisphosphonates (e.g., pamidronate, zalendromic acid), and the radiopharmaceuticals (strontium-89, samarium-153-lexidronan) are effective. Bisphosphonates also help patients with bone bone due to Paget's disease. The treatment of low back pain of nonmalignant origin requires a combination of pharmacologic, nonpharmacologic, rehabilitative, psychological, and occasionally surgical and anesthetic strategies.

8. What problems may occur in elderly patients using NSAIDs?

Renal insufficiency, peptic ulcer disease, bleeding diatheses, and exacerbation of fluid retention in patients with cirrhosis or congestive heart failure. Renal function should be assessed 1 or 2 weeks after initiation of the NSAID.

9. What agents are helpful for patients with neuropathic pain?

Tricyclic antidepressants (amitriptyline, nortriptyline), anticonvulsants (phenytoin, carbamazepine, gabapentin), capsaicin, and steroids are nonopioid analgesics with particular efficacy in relieving moderate or severe neuropathic pain. Gabapentin is the agent of choice.

Postherpetic neuralgia, which occurs in 1–2% of geriatric patients each year, is not very responsive to opioid medications. Gabapentin is the agent of choice. Start at 100 mg orally 3 times/day and escalate by 100 mg/day every week to an effective dose. Nortriptylin is second line, starting at 10 mg orally at bedtime. Topical capsaicin (0.075%), TENS devices, and nerve block or lysis are also useful.

Trigeminal neuralgia, which occurs mostly in geriatric patients, responds to the anticonvulsant carbamazepine (Tegretol) or baclofen. Tegretol is started at 100 mg twice daily, with careful monitoring for decreases in the white blood cell count. Doses need to be increased very slowly, as tolerated and needed to a target of ≤ 1400 mg/day. Baclofen doses increase from 5 mg 3 times/day to as high as 50 mg 3 times/day, if needed. Facial nerve decompressive surgery is elective for a small group of patients unresponsive to pharmacotherapy.

10. How can compliance with an opioid prescription be optimized?

Opioid analgesics are the mainstay of therapy for patients with moderate to severe pain of any type, whether of malignant or nonmalignant origin. Education of the patient and family is often required to dispel the misconceptions about opioid therapy. The fear of addiction is a common cause of inadequate dispensing of opioids and a barrier to their acceptance by patients. The physician can increase compliance by providing a full explanation of the differences between addiction and physical dependence, along with reassurance that patients with malignancies who take opioids do not become addicts. Patients also may fear that if they take opioid medications for moderate pain, these agents will no longer be effective if more severe pain occurs. A functional goal of therapy, such as returning to a favorite hobby or reinstituting normal activities of everyday life, may enable the patient and family to accept the opioid.

11. Which opioid medications should be used in elderly patients?

A wide variety of medications are available for use by the oral, transmucosal, rectal, transdermal, or parenteral route. These include the short-acting agents codeine, hydrocodone, oxycodone, hydromorphone, and morphine and the longer-acting agents methadone, transdermal fentanyl, and morphine or oxycodone in sustained-release preparations. Oxycodone or hydrocodone (5 mg/pill) are the opioids in the combination agents with acetylsalicylic acid, acetaminophen, and NSAIDs.

The choice of agent should be dictated by the frequency and type of the pain being treated. **Intermittent, moderate to severe pain** lasting hours to several days is amenable to oral short-acting (3–4 hr) analgesics with appropriate potency. **Severe pain** of relatively constant intensity should be treated with oral long-acting oxycodone or morphine preparations (given every 8–12 hrs) or fentanyl, absorbed through a transdermal patch (renewed every 72 hours). Meperidine is the least useful opioid for patients with long-lasting moderate to severe pain. It provides pain relief for only about 1–2 hours, and its metabolite can cause seizures. Because of its long half-life, methadone is problematic in elderly patients.

Combinations of a nonopioid analgesic along with an opioid (e.g., Percodan) are very useful, even for patients with moderate somatic or visceral pain of nonmalignant origin. Patients with pain of bony origin, such as severe osteoarthritis or rheumatoid arthritis, are ideal candidates for these agents.

12. How is physical dependence different from addiction?

In a patient with physical dependence, "Physiologic adaptation of the body to the presence of opioid is required to maintain the same level of analgesia," whereas in addiction (psychological dependence), there is a "pattern of compulsive drug use characterized by a continual craving for an opioid and the need to use the opioid for effects other than pain relief."[11]

Fewer than 1% of people who use opioids for pain become addicted to them. They may continue to need them to keep their pain at a tolerable level and may even develop a physiologic dependence, but they will not start stealing TV sets. They will not begin to crave the drugs or seek them to "get high."

13. What other routes are available for patients who cannot take opioids orally?

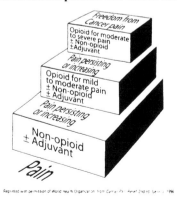

Reprinted with permission of World Health Organization from Cancer Pain Relief, 2nd ed. Geneva, 1996

World Health Organization Analgesic Ladder

Equianalgesic and Opioid Starting Doses for Opioid-Naïve Adults and Children

Drug	Equianalgesic Dose Oral (Compared to 30 mg PO Morphine)	Usual Starting Dose PO <50 kg	Usual Starting Dose PO >50 kg	PO:IV/SC Ratio	Equianalgesic Dose Parenteral (Compared to 10 mg IV Morphine)	Usual Starting Dose IV/SC <50 kg	Usual Starting Dose IV/SC >50 kg	Biologic Half-Life (Hours)
Codeine	190 mg ("usual" maximum dose is 120 mg)	0.5–1 mg/kg q 3–4 hours	15–30 mg q 3–4 hr	1.5:1.0 SC **Not to be given IV.**	130 mg (usual maximum dose is 60 mg)	0.25–0.5 mg/kg q 3–4 hr SC **Not to be given IV.**	60 mg Q 3–4 hrs SC. **Not to be given IV.**	2.5–3
Hydrocodone (as in Vicodin)	30 mg (Clinical experience suggests lower potency.)	0.1 mg/kg q 3–4 hours	5–10 mg q 3–4 hr	Not available in parenteral form	N/A	N/A	N/A	3–4
Oxycodone (as in Percocet, Tylox)	20 mg	0.1–0.2 mg/kg q 3–4 hours	5–10 mg q 3–4 hr	Not available in parenteral form	N/A	N/A	N/A	2–3
Morphine	30 mg	0.15–0.3 mg/kg q 3–4 hours	5–10 mg q 3–4 hr	3:1	10 mg	0.05–0.1 mg/kg q 3–4 hr	5–10 mg q 3–4 hr	2.5–3
Hydromorphone (Dilaudid)	7.5 mg	0.05 mg/kg q 3–4 hours	1–2 mg q 3–4 hr	5:1	1.5 mg	0.02–0.07 mg/kg q 3–4 hr	1–1.5 mg q 3–4 hr	2–3
Oxymorphone (Numorphan)	N/A	N/A	N/A	5 mg PR equianalgesic with 1 mg IV	1 mg	0.02 mg/kg q 3–4 hr	1 mg q 3–4 hr	1.5
Fentanyl Intravenous (Caution-Rapid infusion may cause chest wall rigidity)	N/A	N/A	N/A	N/A	**Single dose:** 100 mcg **By infusion:** 100 mcg/h = 2.5 mg/h morphine	0.5–1.5 mcg/kg q 30 min	25–75 mcg q 30 min	IV: 3–12 hours TD: 18–24 hours (elimination half-life) TD IV Ratio=1:1 (Based on clinical experience)

NA = not available TD = Transdermal

Notes

1. When converting from one short half-life opioid to another, reduce the dose of the new opioid by 25%–50% of the equianalgesic dose (because of incomplete cross-tolerance), then titrate as required.
2. Usual starting doses often are empiric and NOT necessarily calculated according to equianalgesic principles (e.g., the usual starting dose for hydromorphone may be 2 mg PO even though the parenteral: oral ratio = 1:5).
3. For infants <6 months of age, use 1/4 of the usual starting dose, then titrate to effect.
4. Transdermal fentanyl not recommended for use in opioid-naïve patients.
5. Conversion to a long-acting preparation is recommended after dose titration achieves pain relief.

Modified from Memorial Sloan-Kettering Cancer Center Pain Service

14. How is a patient converted from oral or parenteral morphine to a transdermal fentanyl patch?

The table provides information on converting dosages. For example, a patient who has been receiving 1000 mg of sustained-release morphine every 12 hours should be given a 100-μg fentanyl patch ($100 \times 2 = 200$ mg oral morphine dail corresponding to a 100-μg fentanyl patch). A patient on a morphine drip of 2 mg/hr should be started on 75 μg of fentanyl (2 mg/hr $\times$ 24 hrs = 48 mg parenteral morphine daily corresponding to 75 μg of fentanyl).

Dosage Conversions[4]

FENTANYL (μg/hr)	MORPHINE (mg/day)	
	PARENTERAL	ORAL
25	17	50
50	33	100
75	50	150
100	67	200
125	83	250
150	100	300

15. In addition to NSAIDs, which medications can add to the pain-relieving effect of the opioids and thereby minimize the dose needed?

Gabapentin and tricyclics are effective for neuropathic pain. Side effects of gabapentin include somnolence and peripheral edema. Low doses of tricyclic antidepressants (TCAs, such as despiramine, 10 mg given at bedtime) are well-tolerated and are effective within 2–3 days. Although despiramine has the fewest anticholinergic side effects of the TCA class, it should not be given to patients with known glaucoma, urinary retention, or first-degree heart block. Side effects (usually associated with amitriptyline) may include autonomic effects, which can be mild (dry mouth, constipation) or more severe (postural hypotension, glaucoma, or urinary retention).

16. How should the constipation and sedation associated with opioids be managed?

Laxatives must be given routinely, not on an as-needed basis, to patients treated with any opioids. Bowel irritants such as Senokot, resins such as lactulose, or polyethylene glycol grannules (Miralax) are the most effective agents. Docusate is not effective, and fiber only exacerbates the problem.

Long-acting benzodiazepines (e.g., Valium), barbiturates, and chloral hydrate are not recommended as sleep medications for patients receiving opioids, because they produce excessive daytime sedation. When possible, medications that produce sedation as a side effect (e.g., cimetidine or diphenhydramine) should be discontinued.

Sedation or confusion induced by opioids may resolve if a different opioid is used. Use the opioid equianalgesic table and decrease the equianalgesic dose of the new agent to allow for incomplete cross-tolerance. If this is ineffective, dextroamphetamine or methylphenidate (Ritalin, 2.5–10 mg orally with breakfast and lunch) will decrease sedation. Doses can be slowly escalated as needed. The amphetamine can be important in helping patients be as alert and pain-free as possible for an important event, such as a child's wedding or an important anniversary. Methylphenidate is contraindicated in patients with cardiac disease, as serious arrhythmias may occur. Patients may also become overstimulated or anxious and develop insomnia, paranoia, or confusion. Paradoxically, however, many elderly patients with depression respond well to similar doses of methylphenidate, with increased appetite and a better sense of well-being.

Naloxone reverses opioid-induced respiratory and CNS depression, but caution should be exercised before administering naloxone to a patient chronically receiving opioids: severe withdrawal may be precipitated. In such patients, rather than administering the usual 0.4-mg/ml dose, dilute the 0.4 mg of naloxone into 10 ml of saline, and give only enough to reverse respiratory depression, not enough to awaken the patient.

17. Define and describe the term *palliative sedation.*

Rare patients who are within days to weeks of death and who have distressing symptoms that cannot be controlled in any other way may require sedation to unconsciousness. This practice is called "palliative sedation." Expert palliative care, psychiatric, and pastoral care consultation should be obtained. If they are unable to provide sufficient relief, the primary physician should next consult extensively with the family and patient and obtain their informed consent to the sedation. Hospital admission for palliative sedation is not required if adequate personnel can be provided in the home or long-term care facility. Under the physician's direction and close nursing monitoring, phenobarbital as a suppository or intravenous pentobarbital, lorazepam or midazolam infusions will induce sedation adequate to relieve the symptoms. Parenteral or enteral feedings and hydration usually are not provided but can be if required to fulfill the goals of the patient and their families.[3]

18. Discuss the special problems presented by opioids and adjuvants in the elderly.

Pharmacokinetics both of opioids and psychotropic adjuvant medications are altered in the elderly. Elderly patients (age 70–89) have decreased opioid clearance, which leads to a prolonged duration of effect. Effective doses are one-half to one-quarter of those needed in younger patients. Long-acting agents such as methadone, sustained-release oxycodone or morphine, or fentanyl patches should be used with caution in the frail elderly, as the drug may accumulate and cause excessive toxicity. Drugs with short half-lives are preferred, and initial doses should be half those used with younger patients. The acute urinary retention due to opioids (especially in patients with prostatic hypertrophy) and hypotension and tachycardia caused by TCAs can be more frequent and of more clinical severity in this population.

19. What are the special problems of pain control in patients with dementia?

Little is known about the problem of giving pain medications to elderly patients with dementia. However, patients with AIDS dementia have been found to be much more sensitive to the adverse side effects of opioids. Sedation and confusion have been especially troublesome but have responded to psychostimulants such as methylphenidate or to antipsychotics such as haloperidol without diminution of the pain relief. It may be reasonable, therefore, to add psychostimulants or antipsychotic agents in appropriate elderly demented patients who develop these side effects from the opioids used to control their pain. Whenever possible, nonpharmacologic therapies, such as relaxation, hypnosis, or other cognitive therapies, should be used.

20. What are the common mistakes and misperceptions in treating pain in the elderly?

1. Failure to use a quantitative pain scale and assess pain routinely and the assumption that cognitively impaired patients cannot give accurate pain assessments.

2. Use of NSAIDs in patients with significant risk of toxicity in an effort to avoid opioid use. NSAIDs should be used with caution, if at all, in elderly patients with a history of gastrointestinal intolerance or bleeding, renal insufficiency, hypertension, congestive heart failure, or cirrhosis.

3. Failure to prescribe opioids for patients whose pain levels are moderate or severe, whether the pain is of malignant or nonmalignant origin.

4. Failure to provide an aggressive routine laxative regimen to prevent opioid-induced constipation.

5. Failure to discontinue medications that contribute to sedation and thereby limit tolerable opioid dose.

BIBLIOGRAPHY

1. AGS Clinical Practice Committee: Management of cancer pain in older patients. J Am Geriatr Soc 45:1273–1276, 1997.
2. AGS Panel on Chronic Pain in Older Persons: The management of chronic pain in older persons. J Am Geriatr Soc 46:635–651, 1998.

3. American Pain Society: Principles of Analgesic Use in the Treatment of Acute Pain and Cancer Pain, 4th ed. American Pain Society, 1999.

4. Cherny NI, Coyle N, Foley KM: Guidelines in the care of the dying cancer patient. Hematol Oncol Clin North Am 10:261–286, 1996.

5. Eisenberg E, Berkey CS, Carr DB, et al: Efficacy and safety of nonsteroidal antiinflammatory drugs for cancer pain: A meta-analysis. J Clin Oncol 12:2756–2765, 1994.

6. Ferrell BA: Pain evaluation and management in the nursing home. Ann Intern Med 123:681–687, 1995.

7. Ferrell BR, Ferrell BA (eds): Pain in the Elderly. Seattle, IASP Press, 1996.

8. Ferrell BR: Patient education and nondrug interventions. In Ferrell BR, Ferrell BA (eds): Pain in the Elderly. Seattle, IASP Press, 1996, p 35.

9. Forman WB: Opioid analgesic drugs in the elderly. Clin Geriatr Med 12:489–500, 1996.

10. Gloth FM: Concerns with chronic analgesic therapy in elderly patients. Am J Med 101(Suppl 1A):19S–24S, 1996.

11. Jacox A, Carr DB, Payne R, et al: Management of Cancer Pain: Clinical Practice Guideline No 9. Washington, DC, UPHS, AHCPR, 1994, AHCPR publication 94-0592.

12. Kost RG, Straus SE: Postherpetic neuralgia—pathogenesis, treatment, and prevention. N Engl J Med 335:32–42, 1996.

13. Levy MH: Pharmacologic treatment of cancer pain. N Engl J Med 335:1124–1132, 1996.

14. Lipman AG: Analgesic drugs for neuropathic and sympathetically maintained pain. Clin Geriatr Med 12:501–515, 1996.

15. Parmelee PA: Pain in cognitively impaired older persons. Clin Geriatr Med 12:473–487, 1996.

16. Portenoy RK: Adjuvant analgesics in pain management. In Doyle D, Hanks G, MacDonald N (eds): Oxford Textbook of Palliative Medicine, 2nd ed. New York, Oxford University Press, 1997, p 361.

16. NUTRITION

Marie Bernard, MD

1. Name the most common nutritional problem among elderly individuals.

In studies of elderly individuals in hospitals and nursing homes, **protein-calorie malnutrition** is found in 30–50% of the population. Borderline protein-calorie malnutrition is common in elderly outpatients. Multiple epidemiologic studies have demonstrated that elderly individuals commonly consume less than two-thirds of the recommended daily allowance (RDA) for multiple nutrients. This, combined with the effects of accumulated illnesses, medications, and social circumstances, depletes body caloric reserves for the stress of acute illness or surgery. Thus, with hospitalization, elderly individuals often have developed protein-calorie malnutrition and its associated morbidity and mortality. Elderly outpatients are much less likely to have overt malnutrition, unless they are recuperating from an acute illness.

2. Why do many elderly have reduced calorie intakes?

A number of factors contribute to elderly individuals' becoming protein-calorie malnourished:

1. As one ages, the senses of smell and taste diminish, thus rendering foods less palatable.

2. Accumulated illnesses and medications may suppress the appetite or impair the absorption of nutrients.

3. Many elderly individuals suffer from functional problems, making it difficult to get proper access to food or to prepare food properly.

4. Many elderly individuals suffer from social factors, such as decreased income, social isolation, and depression, that impair their ability to obtain food or their desire to consume it.

All of these factors combine to lead to suboptimal intake among elderly individuals, often leading to protein-calorie malnutrition upon their presentation to a hospital or long-term care institution.

Risk Factors for Poor Nutritional Status

Inappropriate food intake	Dependency/disability	Chronic medication use
Poverty	Acute/chronic diseases	Advanced age
Social isolation	or conditions	

Modified from The Nutrition Sceening Initiative, a project of the American Academy of Family Physicians, The American Dietetic Association and the National Council on the Aging, Inc., and funded in part by a grant from Ross Laboratories, a division of Abbott Laboratories.

3. How does malnutrition affect outcome of care in the elderly?

In protein-calorie malnourished patients, the length of stay in the hospital, cost of hospital care, and mortality are all 30–100% greater than in normally nourished individuals. Malnourished elderly outpatients also have poorer health and greater morbidity than normally nourished individuals. Morbidity associated with protein-calorie malnutrition includes increased infections, longer recovery time for wound healing, and less recovery of function.

4. When should you evaluate the nutritional status of elderly individuals? How?

Nutritional assessment can be difficult in elderly patients because aging and disease cause decreases in lean body mass that can mimic those seen with malnutrition. Although weight loss is seen with aging, recent unintentional weight loss—especially if it is > 5–10% of one's usual weight or > 10 lbs in 6 months—is significant.

An expert panel of nutritionists and gerontologists has developed a consensus regarding the nutritional assessment of elderly individuals. Their Nutrition Screening Initiative provides the first generally agreed-on standards for determining the nutritional status of elderly individuals. They also recommend proper interventions once risk factors for malnutrition are identified.

5. When should nutritional intervention be initiated for elderly individuals?

Most experts would not advise allowing a thin, frail, elderly person to go for 10 days with suboptimal intake. There are no firm guidelines, but the more underweight the patient and the greater the metabolic stress (particularly if the albumin level is < 3.5 gm/dl), the earlier nutritional intervention should be considered. Early identification of patients with intake significantly below 1000 kcal/day is therefore necessary.

A registered dietitian often is helpful in guiding the assessment of the nutritional needs of hospitalized or institutionalized elderly individuals and in assessing how closely spontaneous intake approximates those needs. This task is more difficult in ambulatory elderly. However, the guidelines of the Nutrition Screening Initiative for the Level 1 screen may help in identifying elderly individuals at risk for borderline intake.

Medicare does not pay for a home nutritional assessment. However, such assessments can be performed easily by a number of individuals.

- Checklists of risk factors can be administered by lay persons or home health aides. These should be considered for every elderly individual.
- Level I screens can be performed by nurses, social workers, and other health professionals in regular contact with elders. This screen should be performed if an elder is found to be at risk of nutritional deficiency, based on responses to the checklist.
- The Level II screen is intended for physicians to evaluate elderly individuals who appear nutritionally deficient based on the checklist and Level I screen.

(See figures on pages 84–87.)

6. What is unique about providing dietary supplements to elderly individuals?

Supplementation of the diet with enteral formulas is the first intervention to be provided (after problems with depression, social isolation, and/or difficulties with access to food have been addressed). Unfortunately, no medications have been identified that are clearly beneficial in stimulating appetite in the elderly. Food supplements have limited benefit in many elderly, due to the development of early satiety and/or taste fatigue. In addition, many elderly substitute enteral formulas intended for diet supplementation for their usual intake, thus deriving no net benefit from the intervention. In cases when spontaneous and supplemented intake cannot bring calorie and protein intake to goal levels, nutritional support via a nasoenteric or enteric tube is indicated.

7. How are the enteral nutrition formulas classified?

A plethora of formulas is available for nutritional support of the elderly. Each formula claims special properties that purportedly benefit diverse populations. However, based on review of the literature, there are few indications in the elderly for specialized formulas.

Formulas can be classified according to **protein form** as polymeric (blenderized), elemental, or free amino acids. Polymeric formulas are preferable to elemental formulas for simple diet supplementation, because they are more palatable. Polymeric formulas appear to be better tolerated in most elderly than elemental or amino acid formulas, which are more costly and unnecessary in most instances. The source of the protein does not appear to affect tolerance of feedings, with the exception of milk-based formulas. (The elderly have a higher prevalence of lactase deficiency than younger individuals, making milk-based formulas poorly tolerated by many.) Formulas that are high in osmolality and/or fiber do not appear to influence the occurrence of diarrhea. A study with a very small number of patients suggests that elemental formulas are beneficial for diarrhea in hypoalbuminemic patients because of their easier absorption. (See table, top of next page.)

8. How is an appropriate formula selected?

In general, the elderly require 0.8–1.0 gm protein and 25 kcal/kg body weight. Patients recuperating from hip fracture or major surgery may have higher protein needs, up to 1.0 gm/kg body weight. Thus, you should select a formula that provides an appropriate quantity of calories and protein over the course of 24 hours in an isosmolar form or more concentrated form if there are concerns regarding fluid retention. Formulas that have a mixture of carbohydrate, long-chain

Enteral Formula Comparison Chart

	BLENDERIZED		ELEMENTAL	FIBER-CONTAINING		LACTOSE-FREE
Product	Compleat Regular	Vitaneed	Travasorb	Enrich	Ensure Plus	Isocal
Cal/ml	1.07	1.0	1.0	1.1	1.5	1.06
mOsm/kg water	450	300	560	480	690	270
Calories to meet 100% RDA for vitamins and mineratls	1600	1500	2000	1530	2130	2000
Flavors	Natural food	Natural food	Unflavored	Varied	Varied	Unflavored
Cal/protein per 8-oz can	250/9	250/8	250/11	250/9	360/13	250/8

triglycerides, and intact protein (i.e., formulas that mimic real food) are usually well-tolerated. Although the elderly have a high prevalence of disorders of the GI tract that can affect fat absorption, data suggest that many elderly individuals can tolerate enteral formulas with as much as 67% of calories provided as fat.

In intensive care unit patients, a low non-protein calorie to nitrogen ratio (e.g., 97:1) may be beneficial in promoting nitrogen retention. In metabolically stable patients, there also may be a role for providing more nitrogen-dense formulas to compensate for the fact that patients often do not receive the full amount of enteral nutrition prescribed (e.g., due to technical difficulties, cessation of feedings for diagnostic testing).

9. Is nutritional intervention effective in elderly individuals?

Few studies actually have demonstrated the efficacy of nutritional intervention in this or any age group. One study evaluated a group of 122 "thin" and "very thin" elderly women with hip fractures. In the randomized, controlled trial, 1000 cal and 28 gm of protein were provided by overnight tube feeding, in addition to a regular diet throughout the day. This intervention led to more rapid ambulation than in control patients. Another study demonstrated similar benefit of simple oral supplementation in 59 elderly hip fracture patients. In a prospective, controlled trial, the daily addition of 250 cal and 20 gm of protein to the usual diet resulted in fewer hospital complications, increased mobility, and fewer nursing home placements at 6-month follow-up than in the controls.

Several studies of long-term feedings in chronically ill elderly in nursing homes have failed to show the benefits demonstrated in shorter studies of elderly who have undergone surgical procedures. However, many of the long-term evaluation studies are retrospective, without clear documentation of the degree to which nutritional needs were matched with the nutrition support provided.

In sum, nutritional deficits would appear to be reversible in many cases. Adverse outcomes associated with malnutrition in the elderly are well-documented. Thus, the potential benefits of nutritional intervention appear worthy of the effort.

Benefits and Risks of Enteral Nutritional Support

BENEFITS	RISKS
Nutritional repletion	Aspiration pneumonia
Hydration	Diarrhea
Decreased morbidity	Tube displacement
Decreased mortality	Clogged tube
Fewer complications than parenteral therapy	Electrolyte disturbance
Lower cost than parenteral therapy	Infection of feeding formula

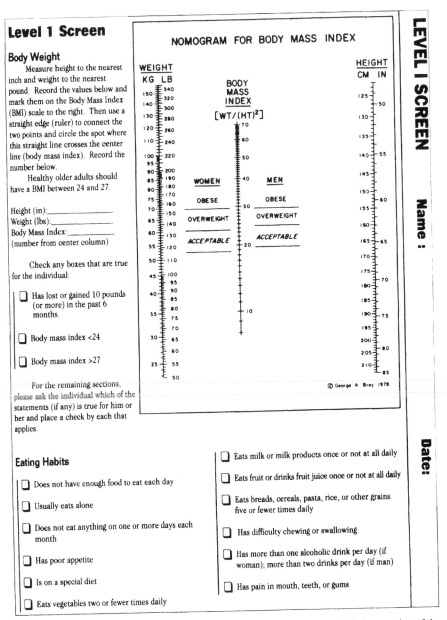

Level 1 Screen

Body Weight

Measure height to the nearest inch and weight to the nearest pound. Record the values below and mark them on the Body Mass Index (BMI) scale to the right. Then use a straight edge (ruler) to connect the two points and circle the spot where this straight line crosses the center line (body mass index). Record the number below.

Healthy older adults should have a BMI between 24 and 27.

Height (in):_____
Weight (lbs):_____
Body Mass Index:_____
(number from center column)

Check any boxes that are true for the individual:

☐ Has lost or gained 10 pounds (or more) in the past 6 months.

☐ Body mass index <24

☐ Body mass index >27

For the remaining sections, please ask the individual which of the statements (if any) is true for him or her and place a check by each that applies.

NOMOGRAM FOR BODY MASS INDEX

WEIGHT
KG LB

BODY MASS INDEX
[WT/(HT)²]

WOMEN   MEN

OBESE   OBESE

OVERWEIGHT   OVERWEIGHT

ACCEPTABLE   ACCEPTABLE

HEIGHT
CM IN

© George A Bray 1978

LEVEL I SCREEN   Name:

Date:

Eating Habits

☐ Does not have enough food to eat each day

☐ Usually eats alone

☐ Does not eat anything on one or more days each month

☐ Has poor appetite

☐ Is on a special diet

☐ Eats vegetables two or fewer times daily

☐ Eats milk or milk products once or not at all daily

☐ Eats fruit or drinks fruit juice once or not at all daily

☐ Eats breads, cereals, pasta, rice, or other grains five or fewer times daily

☐ Has difficulty chewing or swallowing

☐ Has more than one alcoholic drink per day (if woman); more than two drinks per day (if man)

☐ Has pain in mouth, teeth, or gums

The level I and II screens. Reprinted with permission of the Nutrition Screening Initiative, a project of the American Academy of Family Physicians. The American Dietetic Association, and the National Council on the Aging, Inc., and funded in part by a grant from Ross Laboratories, a division of Abbott Laboratories.
(Figure continues on following pages.)

It should be noted that enteral therapy cannot be relied upon to meet the full hydration needs of a patient. If enteral feedings are the sole source of nutrition and hydration, 500–1000 cc of free-water supplementation also must be provided, depending on the patient's clinical condition

A physician should be contacted if the individual has gained or lost 10 pounds unexpectedly or without intending to during the past 6 months. A physician should also be notified if the individual's body mass index is above 27 or below 24.

Living Environment

☐ Lives on an income of less than $6000 per year (per individual in the household)

☐ Lives alone

☐ Is housebound

☐ Is concerned about home security

☐ Lives in a home with inadequate heating or cooling

☐ Does not have a stove and/or refrigerator

☐ Is unable or prefers not to spend money on food (<$25-30 per person spent on food each week)

Functional Status

Usually or always needs assistance with (check each that apply):

☐ Bathing

☐ Dressing

☐ Grooming

☐ Toileting

☐ Eating

☐ Walking or moving about

☐ Traveling (outside the home)

☐ Preparing food

☐ Shopping for food or other necessities

If you have checked one or more statements on this screen, the individual you have interviewed may be at risk for poor nutritional status. Please refer this individual to the appropriate health care or social service professional in your area. For example, a dietitian should be contacted for problems with selecting, preparing, or eating a healthy diet, or a dentist if the individual experiences pain or difficulty when chewing or swallowing. Those individuals whose income, lifestyle, or functional status may endanger their nutritional and overall health should be referred to available community services: home-delivered meals, congregate meal programs, transportation services, counseling services (alcohol abuse, depression, bereavement, etc.), home health care agencies, day care programs, etc.

Please repeat this screen at least once each year—sooner if the individual has a major change in his or her health, income, immediate family (e.g., spouse dies), or functional status.

and the tonicity of the formula. Additionally, although enteral feedings have fewer complications and lower cost than parenteral feedings, there are risks associated with enteral nutritional therapy, including aspiration pneumonia and diarrhea. Tube displacement and clogging can become significant clinical issues for patients with gastrostomies and jejunostomies. Unmonitored patients on enteral feedings can develop a vast array of electrolyte disturbances, generally relating to insufficient free water accompanying the feedings. Patients receiving enteral feedings that are mixed from powders are at risk for receiving infected feedings if good aseptic technique is not maintained or if feedings are allowed to hang for more than 24 hours. This is potentially problematic for frail older individuals with impaired immune responses.

10. What type of enteral feeding tube is preferable for short-term use in elderly patients?

Patients anticipated to require enteral nutrition support for a short time should have a **small-bore, pliable, nasoenteric tube** placed. These are often weighted to facilitate placement and identification by x-ray. Before feedings are initiated, the tube tip must be confirmed to be in the stomach, either by aspiration of gastric contents or by x-ray. Inadvertent placement of the feeding tube into the tracheobronchial tree may not induce coughing in the elderly. Nasoenteric tube malposition may occur in up to 1.3% of the population receiving tube feedings, and as many as 35% of tube-fed patients may have clogged tubes. Such clogging may be resolved with water or

Level II Screen

Complete the following screen by interviewing the patient directly and/or by referring to the patient chart. If you do not routinely perform all of the described tests or ask all of the listed questions, please consider including them but do not be concerned if the entire screen is not completed. Please try to conduct a minimal screen on as many older patients as possible, and please try to collect serial measurements, which are extremely valuable in monitoring nutritional status. Please refer to the manual for additional information.

Anthropometrics

Measure height to the nearest inch and weight to the nearest pound. Record the values below and mark them on the Body Mass Index (BMI) scale to the right. Then use a straight edge (paper, ruler) to connect the two points and circle the spot where this straight line crosses the center line (body mass index). Record the number below; healthy older adults should have a BMI between 24 and 27; check the appropriate box to flag an abnormally high or low value.

NOMOGRAM FOR BODY MASS INDEX

BODY MASS INDEX [WT/(HT)^2]

WEIGHT KG LB

HEIGHT CM IN

WOMEN | MEN
OBESE | OBESE
OVERWEIGHT | OVERWEIGHT
ACCEPTABLE | ACCEPTABLE

© George A Bray 1978

LEVEL II SCREEN   Name: Date:

Height (in):_____
Weight (lbs):_____
Body Mass Index
(weight/height^2):_____

Please place a check by any statement regarding BMI and recent weight loss that is true for the patient.

☐ Body mass index <24

☐ Body mass index >27

☐ Has lost or gained 10 pounds (or more) of body weight in the past 6 months

Record the measurement of mid-arm circumference to the nearest 0.1 centimeter and of triceps skinfold to the nearest 2 millimeters.

Mid-Arm Circumference (cm):_____
Triceps Skinfold (mm):_____
Mid-Arm Muscle Circumference (cm):_____

Refer to the table and check any abnormal values:

☐ Mid-arm muscle circumference <10th percentile

☐ Triceps skinfold <10th percentile

☐ Triceps skinfold >95th percentile

Note: mid-arm circumference (cm) - [0.314 x triceps skinfold (mm)]= mid-arm *muscle* circumference (cm)

For the remaining sections, please place a check by any statements that are true for the patient.

Laboratory Data

☐ Serum albumin below 3.5 g/dl

☐ Serum cholesterol below 160 mg/dl

☐ Serum cholesterol above 240 mg/dl

Drug Use

☐ Three or more prescription drugs, OTC medications, and/or vitamin/mineral supplements daily

pancreatic enzyme. At least one case report has described an elderly individual post-stroke who became an obligate nasal breather, leading to an inability to tolerate nasoenteric feedings.

11. Which type of enteral feeding tube is preferrable for long-term use?

In an individual who may require feedings for a prolonged period, **percutaneous endoscopic gastrostomy** (PEG) is the preferred method of feeding. **Surgical gastrostomies** are reserved for

Clinical Features

Presence of (check each that apply):

☐ Problems with mouth, teeth, or gums

☐ Difficulty chewing

☐ Difficulty swallowing

☐ Angular stomatitis

☐ Glossitis

☐ History of bone pain

☐ History of bone fractures

☐ Skin changes (dry, loose, nonspecific lesions, edema)

Percentile	Men 55-65 y	Men 65-75 y	Women 55-65 y	Women 65-75 y
Arm circumference (cm)				
10th	27.3	26.3	25.7	25.2
50th	31.7	30.7	30.3	29.9
95th	36.9	35.5	38.5	37.3
Arm muscle circumference (cm)				
10th	24.5	23.5	19.6	19.5
50th	27.8	26.8	22.5	22.5
95th	32.0	30.6	28.0	27.9
Triceps skinfold (mm)				
10th	6	6	16	14
50th	11	11	25	24
95th	22	22	38	36

From: Frisancho AR. New norms of upper limb fat and muscle areas for assessment of nutritional status. Am J Clin Nutr 1981; 34:2540-2545. © 1981 American Society for Clinical Nutrition.

Eating Habits

☐ Does not have enough food to eat each day

☐ Usually eats alone

☐ Does not eat anything on one or more days each month

☐ Has poor appetite

☐ Is on a special diet

☐ Eats vegetables two or fewer times daily

☐ Eats milk or milk products once or not at all daily

☐ Eats fruit or drinks fruit juice once or not at all daily

☐ Eats breads, cereals, pasta, rice, or other grains five or fewer times daily

☐ Has more than one alcoholic drink per day (if woman); more than two drinks per day (if man)

Living Environment

☐ Lives on an income of less than $6000 per year (per individual in the household)

☐ Lives alone

☐ Is housebound

☐ Is concerned about home security

☐ Lives in a home with inadequate heating or cooling

☐ Does not have a stove and/or refrigerator

☐ Is unable or prefers not to spend money on food (<$25-30 per person spent on food each week)

Functional Status

Usually or always needs assistance with (check each that apply):

☐ Bathing

☐ Dressing

☐ Grooming

☐ Toileting

☐ Eating

☐ Walking or moving about

☐ Traveling (outside the home)

☐ Preparing food

☐ Shopping for food or other necessities

Mental/Cognitive Status

☐ Clinical evidence of impairment, e.g. Folstein<26

☐ Clinical evidence of depressive illness, e.g. Beck Depression Inventory>15, Geriatric Depression Scale>5

Patients in whom you have identified one or more major indicator (see pg 2) of poor nutritional status require immediate medical attention; if minor indicators are found, ensure that they are known to a health professional or to the patient's own physician. Patients who display risk factors (see pg 2) of poor nutritional status should be referred to the appropriate health care or social service professional (dietitian, nurse, dentist, case manager, etc.).

individuals at risk of complications with PEG placement (e.g., morbid obesity, esophageal obstruction, bleeding diathesis). Both procedures are associated with minimal complications. Morbidity and mortality associated with placement of these tubes may be due to the frail state of elders generally selected for this form of feeding. Occasionally, life-threatening complications of gastrostomies may arise, such as wound dehiscence, sepsis, or peritonitis.

Percutaneous endoscopic gastrojejunostomies and surgical jejunostomies have been recommended in the past to limit problems with aspiration pneumonia, but these procedures do not necessarily limit aspiration. They are associated with a number of complications, such as bleeding, infections, and wound dehiscence.

12. How should enteral feedings be provided to the elderly?

Continuous enteral feedings are most commonly provided for individuals receiving naso-enteral feedings and often for individuals receiving gastrostomy or jejunostomy feedings. Continous feedings are more easily administered through small-bore tubes than intermittent feedings. They also may decrease nausea, vomiting, and diarrhea. They have in the past been thought to be associated with a lower risk of aspiration pneumonia than intermittent feedings, but more recent data challenge this assumption. Data suggest that intermittent feedings allow for better protein synthesis than do continuous feedings. However, at present, no conclusive evidence shows that one form of feeding should be preferred over another.

Continuous feedings are generally administered starting at 25–50 ml/hr and progressively increased to 100–125 ml/hr, depending on the predicted caloric needs of the individual and the caloric density of the formula. Intermittent feedings are generally started at 200 ml four times daily and progressively increased to as much as 400–500 ml every 4–6 hours, depending on caloric needs. Formulas with a high tonicity are often diluted initially and then progressively increased to full strength and eventually full volume.

13. What is the most dangerous complication of tube feeding in elderly individuals?

Aspiration pneumonia is the one complication that can lead to mortality. In the literature, its incidence ranges from 3–33%. In the past, experts believed that this complication could be limited by continuous feedings (which limit the volume of fluid in the stomach at any one time) and by feedings below the pyloric junction. However, more recent studies suggest that continuous feedings may in fact increase the risk of aspiration pneumonia. Risk factors for pneumonia associated with tube feedings appear to be a history of pneumonia, esophagitis, and/or advanced age. The present literature suggests that gastrostomies and jejunostomies do not necessarily protect against the development of aspiration pneumonia.

All elderly patients, and especially those at high risk, should be monitored for clinical signs of aspiration, such as shortness of breath, rales, increased leukocyte count or shift, or simple confusion in a previously alert individual. If possible, avoid continuous tube feedings in individuals at risk for aspiration (i.e., with a prior history of aspiration or stroke).

14. What is the most common problem associated with tube feeding in elderly individuals?

Diarrhea. The development of diarrhea is particularly risky in the elderly, because it can predispose to skin irritation and the development of pressure ulcers. Risk factors for diarrhea in tube-fed patients include low serum albumin, antibiotic usage, hypertonicity of the formula, or low fiber content of the formula. However, several studies have disputed the role of low serum albumin level, tonicity of the formula, and fiber content of the formula. The major risk factor appears to be antibiotic usage.

15. Can frail elderly become infected as a result of contaminated tube feedings?

Studies have shown that manipulation of formulas (e.g., mixing of powdered formulas) leads to contamination. However, contamination does not appear to be related to the development of diarrhea or sepsis. One series found that pneumonia developed in 2 patients out of 24, with the organism found in respiratory secretions being the same organism found in the enteral formula. In this study, similar organisms were also found on the hands of nurses caring for these patients. Several other studies have had similar findings.

BIBLIOGRAPHY

1. Casper RC: Nutrition and its relationship to aging. Exp Gerontol 30:299–314, 1995.
2. Dwyer J: Nutrition Screening Initiative. Washington, DC, Nutritional Screening Initiative, 1991.

3. Evans WJ, Cyr-Campbell D: Nutrition, exercise, and healthy aging. J Am Diet Assoc 97:632–638, 1997.
4. Finucane TE, Christmas C, Travis K: Tube feeding in patients with advanced dementia. A review of the evidence. JAMA 282:1365–1370, 1999.
5. Gariballa SE, Sinclair AJ: Nutrition, aging and ill health. Br J Nutr 80:7–23, 1998.
6. Howard L, Malone M: Clinical outcome of geriatric patients in the United States receiving home parenteral and enteral nutrition. Am J Clin Nutr 66:1364–1370, 1997.
7. Johnson K, Bernard M: Vitamin nutrition in the elderly. Clin Geriatric Med 18(4):773–800, 2002.
8. Morley JE, Glick Z, Rubenstein LZ: Geriatric Nutrition: A Comprehensive Review, 2nd ed. Philadelphia, Lippincott Williams & Wilkins, 1995.
9. Safadi BY, Marks JM, Ponsky JL: Percutaneous endoscopic gastrostomy. Gastrointest Endosc Clin North Am 8:551–568, 1998.

17. CONSTIPATION

William F. Edwards, MSN, RN, CS, CRNP

1. What is constipation?

From a medical perspective, constipation is often defined as a frequency of < 3 bowel movements a week. From the individual's perspective, constipation can mean that stools are difficult to expel, too hard, or too small, or there may be a sensation of incomplete evacuation or bloating. Although it is important to teach the patient about normal bowel function, successful management requires that the clinician also respect the patient's concerns.

2. Is constipation a normal part of aging?

The frequency of bowel movements in healthy older populations is essentially the same as it is in the younger population. Despite this fact, the use of laxatives is more common in the elderly, even if they are not having infrequent stools.

3. List the causes of constipation.

For most elderly individuals, there are likely to be multiple contributing factors:

Dietary
Inadequate caloric intake
Poor fluid intake
Low-fiber diet
High-fat diet
Refined foods
Poor dentition
Swallowing problems
Tube feedings

Psychological
Depression
Confusion
Emotional stress

Functional
Inadequate toileting
Poor bowel habits
Weakness
Immobility/lack of exercise

Colonic/anorectal disorders
Ischemia
Postsurgical obstruction
Rectocele or rectal prolapse

Colonic/anorectal disorders *(cont'd.)*
Tumors
Volvulus or megacolon
Barium or bezoars
Fissures or hemorrhoids
Fistula or abscess
Radiation fibrosis
Stricture
Prostatic enlargement
Diverticulosis

Neurogenic disorders
Spinal cord lesions
Parkinson's disease
Cerebrovascular accidents
Dementia

Endocrine/metabolic disorders
Diabetes
Hypothyroidism
Hyperparathyroidism
Hypokalemia
Hypercalcemia

4. What medications can cause constipation?

Aluminum: antacids (Amphojel, ALternaGEL), sucralfate
Anticonvulsants: phenytoin, carbamazepine, phenobarbital
Antidepressants: amitriptyline, nortriptyline, venlafaxine
Antihistamines: diphenhydramine, chlorpheniramine
Antihypertensives: acebutolol, prazosin
Antilipemics: cholestyramine, colestipol
Antiparkinsonian drugs: bromocriptine, Sinemet, amantadine, benztropine, pramipexole
Antipsychotics: haloperidol, risperidone

Antispasmodics: oxybutynin, opiate or barbiturate compounds
Bismuth: Pepto-Bismol, Rectacort
Calcium: antacids (Tums), supplements (calcium carbonate)
Calcium channel blockers: verapamil, nifedipine
Diuretics: hydrochlorothiazide, furosemide, indapamide
Ganglionic blockers: trimethaphan
Iron supplements
Laxative misuse
Nonsteroidal anti-inflammatories: naproxen, sulindac, ketoprofen
Opiates: codeine, morphine, oxycodone
Phenothiazines: thioridazine, chlorpromazine, perphenazine
Sedatives: diazepam, flurazepam, thiothixene

5. Do all individuals complaining of constipation require a complete evaluation?

Individuals with a precipitous change in bowel habits (including the caliber or characteristics of the stool) require a thorough evaluation. For those with a history of constipation > 2 years, the focus should be on management. In obtaining the history, you must find out how the patient defines constipation and whether the patient has had a change in bowel function or is dealing with a long-term problem. Many elderly were reared with the idea that daily movements were essential to good health and that failure to move the bowels led to the buildup of dangerous toxins.

6. What other aspects of the history are most important?

- In patients with recent onset of constipation, the history should focus on excluding underlying causes such as malignancy, intestinal obstruction, or irritable bowel syndrome.
- Exacerbation or complications of a known illness must be considered.
- A thorough evaluation of recent changes in diet, medications, emotional state, and level of activity is warranted.
- In evaluation of the diet, total caloric intake, fiber content, and fluid intake should receive special attention.
- The clinician needs to inquire about problems related to chewing and swallowing.
- It is essential to evaluate the patient's complaint of constipation as thoroughly as possible.
- The color, amount, consistency, frequency, size, and symptoms experienced during defecation are key components of the history (see chart, next page).
- Brief screening tests for cognitive function and mood assist the clinician in detecting nonphysiologic causes of constipation.

7. Is a complete physical examination necessary in evaluating the patient with constipation?

If the patient is not known to the clinician, a complete physical exam is needed to rule out systemic causes. For most patients, the focus is on examination of the mouth, abdomen, and anorectal area and assessment for dehydration. The **oral** examination focuses on adequacy of dentition and detection of any lesions or tumors. The **abdomen** is examined for bowel sounds and detection of pain or localized masses. The **anorectal area** is evaluated for sphincter muscle tone; presence of stool in the vault; lesions such as hemorrhoids, strictures, fistulas, or masses; and prostatic enlargement. A neurologic examination can identify common systemic causes of constipation.

8. How do you decide when to do additional diagnostic testing?

If the symptom of constipation began < 2 years ago or if the patient has pain or any evidence of rectal bleeding, colonoscopy or sigmoidoscopy and barium enema are mandatory. In addition to detecting cancer, endoscopy also can reveal the presence of diffuse dark pigmentation, melanosis coli, which is caused by chronic use of laxatives such as cascara, senna, and aloe.

If the patient has liquid stool leakage or symptoms of impaction with an empty rectal vault, abdominal x-rays can detect a high impaction or other signs of obstruction. Additional diagnostic testing, such as colonic transit time and motility studies, is needed only if the patient does not

Bowel Movement Log

Instructions: (1) Write the date (even if your bowels do not move) and time (if they did move or if you tried to have a B.M.). (2) If "No" the remainder of the row is blank. If "Yes" indicate: **amount** (small = less than 1 cup; medium = 1–2 cups; large = more than 2 cups); **diameter** (narrow = ½ inch or less; medium = ½ to 1¼ inches; wide = more than 1¼ inches); **consistency** (loose = unformed or watery; soft = partly formed; firm = well formed; hard = small pellets or very firm stool with visible lines like hard pieces stuck together); **color** (light, medium, or dark brown; black; green, etc.). Indicate whether you needed to use a **laxative, suppository, enema,** or your **finger** in order to have a bowel movement and whether you had symptoms such as **bloating,** a sensation of **not emptying** your bowel, or if you had to **strain** or had **pain** when moving your bowels.

Date/Time	B.M.? Yes or No (Y/N)	Amount (S, M, L) Small, Medium, Large	Diameter (N, M, W) Narrow, Medium, Wide	Consistency (L, S, F, H) Loose, Soft, Firm, Hard	Color	Laxative Suppository or Enema? (L, S, E)	Use finger to remove stool? (Y, N)	Symptoms (B, NE, S, P) Bloating, Not Emptying, Straining, Pain

respond to treatment for constipation. Blood work should include a complete blood count (CBC), electrolytes, glucose, and thyroid studies.

9. Are any serious complications associated with constipation?

Fecal impaction is the major complication, and it can be life-threatening. Fecal impaction can cause cognitive problems, malaise, fatigue, urinary retention, bowel and urine incontinence, anal fissure, hemorrhoids, stercoral ulcer, and intestinal obstruction. Watery diarrhea can occur around impacted stool, leading to use of antidiarrheal agents and further complicating the problem. A mass of stool in the rectum can impair sensation and lead to the need for larger volumes of stool to stimulate the urge to defecate. Constipated patients, especially those who have chronically abused laxatives, can develop **megacolon** and **volvulus**. Straining during defecation affects cerebral and coronary circulation and can cause **transient ischemic attacks** and **syncope**, especially in the frail elderly. Finally, chronic constipation is a risk factor for **colon** and **rectal carcinoma**.

10. Discuss approaches to treating constipation.

The treatment of constipation is individualized for each patient according to the identified causes. The clinician must balance the need to make changes slowly with the patient's desire to get results quickly (as evidenced by the $725-million/year laxative industry). Patient outcome goals might include the passage of a soft formed stool at least 3 times a week without straining and the avoidance of complications associated with constipation.

1. The first step in managing constipation is to stop or switch any medications that may be contributing, including laxatives.

2. It is best to start a bowel program with an empty colon, which may require the use of enemas or even manual disimpaction. Aside from avoiding soap suds, there is no consensus on the best type of fluid to use for enemas. In patients who may require a series of enemas, normal saline is probably best. The temperature should be about 105°F, and the amount should not exceed 500 ml. For occasional use, the popular sodium phosphate enema is usually safe, but the amount should not exceed 120 ml.

3. Healthy bowel function requires an adequate **fluid intake**. If there are no fluid restrictions because of renal or cardiac problems, 2 to 3 liters/day is an appropriate goal. This needs to be done gradually to improve compliance. Water is the ideal fluid—caffeinated beverages and some fruit juices can cause diuresis, which can exacerbate constipation.

4. **Dietary fiber** should also be increased. This is done gradually to avoid unpleasant bloating and gas pains and to give the patient's colon a chance to adapt. The amount of additional fiber required to improve bowel function varies greatly, from 6 to 30 gm.

5. Regular **exercise** is an important component of healthy bowel function. Ambulatory patients should be encouraged to walk for 20 minutes daily. Even those elderly individuals who are bed- or chair-bound can benefit from an exercise program that involves turning from side to side, twisting the trunk, or exercising the arms.

6. The clinician should instruct the patient in the importance of establishing a **routine** that promotes normal bowel function. This includes taking advantage of the gastrocolic reflex, which for most individuals is most pronounced after breakfast or supper. Many individuals find it helpful to have a warm drink with breakfast. It is important that the patient have a private opportunity for about 10 minutes each day to attempt to have a bowel movement. It is also important to emphasize the need to respond as soon as possible to any urge to defecate. Proper position also facilitates bowel function. Squatting is the best position, but this is often not possible for the elderly who require high toilet seats. The squatting position can be emulated in these cases by using a foot stool. The patient should be instructed to lean forward and use the hand to apply firm pressure on the lower abdomen.

7. Institutionalized patients require close monitoring. It is not adequate simply to mark whether or not the person's bowels moved. It is important to note the amount, color, and consistency of the stool. Each care plan should include information about the individual's usual bowel habits, including the time of day that is most conducive to normal evacuation.

Comparison of Laxatives, Suppositories, and Enemas

LAXATIVES	USUAL DAILY DOSE	ONSET OF ACTION	COMMENTS/CONSIDERATIONS
Bulk laxatives			
Psyllium	1 tbls up to 3 times/day	12–72 hr	Good for long-term use in ambulatory
(Metamucil)	1 tbls up to 3 times/day	12–72 hr	individuals who maintain adequate
Methylcellulose			fluid intake. Psyllium can lower cho-
(Citrucel)	2–4 tabs every day	12–72 hr	lesterol, and methylcellulose and cal-
Polycarbophil			cium polycarbophil are less likely to
(FiberCon)			cause gas pain.
Hyperosmolar laxatives			
Lactulose	15–30 ml tid-qid	24–48 hr	Effective in ambulatory and immobile
(Chronulac)			patients. Safe for diabetics and pa-
Sorbitol	15–30 ml tid-qid	24–48 hr	tients with renal failure. Sorbitol costs
Polyethylene glycol	17 gm qd	48–96 hr	10% as much as lactulose with the
(Miralax)			same efficacy. Polyethylene glycol is
			more effective and less expensive than
			lactulose, with fewer side effects.
Stimulant laxatives			
Senna (Senokot)	2 tabs every day to 4 tabs 2 times/day	8–12 hr	Castor oil and aloe should be avoided. Senna is safe for long-term use in the
Bisacodyl	10–30 mg at bedtime	6–12 hr	elderly and is a good choice for slow-
(Dulcolax)			transit constipation that does not
Cascara	1 tab or 5 ml at bedtime	8–12 hr	respond to sorbitol.
Saline laxatives			
Magnesium	5–30 ml every day, 2	1–3 hr	Commonly prescribed in hospitals
hydroxide (milk	times/day		because they empty the bowel in a
of magnesia)			few hours. Can cause electrolyte im-
Magnesium citrate	200 ml every day	1–3 hr	balance; magnesium levels should be
			monitored if used regularly. Avoid
			magnesium- and aluminum-contain-
			ing products in patients with renal in-
			sufficiency. May be useful in patients
			with colonic hypomotility if stimulant
			agents are no longer effective.
Emollient laxatives			
Mineral oil	15–45 ml	6–8 hr	Avoid mineral oil in the elderly be
Docusate salts	100 mg 2 times/day	12–72 hr	cause of the risk of aspiration, inter-
(Colace)			ference with absorption of fat-soluble
			vitamins, and risk of leakage through
			anal sphincter. Stool softeners are
			popular, but there is little evidence for
			their efficacy. They should be avoided
			in patients with a large amount of soft
			stool in their rectum. Adding 8 ounces
			of water to the diet probably is more
			effective.
Suppositories			
Bisacodyl	10 mg suppository	5–30 min	For occasional use when stool is pre-
suppositories			sent in rectum. May cause cramping
Glycerin	3–4 gram suppository	15–60 min	and local irritation.
suppositories			

(Cont'd.)

Comparison of Laxatives, Suppositories, and Enemas (Continued)

LAXATIVES	USUAL DAILY DOSE	ONSET OF ACTION	COMMENTS/CONSIDERATIONS
Enemas			
Soap-suds	500 ml	2–15 min	Reserve for constipation that does not
Mineral oil	100–250 ml	2–15 min	respond to other approaches. Soap-
Phosphate (Fleet)	100–250 ml	2–15 min	suds enemas can cause damage to
Tap water	500 ml	2–15 min	rectal mucosa and should be avoided.
Normal saline	500 ml	2–15 min	Mineral oil may be helpful for acute
			disimpaction. Phosphate enemas are
			generally well-tolerated with occa-
			sional use but can cause hyperphos-
			phatemia. Normal saline or tap water
			is probably the safest for the elderly.

11. What are the most effective ways of adding fiber to the diet?

The best way to add fiber is by making subtle changes in the diet. The changes should be made gradually to avoid gas pains and bloating, which can occur with fiber. Switching to **whole-grain breads** and to **cereals** high in fiber may be the only change some individuals need to make. Lessons in label reading are often necessary because prominently advertised "wheat" breads are often not made of whole wheat.

Many brans have become popular, but wheat bran is the most effective type for promoting bowel function. For individuals who prefer hot cereals, wheat bran may be mixed in with the cereal. Institutional food is often low in fiber, and residents of such facilities may benefit from a **fiber supplement**. Supplements made from 2 parts wheat bran (sometimes given in the form of 100% bran cereal, which is more palatable but less effective than crude bran), 2 parts applesauce, and 1 part prune juice have been effective. The starting dose is 30 ml daily, and it costs significantly less than laxatives.

The common advice "eat more fruits and vegetables" may not be sufficient to add enough insoluble fiber to the diet. A dietary consultation may be appropriate to help an individual make changes that take into consideration traditional eating habits, cost, dentition, and taste.

12. Are there any precautions associated with adding fiber to the diet?

1. Fiber should not be added to the diets of individuals with **megacolon**. In fact, such patients should be on a fiber-restricted diet and may need to be managed with enemas.

2. Some elderly individuals are at risk for development of **bezoars**. Bezoars are hard, dense masses of fibrous materials that can cause irritation in the stomach or obstruction in the intestines. Individuals with poor dentition, history of surgery for peptic ulcer disease, or stomach cancer are at greater risk for bezoars.

3. Fiber should be avoided in patients with **intestinal stricture**.

4. Increased fiber can pose a hazard for **bed-bound patients** by increasing bulk in a colon that is already distended.

These exceptions aside, most elderly individuals who make dietary changes gradually to increase fiber will have no problem. Individuals who use fiber supplements should be told not to expect overnight results. They also should not double-up on supplements because this can cause diarrhea or even obstruction. The latter is most likely to occur if the patient does not drink enough water.

13. What is the role of laxatives in the management of constipation?

For most patients, laxatives and enemas should not be a part of routine bowel management but should be used only occasionally to prevent the complications associated with constipation. Individuals who have used laxatives for years will require education about the harmful effects of laxatives and their role in causing constipation. However, patients with megacolon or with a medical condition that requires that they avoid straining may need to use laxatives or enemas.

14. What considerations influence choice of laxatives?

The choice of laxative is determined by:

- The cause of the problem
- Nature of the constipation (is the stool hard or soft, high in the colon or in the rectum?)
- Other medical conditions
- Other medications the patient may be taking
- Cost of treatment
- Patient preference

15. Describe the different types of laxatives and considerations in their usage.

1. **Psyllium-based supplements** offer the benefit of lowering cholesterol, whereas **methylcellulose** and **calcium polycarbophil** are less likely to cause gas pain.

2. **Hyperosmolar laxatives** are effective in both the amulabory elderly and those in nursing homes. Sorbitol is much less expensive than lactulose and just as effective. Polyethylene glycol (Golytely) is often used for bowel preparation before colonoscopy or barium enema. Polyethylene glycol 3350 is available as a powder (Miralax) to treat constipation. Once daily dosing is more convenient than lactulose or sorbitol. It has been used in nursing home residents to treat impaction and is more effective, less expensive, and has fewer side effects than lactulose.

3. **Stimulant laxatives** are popular because of their efficacy, but many have toxic long-term effects and can damage the colon and cause electrolyte imbalance. Senna is safe for the elderly and did not cause problems in individuals over age 80 who used it daily for 6 months. Senna is a good choice for patients with more resistant slow-transit constipation who do not respond to sorbitol.

4. **Saline laxatives** are the most commonly prescribed laxatives in hospitals because they empty the bowel within a few hours. These products can cause electrolyte imbalance and magnesium levels should be monitored if a magnesium-based product is used regularly. Products containing aluminum or magnesium should be used with caution in individuals with poor renal function. Saline laxatives are useful for patients with colonic hypomotility if stimulant agents are no longer effective.

5. **Emollient laxatives** include mineral oil and docusate salts. Mineral oil should be avoided in the elderly because of the risk of aspiration, interference with absorption of fat-soluble vitamins, and risk of leakage through the anal sphincter. Stool softeners are popular, but studies of patients receiving them have shown no change in stool weight or water content, no increase in frequency of bowel movements, and no change in colonic transit time. They are especially ineffective in patients who have a large amount of soft stool in the colon. Stool softeners are often recommended in bed-bound patients with hard dry stool, in patients who must avoid straining, and as an adjunct to bulk agents. For most individuals, adding 8 oz of water to their daily intake would probably be more effective.

6. **Bisacodyl** and **glycerin suppositories** are appropriate for occasional use when stool is present in the rectum and are usually effective within an hour. They may cause cramping and local irritation. **Enemas** should be reserved for constipation that does not respond to other approaches.

BIBLIOGRAPHY

1. Ahlquist DA, Camilleri M: Diarrhea and constipation. In Braunwald E, Fauci AS, Kasper DL, et al (eds): Harrison's Principles of Internal Medicine, 15th ed. New York, McGraw-Hill, 2001, pp 241–249.
2. De Lillo AR, Rose S: Functional bowel disorders in the geriatric patient: Constipation, fecal impaction, and fecal incontinence. Am J Gastroenterol 95:901–905, 2000.
3. Glia A, Lindberg G, Nilsson LH, et al: Clinical value of symptom assessment in patients with constipation. Dis Colon Rectum 42:1401–1408, 1999.
4. Harari D: Constipation in the elderly. In Hazzard WR, Blass JP, Ettinger WH, et al (eds): Principles of Geriatric Medicine and Gerontology, 4th ed. New York, McGraw-Hill, 1999, p 1491.
5. Thompson WG, Longstreth GF, Drossman DA, et al: Functional bowel disorders and functional abdominal pain. Gut 45(Suppl 2):II43, 1999.

18. ELDER ABUSE, NEGLECT, AND EXPLOITATION

Elizabeth Capezuti, PhD, RN

1. What constitutes elder abuse and neglect?

- **Physical abuse** is the infliction of bodily injury and may be manifested by lacerations, fractures, soft-tissue trauma, burns, or bruises.
- **Sexual abuse** is any form of intimate sexual activity without consent. This includes sexual activity with those unable to give adequate consent, such as those with dementia or the older mentally retarded person.
- **Emotional or psychological abuse** is the infliction of mental anguish, such as intimidation by yelling, insulting, threatening, or silence.
- **Financial exploitation** is the misuse of an older person's funds or assets without his or her explicit knowledge or consent. It may take many forms, such as the withdrawal of small amounts of money from banking accounts or the overcharging for grocery shopping or housekeeping by persons providing these services.
- **Caregiver neglect** is the malicious neglect by a caregiver of an older person's needs, whether for retaliation, disinterest, or financial incentives. Examples include inadequate provision of nutrition and the misuse of medications, such as oversedation with tranquilizers.
- **Self-neglect** is disregard of one's personal well-being and home environment.

2. What is the significance of elder mistreatment?

Elder mistreatment is associated with significantly decreased survival after controlling for other factors associated with increased mortality. One to 2 million older Americans are mistreated annually. To date, there has been only one population-based survey conducted, which found a prevalence of 32/1000 older persons. According to the National Elder Abuse Incidence Study, there were approximately a half million new cases of elder mistreatment in 1996.

3. What causes elder abuse?

Physical abuse and financial exploitation are usually due to the psychopathology of the perpetrator and have little to do with the older person's characteristics. Perpetrators (family members or nonrelatives) are more likely to abuse alcohol or drugs, to be mentally ill, and/or to be financially dependent on the older person.

Neglect of an older individual due to lack of information or resources, usually referred to as "passive neglect," is not considered mistreatment. It often is seen when the caregivers have their own physical or mental handicaps. Adult children may be developmentally disabled or mentally ill or may be elderly themselves and, as a result, unable to provide sufficient care. Passive caregiver neglect may be rectified by providing education and community supports.

Active caregiver neglect, which implies malicious intent, has not been demonstrated to be due to the stress and burdens of providing care to an older person. These caregivers also are likely to have substance abuse issues, have serious untreated mental illness, or be financially dependent on the older person. Caregivers who are socially isolated and lack social supports (family, friends, or community-based services) or those with a history of violence, such as spousal abuse, also have been implicated.

Victims and perpetrators of any type of mistreatment are found in all socioeconomic groups.

4. What leads to self-neglect?

The exact cause of self-neglect is often difficult to determine. In some cases, there appears to be a mental health problem, such as chronic schizophrenia, depression, or dementia. In other cases, the older person demonstrates no deficits in cognitive functioning but is fearful of "outsiders." These older persons may be reclusive, suspicious, and territorial. The key to successful intervention with this type of elder is to establish a trusting relationship that allows the older person to feel in control. This is usually best handled by case managers in private or county social service agencies, who can provide long-term follow-up.

5. Discuss the role of mental status assessment in the evaluation of elder mistreatment.

Mental status assessment, especially cognitive functioning, is an essential component of the evaluation; it is necessary to determine if the person is able to make a decision to remain in an abusive relationship with a perpetrator or remain in a self-neglecting situation. Furthermore, new onset of confusion has been found to be a significant risk factor for elder mistreatment. Accusations of abuse should be assessed within the context of other psychiatric symptoms, such as delusions and hallucinations, which may or may not lend credence to the allegations. Displays of paranoia or anxiety in the presence of the suspected perpetrator may be related to fear, thus leading to inquiries of other family members or friends to provide further information about the relationship. The older person presenting with new onset of disorientation, confusion, or extreme lethargy may be the victim of oversedation. Depression can be the cause of self-neglect or may indicate resignation to an abusive situation.

6. What are the physical findings of physical abuse?

Physical abuse should be considered when investigating the underlying cause of any injury. Identification of physical abuse, however, is often complicated by normal age changes that may mimic trauma. In senile purpura, even gentle handling of an older person's skin may result in bruising because of capillary fragility. Bilateral **bruises** of the upper arms, however, are more likely to result from forcibly holding, grabbing, or shaking a person. **Fractures, dislocations, and sprains** need to be explored within the context of other suspicious signs and symptoms of abuse. **Imprint injuries** (bruises that retain the shape of the object, such as a belt buckle, hand, or iron) are strong physical indicators of abuse. A person physically restrained may have **rope burns** or marks on the ankles or wrists. **Burns** in an unusual location, such as cigarette burns on the back, are highly significant. **Spotty absence of hair**, contrary to the typical temporal pattern of balding in aging men, may be due to vigorous hair-pulling.

7. List the chief indicators of neglect.

- Malnutrition
- Dehydration
- Pressure ulcers
- Contractures
- Oversedation
- Poor hygiene
- Urine burn excoriations
- Manifestations of inadequately treated medical problems (i.e., unfilled prescriptions and recurrent urinary tract infections)

One indicator alone cannot confirm a diagnosis of mistreatment, but a suspicious history with a recurrent presentation of signs should raise the clinician's suspicions of mistreatment. Many signs of neglect also can be attributed to common age-related health problems. For example, malnutrition may be explained as the older person's lack of appetite, just as poor personal hygiene may be attributed to one's refusal to be bathed. Therefore, care must be exercised not to be overly accusatory and threaten your relationship with the caregiver.

8. What should be emphasized in interviewing possible victims and perpetrators of mistreatment?

The interview should proceed from the least threatening questions to a more directed inquiry. The history of a presenting physical injury needs to be evaluated for **inconsistencies** and the following questions should be addressed:

- Could the injury actually have occurred in the manner in which the suspected abuser or victim has explained?
- Is the individual bed-bound and seeking treatment for several fractures?
- Did the person "fall down the stairs" and present with bilateral upper arm bruising?

If possible, interview the victim separately from the caregiver. However, do not always expect to get a different story than the suspected abuser's story, because the victim may have been coached or threatened before being brought in for treatment.

When evaluating an injury or signs of deteriorating health (e.g., malnutrition, dehydration, multiple pressure sores), the **index of suspicion** is raised when the elderly individual is taken to an emergency department or family physician located far from home. This occurs when the family or caregiver believes the staff in the local emergency department or the physician has become suspicious of the home situation. It also is suspect when someone other than the primary caregiver brings the person to the physician's office or emergency department and knows little of the older person's health status, medications, and so forth. The inability to answer questions may be a way to block the physician's probing of the cause of an injury or of inadequate care. Any individual who is brought in for treatment late in the illness process or who repeatedly needs treatment despite a previously well-thought-out discharge plan should be evaluated for needed in-home supports or breakdown of a current home care system.

9. What type of situations should alert the clinician to the possibility of financial exploitation?

If a cognitively intact individual is unaware of his or her own financial situation or there is an apparent discrepancy between financial resources and lifestyle, the clinician may want to probe further or to refer to a social worker. In the latter instance, be aware that lifestyle preferences and income may be incongruent, particularly as some individuals may not be willing to spend money on necessary services. On the other hand, some individuals in the early stages of dementia often will lose the ability to manage their money. Without intervention in these situations, bills may go unpaid, Social Security checks uncashed, and available money squandered.

10. What resources are available for intervention?

Currently, every state has an adult protective services (APS) system, which, in addition to investigating suspected cases (usually with a home visit), provides special services for the victims of mistreatment. Provisions for emergency shelter, home care, food, and transportation, as well as legal counsel and evaluations by health care providers, may be provided, depending on each state's funding of APS. The amount of involuntary intervention by protective service workers also depends on individual state laws. A website providing links to individual state protective service systems can be found at www.elderabusecenter.org/link/apsstate.htm.

Geriatric and geropsychiatric programs in hospitals and outpatient offices are familiar with the problems of elder mistreatment. If such specialized services are not available, hospital social work departments, local area agencies on aging, and visiting nurses associations can provide coordination and referral services.

Many police departments and district attorney's offices have special domestic violence units to handle cases of abuse or neglect.

11. Are physicians mandated to report suspected elder mistreatment?

In 42 states and the District of Columbia physicians are required to report suspected mistreatment of elders residing in the community to APS. With few exceptions, the mistreatment need only be suspected, not fully substantiated. Many mandatory and voluntary reporting statutes grant immunity from civil and criminal liability to those who report in good faith. States without mandatory reporting laws (as of 2003) include Colorado, Illinois, New York, New Jersey, North Dakota, Pennsylvania, South Dakota, and Wisconsin. The primary functions of physicians in suspected cases referred to APS are to document the physical findings and to provide a judgment about the older person's decision-making capacity.

The Joint Commission on the Accreditation of Health Care Organizations requires hospital emergency departments to provide personnel training in the detection and management of the problem. Moreover, emergency departments must develop protocols to deal with cases of mistreatment that address the collection of evidence, the documentation of examinations, and the treatment provided. A current list of community agencies for referral for services should also be readily available. These agencies can provide both immediate and long-term support for victims of elder mistreatment.

12. How does institutional mistreatment differ from mistreatment that occurs in the community?

The various types and manifestations of mistreatment are the same, but the location and responsibility of the perpetrator are chief differences. Institutional mistreatment can occur in hospitals, nursing homes, or board-and-care facilities. The perpetrator may be an individual staff member who physically or sexually abuses a patient, or the perpetrator may be an institutional milieu that discourages the appropriate provision of care. For example, the patients may be physically restrained instead of ambulated because of inadequate staffing levels, thus leading to problems associated with immobility such as contractures and pressure ulcers. Most states require mandatory reporting of physical abuse and financial exploitation to the state health department; several also mandate the reporting of institutional neglect.

Reporting of suspicions of institutional mistreatment should be made to the state ombudsman. The Older Americans Act of 1976 mandated that each state establish ombudsman programs to investigate allegations of mistreatment in nursing homes.

BIBLIOGRAPHY

1. American Medical Association: Diagnostic and Treatment Guidelines on Elder Abuse and Neglect. Chicago, IL, American Medical Association, 1992.
2. Capezuti E, Brush B, Lawson WT: Reporting elder mistreatment. J Gerontol Nurs 23:24–32, 1997.
3. Lachs MS, Pillemer K: Current concepts: Abuse and neglect of elderly persons. N Engl J Med 332:437–443, 1995.
4. Lachs MS, Williams CS, O'Brien S, et al: Older adults: An 11-year longitudinal study of adult protective service use. Arch Intern Med 156:449–453, 1996.
5. Lachs MS, Williams CS, O'Brien S, et al: Risk factors for reported elder abuse and neglect: A nine-year observational cohort study. Gerontologist 37:469–474, 1997.
6. Lachs MS, Williams CS, O'Brien S, et al: The mortality of elder mistreatment. JAMA 280:428–432, 1998.

III. *Office Care of the Geriatric Patient*

19. PERIODIC HEALTH EXAM

Susan Day, MD, MPH

1. Why screen?
Everybody wants to live a long and healthy life. The fundamental principle behind screening is that the quality and duration of an individual's life can be improved by identifying early or asymptomatic disease, by modifying behavior to achieve a more healthy lifestyle, and by maximizing function when disease exists. Interventions for these purposes fall into three categories:

    1. **Primary prevention** is targeted toward identifying and reversing risk factors for disease and promoting behaviors linked to improving quality and length of life. Examples of primary prevention include improved nutrition, exercise, smoking cessation, and accident prevention. Interventions at this stage may involve counseling, immunizations, or chemoprophylaxis.

    2. **Secondary prevention** efforts, including most screening programs, are aimed at identifying and treating disease in the preclinical or asymptomatic phase. Hypertension, osteoporosis, and breast cancer are examples.

    3. **Tertiary prevention** includes measures that prevent complications of existing disease. Cardiac and stroke rehabilitation programs fall into this category, as does the use of beta blockers after a myocardial infarction.

2. In the elderly, for what conditions should we screen?
    1. **The condition must have a significant effect on the quality or quantity of a patient's life**. Screening should be targeted toward identifying conditions associated with significant morbidity or mortality, i.e., the "burden of suffering." In the elderly, the issue of quality of life is particularly important. For example, screening and subsequent treatment of glaucoma or hearing impairment have the potential of not only improving the quality of life but also reducing the risk of potentially debilitating accidents.

    2. **The condition must be treatable**. There must be good evidence that treatment is effective, across a range of patient ages and functional status.

    3. **Early detection and intervention must significantly reduce morbidity and/or mortality**. Advancing detection of disease by 5 years will be useful only if the resulting treatment prevents or delays disease development by more than 5 years *and* the patient has a life expectancy of more than 5 years. Detecting an indolent malignancy in a patient with a limited life expectancy may not be doing that patient a service.

    4. **The incidence of the condition must justify the cost of screening**. Generally, the elderly are a good target population for screening, because many conditions are more common than in younger people. Mass screening for rare conditions is rarely cost-effective. On the other hand, if the pretest likelihood of the condition is high enough, the clinician may opt to initiate treatment without a formal diagnostic test.

3. What makes a good screening instrument?
    1. **The test should be affordable and safe**. Although the elderly may be covered for many tests by Medicare, new tests are often not covered by Medicare and may be quite costly for the patient. The costs, risks, and benefits of both the initial screening test and the subsequent evaluation should be taken into consideration. For example, a whole-body CT scan might not be painful

(or covered by insurance), but follow-up and biopsy of abnormalities could be costly, uncomfortable, and risky.

2. **The instrument should have good test characteristics**. Good screening tests are positive in patients with disease (i.e., have a high sensitivity) and negative in patients who do not have the disease (i.e., have a high specificity). Ideally, a positive test should reflect the presence of disease, with few false positives (a high predictive value positive). A negative test should reassure patients that they do not have the condition (high negative predictive value). Before using a test in an individual patient, it is important to take into consideration the risks and benefits for that person, including the possible psychological effects of a false-positive or false-negative test.

4. What makes screening in the elderly different from screening in younger populations?

1. **The yield of screening interventions is greater in the elderly**. Because of the higher prevalence of disease in this population, more true-positive results will be obtained with a screening test. Of course, these tests may be less specific as well—a positive occult blood stool sample may be due to a spectrum of problems, ranging from benign to malignant.

2. **The measure of an effective screening test differs in the elderly**. Traditionally, screening tests have been subjected to cost-benefit analyses that measure the benefit of a test in "quality-adjusted life years." However, the elderly have a limited number of years left to live, and the benefit from screening is tempered by the presence of comorbid disease and functional status. More qualitative measures as well as measures of functional status are increasingly being used as measures of effectiveness.

3. **The level of intervention is different**. Primary prevention, with lifestyle modification, has the greatest impact on reducing disease for the population as a whole. In older patients, a broad approach to prevention is appropriate. Primary prevention is still crucial; the value of exercise in maintaining functional status, preventing osteoporosis, and reducing the risks of falls is a good example. However, secondary and tertiary prevention interventions become increasingly important. Efforts to maximize functional status in older patients with existing disease may have the greatest effect on the quality and duration of life.

4. **The issue is less often when *to start* screening than when *to stop***. Patients with fewer potential years ahead benefit less from screening. For many common screening tests, guidelines are being generated that recognize the point at which ongoing screening no longer is a benefit to the patient.

5. **Screening recommendations need to be customized for the individual patient**. We all age differently, and part of the physician's task is to tailor the screening program to the individual. Particularly in the elderly, public policy analyses tend to understate the risks and benefits to the individual patient. Take two 75-year-old women, one frail and one robust: an impaired functional status might increase the risks of screening in the first case, whereas the robust woman might benefit from the same recommendations as a 55-year-old.

Patient preferences for treatment also must be considered. Recommendations for screening assume that an individual would pursue treatment. Individuals may have very strong preferences about what treatments they would consider acceptable, and these preferences should be respected. A patient's ability to undergo treatment must also be taken into consideration. If the optimum cancer treatment is too toxic for a given individual, screening is not appropriate unless a less toxic alternative is available.

5. What is the physician's role in screening?

The physician's role in screening has changed dramatically over the past few years due to increased public awareness, media coverage, and internet access. Patients turn to physicians to inform, interpret, and apply guidelines to their particular clinical situation, and physicians must resolve conflicts between different expert groups and sort out recommendations reflecting commercial self-interest. Increasingly physicians are encouraged to apply a model of joint decision making that takes into account patient preference.

Research supports the importance of physician counseling in areas such as smoking cessation and exercise, as well as in performing diagnostic screening procedures such as rectal and breast exams and Pap smears. Other health care personnel also play important roles: for example, nurse-initiated community-based screening for hypertension and breast cancer, counseling by nutritionists, and psychological screening by mental health providers.

6. Why don't physicians comply with screening recommendations?

Physicians give several reasons when asked why they do not carry out the preventive services recommended in their patients:

1. **They are unaware of the recommendations**. Because recommendations change frequently, physicians must be motivated to keep up to date on the frequency and indications for screening.

2. **They do not have the time**. Particularly in the elderly, patients often may have multiple active problems that must be addressed during each interval visit. Procedures such as pelvic or rectal exams, which involve disrobing and sometimes special examination rooms, require additional time. Counseling is also time-consuming, especially if patients and their families wish to discuss and review the recommendations or if the patient has any sensory or cognitive impairments.

3. **They forget**. Despite the best intentions, providers may not remember to include preventive measures into a routine health check, or if they do remember, they forget which measures are due for a given patient.

4. **They disagree with the recommendations**. Physicians sometimes disagree with formal recommendations if these differ from what they were taught or their current practice protocol. Discrepancies among programs endorsed by expert panels and individual providers need to be resolved by careful review of the basis for the recommendations.

7. Why don't patients participate in screening programs?

1. **Misunderstanding about normal aging**. Older patients may accept new symptoms as part of normal aging or consider the development of disease as inevitable.

2. **Cost of screening**. There has been progress in insurance coverage for some preventive health measures, such as flu shots, pneumococcal vaccines, bone mineral density measurements, and mammograms, which are now covered through Medicare. In addition, the participation of the elderly in managed-care systems that emphasize preventive measures has helped to reduce the cost of prevention to the individual. However, the costs (and availability) of transportation and subsequent testing must still be considered.

3. **Fear**. Patients may be reluctant to enter a program that may detect an illness. They may be apprehensive about the actual tests involved. Many patients dread mammograms and sigmoidoscopy because of lack of dignity and discomfort involved or because of negative experiences reported by others.

4. **Access**. Two factors appear crucial to receiving preventive services: health insurance and a usual source of care. The elderly have a higher utilization of preventive services because of Medicare coverage but may not have a usual source of care. Previous physicians may have retired or no longer accept their insurance. Sociodemographic factors, such as race and education, socioeconomic status and residence in a rural community, are known to reduce access, making indigent elderly an important target group for screening efforts.

5. **Misperceptions/lack of information about screening**. Despite increased media coverage, many elderly remain unaware of the value of screening tests in their age group or hold cultural values or beliefs that lead them to be fatalistic about a disease after it has been detected. On the other hand, many older people paradoxically believe themselves to be *less* susceptible to cancer.

8. What do you do when a patient refuses a screening procedure?

If a patient refuses a recommended screening test, you should first be sure that the patient understands the reason screening is being suggested and next explore the patient's reasons. If the refusal is based on misinformation or logistic concerns, these should be addressed. Population-based estimates of disease should be translated into terms relevant to the individual; for example, what is the patient's risk of developing the condition, with and without screening? What are the chances of a false-positive or false-negative test? Does the patient understand the consequences of not participating? If an informed, competent patient refuses a screening test, the physician should respect that decision. The physician's recommendation and reasons for the patient's refusal should be documented on the patient's chart.

9. How can you improve the preventive care your elderly patients receive?

1. Work as a team to screen for preventable disease. Take advantage of community-based programs whenever possible.

2. Educate yourself and your patients about which conditions warrant screening and translate the statistics into terms that have meaning to them. Explore your patients' health beliefs.

3. Integrate screening into routine visits when possible, but do not hesitate to schedule a separate visit if more time is needed.

4. Develop a reminder system and flow sheet that is part of each individual's record.

5. Find out what barriers exist for the individual (health beliefs, language, transportation, cost, need for a companion) and work to fix them.

6. If you are part of a health care organization, work with your practice administrator to implement clinical recommendations.

10. What are the preventive interventions recommended for the general population aged 65 and older?

There are multiple expert panels and guidelines for screening from organizations as diverse as the American Cancer Society and WebMD. The U.S. Preventive Services Task Force used a balanced, evidence-based approach to screening. The following table summarizes the 1996 USPSTF recommendations for asymptomatic individuals 65 years and older. These guidelines are in the process of being systematically updated for the *Guide to Clinical Preventive Services*, 3rd ed., 2000–2003, and are being released incrementally, as they become available. Current recommendations can be found at <http://www.ahrq.gov/clinic/cps3dix.htm>.

Screening
  Blood pressure
  Height and weight
  Fecal occult blood test (annually) and/or sigmoidoscopy every 3–5 years
  Mammography with or without clinical breast exam (every 1–2 years) (women < 69 yr)
  Papanicolaou test (all women who are or have been sexually active and who have a cervix.
    Discontinuation of testing after age 65 if previous regular screening provided consistently normal results).
  Vision screening
  Assess for hearing impairment
  Assess for problem drinking
Counseling
  Substance abuse
    Tobacco cessation
    Avoid alcohol/drug use while driving, swimming, boating
  Diet and exercise
    Limit fat and cholesterol
    Maintain caloric balance
    Emphasize grains, fruits, and vegetables
    Adequate calcium intake (women)
    Regular physical activity
  Injury prevention
    Lap/shoulder belts

Injury prevention (*cont'd.*)
 Motorcycle and bicycle helmets
 Fall prevention
 Safe storage/removal of firearms
 Smoke detector
 Set hot water heater to < 120–130°F
 CPR training for household members
Dental health
 Regular visits to dental care provider
 Floss, brush with fluoride toothpaste daily
Sexual behavior (STD prevention)
 Avoid high-risk sexual behavior
 Use condoms
Immunizations
 Pneumococcal vaccine
 Influenza (annually)
 Tetanus-diphtheria (Td) boosters (every 10 years)
Chemoprophylaxis

BIBLIOGRAPHY

1. Asch DA, Hershey JC: Why some health policies don't make sense at the bedside. Ann Intern Med 122:846–850, 1995.
2. Fox SA, Roetzheim RG, Kington RS: Barriers to cancer prevention in the older person. Clin Geriatr Med 13:79–95, 1997.
3. Hendriksen C, Lung E, Stromgard E: Consequences of assessment and intervention among elderly people: A three year randomized controlled trial. BMJ 289:1522–1524, 1984.
4. Leventhal EA, Prohaska TR: Age, symptom interpretation and health behavior. J Am Geriatr Soc 34:185–191, 1986.
5. Marton CP, Espino DU: Health screening in older women. Am Fam Physician 59:1835–1842, 1999.
6. McAlister FA, Taylor L, Teo KK, et al: The treatment and prevention of coronary heart disease in Canada: Do older patients receive efficacious therapies? The Clinical Quality Improvement Network (CQIN) Investigators. J Am Geriatr Soc 47:811–818, 1999.
7. Oboler SK, Prochazka AV, Gonzales R, et al: Public expectations and attitudes for annual physical examinations. Ann Intern Med 136:625–659, 2002.
8. Prohaska TR, Leventhal EA, Leventhal H, Keller ML: Health practice and illness cognition in young, middle aged, and elderly adults. J Gerontol 40:569–578, 1985.
9. Rubenstein LZ, Josephson KR, Nichol-Seamons M, Robbins AS: Comprehensive health screening of well elderly adults: An analysis of a community program. J Gerontol 41:342–352, 1986.
10. Sackett DL, Haynes RB, Tugwell P: A Basic Science for Clinical Medicine. Boston, Little, Brown, 1985.
11. Soloman LJ, Mickey RM, Rairikas CJ, et al: Three-year prospective adherence of three breast cancer screening modalities. Prev Med 27:781–786, 1998.
12. Sox HC: Preventive health services in adults. N Engl J Med 330:1589–1595, 1994.
13. U.S. Preventive Services Task Force: Guide to Clinical and Preventive Services: An Assessment of the Effectiveness of 169 Interventions. Baltimore, Williams & Wilkins, 1995.
14. Walter LC, Covinsky KE: Cancer screening in elderly patients: A framework for individualized decision making. JAMA 285:2750–2756, 2001.
15. Woolf SH, Atkins D: The evolving role of prevention in health care: Contributions of the U.S. Preventive Services Task Force. Am J Prev Med 20(3S):13–20, 2001.

20. ADVANCE DIRECTIVES

Joel E. Streim, MD

1. What is an advance directive?

A written document, completed by a competent person, that aims to guide health care decisions in the event that the person should become unable to communicate medical preferences or participate in medical decision-making.

2. What are the three different types of advance directives?

Instruction directives indicate the types of treatment or treatment approaches that the person would want in various clinical situations. These typically focus on lifesustaining treatments, though they may also concern less critical treatments. This type of directive may be made informally, through oral instructions given to family members, friends, or caregivers, or formally in a written "living will."

Proxy directives designate someone whom the person wants to make health care decisions on his or her behalf if he or she becomes unable to do so. This is sometimes referred to as a durable power of attorney for health care decisions.

A **values history** may also contain advance directives. This may be a written, audiotaped, or videotaped personal discussion of the person's values and goals. It provides an opportunity to make known one's specific values, beliefs and attitudes regarding life, longevity, quality of life, suffering, the dying process, and death.

3. Explain what is meant by "durable" power of attorney.

When a patient who is still competent designates a proxy decision-maker for health care matters, the patient continues to make autonomous decisions (i.e., without involvement of the proxy) as long as he or she remains competent. Decisions are not made by proxy until the patient becomes incapacitated, at which time the power of attorney "springs" into effect. (This is sometimes called "springing" power of attorney.) From that point forward, the incapacitated person (whose judgment may now be impaired) cannot rescind the proxy appointment; hence, the power of attorney is said to be durable.

4. What does federal law require of patients regarding advance directives?

The Patient Self-Determination Act was passed by Congress as part of the Omnibus Budget Reconciliation Act of 1990 and became federal law in December 1991 (U.S. Public Law 101-508). Under this law, at the time of admission to an acute care hospital or nursing home that participates in Medicare or Medicaid programs, the admitting facility is required:

1. To ask patients if they have executed an advance directive
2. To furnish them with information about advance directives
3. To inform them of their rights under the law to execute such directives if they wish
4. To inform them of their rights to accept or refuse any form of medical treatment

All patients are thereby given the opportunity to make their preferences for future treatment known to their health care providers. However, patients are not required to draft directives or state their treatment preferences, and their eligibility for admission or treatment is not affected by their having or not having an advance directive.

5. Who should be responsible for discussing advance directives with elderly patients?

Although the staff in a hospital or nursing home admissions office may ask patients about their advance directives to comply with federal law, discussions regarding patient values and treatment preferences are probably best accomplished in the context of an ongoing primary care practitioner–patient relationship, as well as between the patient and trusted family members or friends who might later serve as proxy decision-makers.

6. Are patients who are old and frail likely to become upset when a health care provider asks them to consider hopeless situations or terminal illness?

Most patients who are in the late stages of life, including those who are near death, are relieved when someone asks about their concerns regarding the end of life. Most of them also appreciate the opportunity to express their preferences for how their health care is to be managed. The relatively few patients who are anxious about such matters will decline to discuss them or may be so highly defended that they deny such discussions are applicable to them personally.

7. How should the discussion about advance directives be focused?

While there are no established standards for these discussions, some attempts to develop guidelines in recent years have emphasized the need for patients to communicate a set of life values, even more than choices about specific treatments. This is because it is impossible for patients to anticipate all of the possible future illness and treatment situations, coupled with the presumption that a surrogate or proxy decision-maker will be better able to make a decision that reflects what the patient would have chosen for him or herself if that surrogate is well-informed about the patient's overall values. It is not expected that such discussions will be completed in one session. Getting to know a patient's values is a process that occurs over a series of visits and ideally in the context of an ongoing relationship.

Health care providers must appreciate the ways in which religious beliefs, ethnic background, and family values influence health care directives and decisions. It is important to inquire about the patient's cultural and family background and belief system, so that resultant health care choices can be respected and supported even when based on values that differ from those of the provider. Inclusion of close family members or friends in discussions of values and health care preferences is especially helpful, because they are often in the best position to appreciate nuances of the patient's culture and beliefs, to accept those important factors that serve as the foundation for the patient's directives, and to support the patient's choices regarding future health care.

8. Are health care providers and facilities legally bound to follow all advance directives contained in living wills?

No. Not all states have laws that recognize living wills. For those states that now have living will statutes, most only recognize directives that apply to situations in which a person becomes hopelessly or terminally ill; these states stipulate that patients' directives can be implemented only in conformity with existing laws, including those dealing with suicide and euthanasia. When a patient's living will anticipates clinical conditions that are not hopeless or imminently terminal, or when their directives call for health care options that would violate state or federal law, health care providers and facilities are not bound to follow the directives.

Even in situations that do not entail conflict with the law, health care providers sometimes find that a patient's advance directive is in conflict with the provider's personal or professional values. When this occurs, the health care provider or facility has the option of transferring the patient to the care of a provider or facility that can better abide by the patient's wishes.

9. Is there a legal standard for competency to execute an advance directive?

No. While there are legal standards for testamentary capacity and competency to manage one's affairs, there are no specific guidelines for competency to execute an advance directive. All adults are presumed competent to state their treatment preferences and execute an advance directive under the Patient Self-Determination Act, unless a plenary guardian of the person has been appointed under state law.

10. What happens if cognitive impairment prevents an older adult from establishing an advance directive?

Only a small minority of elderly patients with cognitive impairment are ever brought to court and adjudicated incompetent. After a person has been adjudicated incapacitated or incompetent, under most state laws he or she cannot execute valid advance directives in his or her own behalf. The court-appointed guardian of the person then is empowered to make subsequent health care decisions in the patient's behalf. However, if the patient established a power of attorney for health care matters *before* becoming incapacitated, that power of attorney springs into effect at the time the patient is found on *clinical* grounds to be incapacitated. In such cases, a legal determination of incapacity is usually not necessary.

The remainder of cognitively impaired elders retain their full legal rights to issue advance directives in their own behalf. In some cases, they continue to establish advance directives with insufficient comprehension of what they are choosing, or at the other extreme, clinicians or family members may prematurely usurp their right to make their own decisions. In other cases, when clinicians and family members believe that a patient is losing the cognitive capacity to make such decisions, they informally begin to assist in the decision-making process. Patients with some preserved cognitive function may be allowed to continue to participate in that decision-making process, expressing values and preferences that are then taken into consideration as health care providers and family members make final decisions. As cognitive impairment worsens to the point where the patient is no longer able to understand, deliberate, or communicate anything meaningful about future health care choices, an informal decision-maker is designated. Thus, even in the absence of a legally appointed decision-maker, decisions regarding future health care choices are still made, with the patient fully autonomous, partially included, or fully excluded from the process. The law does not dictate how this should be properly accomplished when patients have less than full decision-making capacity.

11. How should the clinician determine a patient's cognitive capacity to create an advance directive?

In the case of clear and total incapacity (e.g., a persistent vegetative state or coma), it is obvious that the patient cannot formulate advance directives, and there is even no legal obligation to inform the patient of their right to do so. However, in all other cases, on admission to hospitals and nursing homes, patients are required by law to be informed of their right to formulate advance directives and are presumed legally competent to establish such directives. This stands in contrast to epidemiologic estimates that approximately 6 million people in the United States have significant cognitive impairment that renders them clinically incapable of making their own health care decisions. However, no formal clinical standards exist for determining when a patient's cognitive impairment precludes them from being capable of formulating an advance directive or, conversely, when the situation safely permits a cognitively impaired patient to participate in this process.

Nevertheless, during discussions regarding the patient's rights and options in formulating advance directives, clinicians have opportunities to appraise the capacity of patients to:

1. Maintain a stable set of values and goals
2. Comprehend the relevant information
3. Reason and deliberate about their choices
4. Appreciate the situation and its possible outcomes
5. Communicate their choices

When the patient's responses during the informing process give the clinician reason to question the patient's decision-making capacity, it is still left to the clinician to judge how best to balance preservation of the patient's right to make autonomous decisions with the obligation of the clinician to protect a vulnerable patient from making flawed decisions that do not truly reflect the patient's values and goals. Many ethicists and legal scholars have suggested that in determining capacity to formulate advance directives, it is preferable for the clinician to err on the side of promoting patient autonomy. However, this debate is not yet resolved.

12. What is the role of ethics committees in disputes about the patient's ability to participate in the formulation of advance directives?

In many situations, clinicians and family members are able to reach a consensus or agreement regarding the extent to which a patient can participate in the formulation of advance directives. However, when a disagreement cannot be resolved among those who share responsibility for the care of the patient, an ethics committee may play a helpful role, and this approach is generally preferable to resorting to remedies through the legal system. Most hospital ethics committees do not render binding decisions but rather serve in a consultative capacity. They focus the goals of the deliberation, clarify the facts of the case, identify values in conflict, and make recommendations for dealing with conflicts to facilitate decision-making. Unfortunately, for patients residing in the community or in long-term care facilities, the availability of ethics committees is limited.

13. Should elderly patients with mild to moderate cognitive impairment be advised to formulate a durable power of attorney even if they are incapable of making a living will?

Yes. Some elderly patients who are already cognitively impaired at the time they choose to formulate an advance directive may not have the capacity to make a living will, but they may still be capable of appointing a health care proxy and should be given the opportunity to do so for legal, ethical, and pragmatic reasons. This important step can avert the need to petition for legal guardianship at a later date when the patient is totally incapacitated. In most states, appointment of a health care proxy is much simpler, less costly, and less time-consuming than establishing a guardianship.

14. What standards or guidelines exist for surrogate decision-making by persons appointed as proxies or guardians?

There are two main ethical standards by which surrogates can make health care decisions on behalf of incapacitated patients. The preferred standard is **substituted judgment**. This directs the surrogate to choose what he or she believes the patient would have chosen. If the surrogate decision-maker has no knowledge of what the patient would want in a given situation, then the surrogate can follow the **best interest principle**. This directs the surrogate to make the choice that is most likely to serve the best interests of the patient. When surrogates are faced with difficult decisions and unclear parameters on which to base their decisions, they can appeal for advice from health care professionals, attorneys, and hospital ethics committees. In some communities, guardianship advisory services have recently been developed.

BIBLIOGRAPHY

1. Diamond EL, Jernigan JA, Moseley RA, et al: Decision-making ability and advance directive preferences in nursing home patients and proxies. Gerontologist 29:622–626, 1989.
2. Gerety MB, Chiodo LK, Kanten DN, et al: Medical treatment preferences of nursing home residents: Relationship to function and concordance with surrogate decision-makers. J Am Geriatr Soc 41:953–960, 1993.
3. Kern SR: Issues of competency in the aged. Psychiatr Ann 17:336–339, 1987.
4. Omnibus Budget Reconciliation Act, 1990. U.S. Public Law 101-508, sect 4206 and 4751.
5. President's Commission for the Study of Ethical Problems in Medicine and Biomedical and Behavioral Research: Making Health Care Decisions, vol 1. Washington, D.C., Government Printing Office, 1982.
6. Singer PA, Siegler M: Advancing the cause of advance directives. Arch Intern Med 152:22–24, 1992.

21. RELIGION AND SPIRITUALITY

Kathleen L. Egan, PhD, and Jennifer M. Kapo, MD

Indeed, throughout history, religion and spirituality and the practice of medicine have been intertwined. As a result, many religions embrace caring for the sick as a primary mission, and many of the world's leading medical institution have religious and spiritual roots.

Mueller, 2001

1. Why do I need to know about spirituality to care for older persons?

Nearly all patients have spiritual lives that help shape their response to illness and to treatment, including treatment decisions. Most want their physicians to be aware of what they consider to be an important dimension of their lives. According to a Gallup poll from 1999, 94% of Americans surveyed reported a belief in God or a higher power, and 60% stated that religion was very important in their lives. Spirituality and religiosity are particularly important to geriatric medicine because the incidence of belief and the importance of religion increase as people age. Many older adults attend religious services, pray, consult clergy, and/or read religious texts regularly. Religious communities often play a pivotal role in an older person's social network, protecting him or her from the morbidities associated with social isolation. Older Americans' spirituality affects their health and healthcare decision-making. Studies demonstrate an inverse relationship between religiosity and psychiatric conditions such as depression and anxiety. Other data, discussed in more detail below, show that patients hold beliefs that would affect their medical decisions if they were to become gravely ill.

2. What is spirituality? What is religiosity?

When chaplains visit hospitalized patients, they often hear statements such as "I don't go to church, but I pray"; "I am spiritual but not religious"; or "I only go to church because my family insists." Claims either of spirituality without religious participation or of religious participation without spiritual involvement indicate that for many persons these are distinct, although overlapping concepts. In a recent review, Mueller offers the following descriptions:

> Religious involvement or religiosity refers to the degree of participation in or adherence to the beliefs and practices of an organized religion . . . Spirituality . . . is a broader concept than religion and is primarily a dynamic, personal, and experiential process. Features of spirituality include quest for meaning and purpose, transcendence (i.e., the sense that being human is more than simple materials existence), connectedness (e.g., with others, nature, or the divine) and values (e.g., love, compassion and justice)."

In the literature about spirituality or religiosity and their relationship to health and illness, spirituality is typically the broader concept that incorporates religiosity. For many persons, the quest for meaning and purpose takes place within a religious context, and in such cases there may be a complete overlap of religiosity and spirituality. Remembering that these concepts are not mutually exclusive, it may be helpful to outline the distinctions between the two concepts:

Religiosity	Spirituality
Social (orientation is outward)	Individual (orientation is inward)
Practiced in community	Practiced individually
Incorporates prescribed ritual	Ritual may be used, but is not prescribed
Involves relationship with an organization (e.g., church, synagogue, mosque)	No institutional involvement necessary
Shared, commonly articulated beliefs	Individually defined, voiced beliefs

Considering both religiosity and spirituality helps us to appreciate the breadth of individual experience and to be cautious about categorizing or judging the importance or role of these qualities in a patient's life. It is usually better to ask the patient than to make unfounded assumptions based on the presence or absence of affiliation with a religious community, ethnicity, or other single patient characteristics. Religiosity and spirituality are also increasingly distinguished for research purposes so that associated variables can be examined for their independent effects. For example, frequent attendance at religious services has often been found to be associated with better health and longer life, but this finding raises the question as to whether the effect is associated with participating in rituals or more with the social support found in a religious community.

3. How does a practitioner learn about a patient's spirituality?

Some health care providers take the initiative and incorporate spirituality screening into the routine medical history. For others, the issue arises informally over the course of caring for the patient. In other cases, issues of spirituality and religion do not arise in the doctor-patient relationship until a serious illness or crisis is encountered. In a published study of screening in outpatients in a pulmonary practice, researchers asked subjects, "If you were seriously ill, would you want your doctor to ask about spiritual issues?" and "Do you have spiritual and/or religious beliefs that affect your medical decisions?" They found that although slightly less than half of respondents reported having beliefs that would affect their medical decisions, a substantial majority wanted their care providers to ask if they had beliefs.

Spirituality screening becomes particularly important when patients are faced with significantly debilitating and life-threatening conditions. Suffering takes all forms, including physical, social, psychological, and spiritual. People often turn to spiritual support systems when faced with their own limitations and mortality. During these times, it may be appropriate and helpful to perform a more detailed assessment. Spiritual assessment questions need to be simple and nonjudgmental as in Pulchalski's template (1999) for using the acronym **FICA**.

F = Faith and belief. Do you have spiritual beliefs that help you cope with stress? What gives your life meaning?

I = Importance. What importance does your faith or belief have in your life? Have your beliefs influenced how you make decisions?

C = Community. Are you a part of a spiritual or religious community? Is there a group of people you really love or are important to you?

A = Address/Action in care: The physician and health team can use this information to decide on the best care plan, whether it be a referral to a chaplain, a spiritual care provider, or simply a notation in the chart to help understand the patient's future needs and potential aids to relieve suffering.

While taking this history, it is fundamentally important to recognize that the patient's wishes and privacy should always be respected. The patient sets the boundaries and should never feel compelled to disclose information about spirituality that he or she wishes to keep confidential. With this information, the physician can facilitate the patient's participation in supportive relationships and activities and be better prepared for the patient's response to news of a difficult diagnosis or prognosis.

4. What are the professional boundaries that physicians should respect?

In discussing a patient's spirituality, it is important for the practitioner to recognize his or her own spirituality and cultural background and the ways in which they affect how the practitioner approaches the conversation. This self-awareness helps prevent the practitioner from becoming judgmental. Clearly it is not appropriate for a physician to proselytize in a professional setting. It would be inappropriate and likely an abuse of the authority of a doctor-patient relationship to challenge a patient's belief or make recommendations for changes in spiritual practices. It is appropriate and potentially helpful to support the patient in spiritual practices, such as meditation, religious services, and prayer, that the patient has identified as a part of his or her own spirituality.

If a practitioner becomes aware of a problem or crisis in a patient's spiritual life, a professional chaplain can be a helpful resource, whether as a consultant for understanding particular spiritual issues or as one to whom the patient can be referred. Knowing how and when to consult a chaplain is important, especially when extensive evaluation and spiritual counseling are needed.

5. What should a doctor do if a patient asks you to pray with him or her?

A basic principle in this situation is to be authentic with the family and patient. If a physician feels that the request is inappropriate or would violate his or her own beliefs, it is important that he or she not feel obligated to participate. However, refusing without offering other support may be taken as disrespect for the patient's faith and leave the family and patient feeling abandoned. Polite refusal coupled with respectful acknowledgement of the significance of the request is appropriate. Other options may include choosing to stand silently while the patient and family pray based on their beliefs and tradition or calling for the chaplain or other clergy to come to the bedside. That said, if the physician is comfortable, it is not inappropriate to share a prayer or moment of silence with the patient and family. The better a physician knows the patient or family, the less likely it is that such a request would come as a surprise or create an awkward situation. However, physician-led prayer is not encouraged.

6. How do religiosity and spirituality shape responses to illness among the elderly?

Awareness of the religious or spiritual resources of patient and family can guide the physician in providing reassurance, emotional support, and referral as well as understanding otherwise puzzling responses to illness and suffering. Consider that a primary function of religion is to provide believers with a framework for understanding suffering and evil. These frameworks are shaped not only by doctrine but also by the culture in which they are developed and thus vary widely. In a more "fatalistic" culture, suffering may be viewed as simply a given of the human situation, giving rise to a stoic response, whereas in other cultures suffering may be seen as a means to spiritual development, as an atonement for sin, or as a punishment, to cite common examples. For many, lessons about good and evil, well-being, and suffering are absorbed early in life from implicit as well as explicit sources. These lessons may lie largely dormant until evoked by a significant threat or crisis.

In the face of illness or crisis, persons who have been actively spiritual or religious are likely to turn to their faith, community, or tradition, especially if they have gained strength and comfort from this source in the past. How they then react to their illness reflects their own understanding and experience of their beliefs and affiliation. For example, a deeply devout Catholic might refuse pain medication, seeing in suffering a welcome opportunity to imitate Christ. Another person who believes in suffering as punishment may want to do everything possible to allay pain or may deny pain and grief. Yet another might take comfort in the belief that suffering is part of a larger design or plan that is ultimately for the good.

Persons who have not been actively spiritual or religious may experience a crisis, especially if past experiences with religion have been negative. For example, one might revert to long-forgotten assumptions of guilt and experience great inner conflict in the midst of suffering. Alternatively, people may recognize a need for spirituality and begin or renew spiritual or religious practice and belief.

Although there are many unifying beliefs, practices, and rituals within major religions, it is easy to overgeneralize on the basis of an identified religion. In fact, great variation within religious groupings such as Judaism, Christianity, Islam, and Buddhism is evident. Among the factors that can make for a very different expression of religiosity are ethnic and racial differences. For example, African-American churches have played a highly significant role in their communities. A recent study indicates that within Christianity in the United States, African-American women are more likely to take emotional and spiritual support from their churches than Caucasian women from theirs.

7. How do religiosity and spirituality shape one's approach to death and dying among the elderly?

Old age is a time of life when people are confronted with many losses in terms of their own health, abilities, and relationships. It is also a life stage when many pressures of work and child-raising are past. There is time for reflection and attention to questions of the meaning of one's life that is mostly in the past. Religion and spirituality are among the resources for supporting such late-life tasks as achieving peace within one's family, forgiving old offenses, and being forgiven in turn. Old age is sometimes a period of great spiritual growth and development.

The approach of death can be the impetus to complete unfinished life business such as transmitting legacies in terms of family stories, values, assurance of love, or financial provision among others. Closure of this kind can greatly assist the individual and family with coming to terms with the anticipated separation and grief. Hopes for an afterlife as well as familiar rituals and prayers can also greatly contribute to a peaceful approach to death that is a comfort to many. At these times, a person may need assistance with pain control or avoiding unnecessary sedation to complete these preparations for dying.

8. Who provides pastoral care? What do they do?

Providers may encounter either community-based clergy, who are typically volunteers or visitors in health care facilities, or professional chaplains, who are increasingly a presence in health care settings. Community-based clergy often visit persons from their own religious communities who are ill and in hospitals, nursing homes, or hospice care. The care that they offer brings the potential benefit of prior relationship with patient and family, serves as a connection with the patient's religious community, and can provide unique comfort. Visits of clergy from patients' own religious communities should ordinarily be encouraged.

Clinical pastoral care chaplains are employed by health care organizations rather than by local churches, denominations, or religious organizations. Although clinical pastoral care chaplains are from many faiths and may be clergy or ministers of a particular denomination, in the health care setting they are bound by a professional code of ethics to serve patients of all faiths and to protect them from any proselytizing. The role of clinical pastoral care chaplains in health care is encouraged by the JCAHO, which states that "patients have a fundamental right to considerate care that safeguards their personal dignity and respects their cultural, psychological and spiritual values."

Clinical pastoral care chaplains are individuals with graduate theological education, endorsement by a faith group, clinical education equivalent to a year of postgraduate training in an accredited program, and demonstrated clinical competency. To be certified by one of several national organizations approved by the JCAHO, chaplains must complete a training program approved by a national accrediting body. Clinical pastoral care chaplains serve in the full range of health care settings, from acute to long-term care and from trauma units and ICUs to nursing homes and home care, hospices, and outpatient units.

Clinical pastoral care chaplains differ from the community-based clergy in training, role as members of the health care team, availability and accessibility within the health care setting, and role as educators, facilitators, and patient advocates within the organization. Because professional chaplains are employed by the health care organization, they are reliably available to all patients and to staff. Their regular presence in the hospital means that they can respond quickly to the acute needs of patients and families, especially those needing to make end-of-life care decisions, or in the immediate time before or after a critical event. The chaplain's role as part of the health care team and close familiarity with the routines and rules of the organization also place him or her in an ideal position to help with the flow of information between patients, families, physicians, nurses, and others. Consider the situation of a family having to make decisions about withdrawing life support to a loved one who is suddenly on the verge of death. The physician may present information about complex concepts such as brain death, outline available choices, and ask for questions. But is more likely that the chaplain can spend the time needed to help family members grasp and come to terms with the issues. Chaplains may also assist families and patients with presenting their concerns and questions to the health care team in a way that expedites resolution and quality care.

Five national health care chaplaincy organizations have collaborated to identify the functions of professional health care chaplains,[3] which are here summarized in the following table.

Functions of Clinical Pastoral Care Chaplains

1. Remind us of the power of faith to heal, sustain, guide and reconcile.*
2. Bridge boundaries among faith groups and protect patients from proselytizing.
3. Provide spiritual care by empathetic listening and understanding the person in distress* by, for example, grief and loss care, risk screening, facilitating issues in organ/tissue donations, crisis intervention, communication with caregivers, referral and linkage to outside resources, and support of staff and the organization in times of stress or crisis.
4. Participate in health care team work such as rounds and charting.
5. Design and lead religious ceremonies such as prayer services, memorials, birth and death rituals.*
6. Lead or participate in healthcare ethics programs.
7. Educate healthcare team and community by interpreting multi-faith and multi-cultural traditions as they impact clinical care.
8. Act as mediator and reconciler, advocate and cultural broker.
9. Assess and refer for complementary therapies.
10. Support research activities.

* Functions often shared by community-based clergy.

Together these activities can be thought of as mobilizing the spiritual resources of patient, family, staff, and organization in the service of healing. The combined efforts of physicians, nurses, chaplains, and other health care professionals can provide care that respects the spiritual as well as physical dimensions of elderly patients.

BIBLIOGRAPHY

1. Mueller P, Plevak DJ, Rummans TA: Religious involvement, spirituality, and medicine: Implications for clinical practice. Mayo Clin Proc 76:1225–1235, 2001.
2. Pulchalski CM: Taking a spiritual history: FICA. Spirit Med Connect 3:1, 1999.
3. VandeCreek L, Burton L: Professional Chaplaincy and its Role and Importance in Healthcare. Association for Clinical Pastoral Education, 2001. Available at www.healthcarechaplaincy.org/publications/publications/white_paper_05.22.01/06.html.

22. VISION LOSS IN THE GERIATRIC POPULATION

Jeff Wick, MD, and Janet DeBerry Steinberg, OD, FAAO

Vision problems are very common in the geriatric population. This chapter is not intended to be full review of ophthalmic diagnosis and disease but rather highlights common problems and issues encountered by primary care physicians who treat geriatric patients.

1. How is vision tested?

The standard way to measure and record vision in the United States is to use a Snellen chart and 20/20 notation. For example, 20/40 means that the person can see at 20 feet what a normal-sighted person would see at 40 feet. The single most important measurement is corrected, distant vision. Each eye must be tested separately. Uncorrected vision, near vision, and color vision are important but secondary concerns in a primary care office.

2. What is meant by "corrected vision"?

The patient should be wearing his or her current spectacle or contact lens prescription. If the patient does not have the correction, record pinhold vision. Pinhole vision removes the refractive component of vision loss, thereby highlighting pathologic loss. All patients with poor vision need a comprehensive ocular evaluation, but evidence of pathologic vision loss mandates a more directed referral.

3. What is significant vision loss?

The answer is not as obvious as it first seems. Normal best-corrected Snellen acuity is 20/20, but changes in the visual field, contrast sensitivity, or the presence of glare may create dysfunction even in the presence of "normal" 20/20 vision. Therefore, a patient's complaint of poor vision should not be ignored even if Snellen acuity is very good. However, as a rule of thumb, most people function quite well when the vision is at least 20/40 in one eye. Snellen acuity of 20/200 or worse or visual fields constricted greater than 20° indicate severe visual impairment and legal blindness in most states.

4. Is vision loss a normal part of aging?

Although the presence of eye pathology increases significantly with age, many elderly people can and do maintain excellent eye health and vision.

5. What are the required components of a comprehensive eye exam?

The physical evaluation of the eye can be conveniently divided into eight parts. Systematic examination and documentation of these eight parts of the eye exam increase thoroughness by the examiner and minimize the chance that an "obvious" problem will be missed or mistreated, even if the examiner is not completely comfortable with ophthalmic disease. The physical components of a full eye exam include attention to the following items:

- Visual acuity: record distant best-corrected Snellen acuity
- External appearance: describe the general appearance of the eye and adnexa
- Visual fields: test by confrontation
- Motility: record movement of each eye
- Pupils: check for anisocoria or an afferent pupil defect
- Tonometry: determine the eye pressure, which is usually between 10 and 21 mmHg

- Slit lamp: check the lids, conjunctiva, cornea, anterior chamber, iris, lens, and anterior vitreous with the slit lamp instrument
- Dilated exam: examine lens, optic nerve, and fundus with direct and indirect ophthalmoscopy

6. How are the eyes dilated? Is dilation safe?

A topical anesthetic, such as proparacaine, is instilled into the eye. A combination of phenylephrine 2.5% and tropicamide 1% dilates the pupil in about 30 minutes, and the effect lasts 4–6 hours in most people. Serious complications from dilation are rare. Precipitation of angle closure, acute hypertension, and dislocation of an intraocular lens have been reported. People with shallow anterior chambers by penlight exam may be at higher risk for angle closure.

7. What are the benefits of dilation?

Dilation allows superior evaluation of the lens, optic nerve, and retina. Cataracts can easily be seen with a direct ophthalmoscope using retroillumination. The direct ophthalmoscope should be held 1 foot from the eye, and the examiner's view inward is about as good as the patient's view outward. The optic nerve and retina are evaluated with a direct or indirect ophthalmoscope, but expert assessment of these structures takes considerable practice and skill.

8. What is a "refractive problem"? What is the difference between pathologic and non-pathologic vision loss?

Vision loss can create dysfunction in daily living regardless of the cause. However, nonpathologic refractive problems such as nearsightedness (myopia), farsightedness (hyperopia), and accommodative insufficiency (presbyopia) are correctable with glasses or contacts. In developed countries, the majority of people develop either myopia or hyperopia at some point in their life. Presbyopia usually occurs in the fifth decade of life and affects 100% of the geriatric population.

9. Must people wear their glasses or contact lenses to prevent eye disease?

An *adult* who chooses not to wear his or her corrective lenses will not damage the eye, but he or she may present a danger to other people in some settings, such as driving.

10. Of what eye diseases should primary care physicians be aware?

Pathologic eye disease is quite common among the geriatric population. Some of the more important eye diseases include?

- **Glaucoma**: a family of diseases causing irreversible, progressive damage to the optic nerve, and subsequent visual field loss. Glaucoma is frequently but not always associated with elevated intraocular pressure. Glaucoma occurs in about 2% of the population, but up to 5% of people have significant risk factors to develop it. About half of the people who have glaucoma are unaware that they have the disease because they do not recognize early visual field loss. Risk factors for the disease include age, family history, and hypertension. Furthermore, glaucoma is more common and severe in African Americans.
- **Diabetic retinopathy**: prolonged elevation of blood glucose creates microvascular abnormalities in the retinal circulation of the eye. The earliest stage is called "background retinopathy" and consists of small microaneurysms, intraretinal hemorrhages, cotton-wool spots, and venous dilation. These abnormal vessels can leak and cause macular edema that may lead to vision loss. The worst form of diabetic eye disease is called proliferative diabetic retinopathy. The relative ischemia in the retina stimulates neovascularization, which is the proliferation of abnormal blood vessels on the surface of the retina, optic nerve, or iris. If untreated, these abnormal vessels may bleed or cause severe glaucoma. Diabetics need routine dilated eye examinations. Patients should control blood glucose and blood pressure to reduce the chance of developing this severe, blinding eye disease.
- **Age-related macular degeneration**: A slow progressive degeneration of the retina. The degeneration occurs in the macula of the retina and therefore causes central vision loss. The peripheral vision is spared unless another disease is present. The "dry" form of the disease

is most common and progresses very slowly. The "wet" form leads to more abrupt and severe vision loss and is associated with formation of abnormal blood vessels and bleeding within the macula. Various treatments have been developed or proposed for this disease but results can be disappointing.

- **Cataracts**: a clouding of the lens of the eye. Cataracts are extremely common and successfully cured with cataract extraction. Cataracts cause a slow loss of vision or contrast sensitivity, or they may create disabling glare or haloes. Because the physiologic stress of cataract surgery is usually small, contraindications to surgery are relatively few even in the elderly.
- **Dry eye**: usually not a vision-threatening condition but may cause considerable discomfort to the patient. This condition is common among the elderly, probably because of a natural decline in tear production and possibly as a side effect of a systemic medication. Antihistamines and antidepressants are the most common offenders.

11. Can glaucoma be excluded by screening for a normal eye pressure?

Public screenings to measure intraocular pressure serve to increase the awareness of glaucoma and may detect a few cases of the disease. However, such methods have high false-positive and false-negative rates. Many people with an ocular pressure above the upper limits of normal do not have glaucoma, whereas many people with "normal" pressures between 10 and 21 mmHg have glaucoma on further examination. Intraocular pressure readings are more important in the treatment of glaucoma but are not a reliable method to screen and detect the disease.

12. What facets of glaucoma treatment should a primary care physician understand?

First of all, many patients take glaucoma medications but forget to mention this fact to their primary care doctor unless specifically asked. A few glaucoma medications, such as beta blockers, have important systemic side effects. Secondly, many pharmaceuticals, including many obtained over the counter, contain sympathomimetic compounds that may aggravate or precipitate certain types of glaucoma. Note, however, that complications from such medicines are uncommon. Thirdly, overly aggressive treatment of hypertension has been associated with progression of glaucoma in some patients. Nocturnal hypotension may be an important factor in glaucoma progression, probably because of relatively poor perfusion of the optic nerve.

13. Does confrontation visual field testing detect glaucoma?

Only if it is relatively advanced with dense, absolute scotomas. A computerized visual field test is far superior.

14. What features help to distinguish the red eye of conjunctivitis from the red eye of glaucoma or another serious eye disease?

The most common cause of a red eye is allergic or viral conjunctivitis. True conjunctivitis does not cause changes in vision unless complicated by corneal disease. Patients complaining of vision loss, pain (as opposed to minor superficial discomfort), or photosensitivity may have a serious ocular disorder and need a full evaluation.

15. Why does vision fluctuate in a diabetic?

Elevation of the blood sugar above 200 mg/dl can cause intumescense of the crystalline lens and a change in the refraction. The vision may take several weeks to stabilize after the sugar is normalized. Unfortunately, such fluctuations in vision cannot be distinguished from the more serious cause of diabetic vision loss, such as macular edema, except by detailed funduscopic evaluation. Metamorphopsia, which is a distortion of vision, is never normal.

16. Are any treatments available for dry age-related macular degeneration?

Although there are no proven treatments for this condition, risk factors can be modified. Patients should stop smoking. Certain vitamin combinations are known to decrease the progression in certain patients.

17. Why do patients need to be screened for macular degeneration?

Patients with appropriate risk factors need to be identified and placed on appropriate vitamin therapy. Patients who are developing the wet form of the disease are at risk for severe vision loss. Laser and surgical treatments can limit vision loss if the pathology is detected soon enough.

18. Do any drops, vitamins, or other medicines prevent cataract progression?

There are no common, generally accepted medical methods to prevent cataract formation. On the other hand, smoking, prednisone use, age, family history, and possibly sunlight exposure are risk factors for cataract formation.

19. Are ophthalmic antibiotics safe?

Antibiotic eye drops can cause systemic anaphylactic reactions just like their oral counterparts. Generally speaking, however, the potential side effects of eye drops are less severe. A more relevant concern is the ineffective use of an antibiotic for an inappropriate condition. Antibiotics, for example, are frequently prescribed for conjunctivitis even though the etiology of this condition is overwhelmingly viral or allergic.

20. Any suggestions for prescribing artificial tears?

Generally, antibiotics are overprescribed and artificial tears are underprescribed or underused. Artificial tears provide real therapeutic benefit in many eye diseases, including conjunctivitis, dry eyes, blepharitis, and many corneal diseases. Furthermore, a properly lubricated ocular surface is more comfortable and less prone to infection. Thin, generic, preservative-containing tears are inexpensive and helpful in mild disease, in which the frequency of use is less than 4 times/day. Thicker, preservative-free, name-brand artificial tears are clearly superior but are more expensive.

21. Should steroid drops ever be prescribed?

Eye drops containing steroids can aggravate an existing infection, mask the symptoms of a serious underlying ocular disorder, cause glaucoma, and accelerate cataract formation. People taking these drops need to be closely monitored and appropriately diagnosed.

22. How should a corneal abrasion be treated?

Abrasions are the most common eye injury encountered by the primary care physician. Complications from infection can be minimized by using a wide-spectrum antibiotic drop or ointment. Cycloplegia helps with discomfort by reducing ciliary spasm but does not aid the healing process. Patching is optional and may not significantly speed the healing process or reduce discomfort. Most uncomplicated abrasions heal in 24–48 hours. An abrasion not healing within this time frame requires ophthalmologic evaluation.

23. How should conjunctivitis be treated?

Bacterial conjunctivitis responds quickly to topical ophthalmic antibiotics. However, bacterial conjunctivitis is relatively uncommon. The common viral conjunctivitis associated with rhinorrhea, cough, sore throat, and/or mild fatigue should not be treated with ophthalmic antibiotics. The antibiotic drops are irritating to the ocular surface and may make the symptoms even worse. Preservative-free artificial tears and time are the preferred treatment. Allergic conjunctivitis is difficult to distinguish from its viral counterpart except that the symptoms typically last for more than 10–14 days and itching is a prominent feature. Topical mast-cell stabilizers and topical antihistamines work well. Oral antihistamines may help some allergic symptoms, such as rhinorrhea, but may worsen the ocular discomfort because they reduce tear production.

24. What is blepharitis?

Blepharitis and its cousin, meibomitis, probably cause more visits to the eye doctor than any other condition. Furthermore, this chronic condition is much more common in the geriatric population. Blepharitis usually causes a mild but persistent burning, foreign-body sensation around the eye. Crusting on the eye lashes, dryness, itching, and mild fluctuations in vision are common. The symptoms tend to wax and wane in severity. Blepharitis is associated with dry eyes and dysfunction of the meibomian glands, producing tears with an abnormal composition of aqueous and lipid. People with dry eyes, acne rosacea, or seborrheic dermatitis, and patients on oxygen therapy have particularly severe blepharitis. Mild blepharitis may be treated with artificial tears, but a referral may be necessary for more symptomatic cases.

25. Give a few examples of eye emergencies that require urgent evaluation.

Sudden changes in vision or onset of pain that cannot be readily explained and treated require urgent referral. Intraocular infection, traumatic rupture of the globe, corneal burn, acute glaucoma, retinal artery occlusion, and retinal detachment are a few examples of entities that require prompt management.

26. My patient needs to be referred for ophthalmologic evaluation. Are there any unique aspects of eye care regarding health insurance and managed care?

The treatment and evaluation of pathologic vision problems, including vision loss, are usually covered by regular health insurance like any disease, but a referral may be necessary. Currently and historically, "routine" exams and refractive conditions are covered only by unique vision care plans or not at all. Hence, the wording of a consult is a nontrivial issue to the patient.

27. What is low vision rehabilitation?

Low vision rehabilitation is a comprehensive, compassionate, multidisciplinary approach to restoring visual function using optical as well as nonoptical devices, along with an educational and counseling program designed to promote visual independence. It is an approach designed to make the best possible use of the patient's remaining healthy vision. Ideally, low vision rehabilitation includes the contribution of a low vision specialist, either an optometrist or ophthalmologist, an occupational therapist, and a social worker.

28. How does low vision rehabilitation work?

Once a patient is referred to a low vision optometrist or ophthalmologist, the evaluation begins with a comprehensive history. A meticulous refraction determines the patient's best possible visual acuity. Then a goal-oriented treatment plan is developed to train the patient in the use of appropriate low vision devices selected to enable the patient to read, write, use the computer as needed, or otherwise fulfill low vision goals. These devices can range from a simple magnifier or prism reading glasses to a complex system of closed-circuit television and computers. Other aspects of the patient's lifestyle are addressed, such as work needs, hobbies, social and recreational needs, and financial and personal needs. Activities of daily living skills are evaluated, and appropriate training to enhance capabilities is given.

29. What optical devices can be used to restore vision?

Optical devices include magnifiers, microscopic lenses, prism reading glasses, telescopes, and electronic devices such as closed-circuit television or camera headsets.

30. What types of nonoptical devices are used?

Nonoptical devices include appropriate and proper illumination, bold-lined writing utensils and paper, and large-print books, magazines, telephone directories and checks. Meal preparation aids include contrasting dishes and utensils. Low vision rehabilitation in no way affects the physical condition of the eye. It cannot make the disease better or worse. The goal of low vision rehabilitation is to capitalize on the healthy remaining vision and use it as effectively and efficiently as possible.

31. What other services are offered?

The patient can be referred for community-based services such as mobility training and home assistance. Most importantly, the patient can be supported and counseled through the grieving process that often accompanies acquired vision loss. Essential to the patient's success is reassurance that continued independence is possible. Referral for psychological counseling and support groups may be made as needed. Family and caregiver counseling may also be required. Most importantly, the patient experiences a more enabling supportive environment.

23. ORAL HEALTH

Ann Slaughter, DDS, MPH

1. Discuss the scope of oral health in the elderly population.

Maintaining healthy teeth does not totally describe the importance of oral health. Oral health is concerned with maintaining the health of the craniofacial complex, teeth, and gums as well as the tissues of the face and head that surround the mouth. Oral, dental, and craniofacial diseases and conditions include tooth loss, diminished salivary functions, oral-facial pain, oral and pharyngeal cancers, mucosal diseases, and functional limitations of prosthetic replacements. These oral health impairments can diminish social inter-actions, self-esteem, and self-image and have a dramatic effect on quality of life. Oral, dental, and craniofacial diseases and conditions disproportionately affect the elderly. Frail elders are particularly vulnerable to increased morbidity due to oral infections.

2. Discuss the relationship between oral health and general health.

The first Surgeon General's Report on Oral Health in the United States was a landmark document that emphasized the interaction between oral health and general health. A general lack of awareness of the links between oral health and overall health status affects health care decisions on an individual, provider, and policy level. This broader focus on oral health reflects a biopsychosocial model and creates new opportunities to promote interdisciplinary partnerships among oral health providers and medical health providers. A paradigm depicting the determinants of health (oral health and general health) is shown in the figure below.

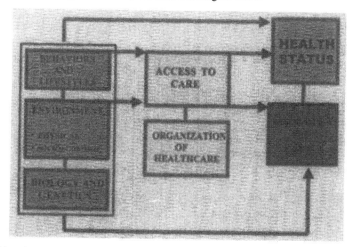

Oral health and general health paradigm. (Adapted by Ann Slaughter, D.D.S., from U.S. Department of Health and Human Services: Oral Health in America: A Report of the Surgeon General. Rockville, MD, National Institute of Dental and Craniofacial Research, National Institutes of Health, 2000.)

3. What key determinants influence oral and general health?

The major factors that determine oral and general health are individual biology and genetics; environmental factors, including physical and socioeconomic aspects; personal behaviors and lifestyle; access to care; and the organization of health care. These factors interact over the lifespan and determine the health of individuals, population groups, and communities.

4. How does the geriatric population fit into the paradigm?

Aging is not a disease, but it does increase susceptibility to disease. The common chronic diseases that affect older adults and medications and treatments to alleviate these conditions can affect the health of the oral cavity. People who have physical or functional disabilities or are medically compromised are at a greater risk for oral diseases. Like medical diseases, dental diseases have strong behavioral, cultural, and social components. Adults over the age of 65 have the highest proportion of out-of-pocket dental expenses; Medicaid and Medicare dental coverage is virtually non-existent. These structural weaknesses in the health care system adversely affect access to care. Conversely, oral health problems can affect overall health. People with diabetes and heart disease are at greater risk for oral infections associated with periodontal disease. The mouth reflects general health and well-being. Many chronic diseases have oral manifestations, which may be the initial signs of clinical disease. All of these factors interact and determine the oral and general health of older adults.

5. Why is oral health a critical component of staying healthy in older adults?

1. Oral health plays a major role in the nutrition of older adults. The elderly are at increased risk for developing nutritional disorders; nutritional deficiencies have oral signs and symptoms. Oral-facial pain caused by infection, trauma, ill-fitting prosthesis, or salivary dysfunction may adversely affect food and fluid intake.

2. The oral cavity is a portal of entry as well as the site of disease for microbial infections that affect general health status. Immunocompromised elders and nursing home elders are at greater risk for general morbidity due to oral infections. Oral diseases give rise to pathogens that can become bloodborne or aspirated into the lungs, leading to life-threatening conditions.

3. Many medications taken to treat systemic conditions can adversely affect the oral cavity and its functions. Polypharmacy is prevalent in the elderly and is also associated with nutritional deficiencies. Salivary dysfunction or dry mouth and taste disorders are common sequelae of many medications taken by older adults (e.g., anticholinergic medications).

6. Summarize the oral signs and symptoms of common nutritional deficiencies in older adults.

Nutritional Deficiencies with Oral Sequelae

MINERAL/VITAMIN DEFICIENCY	ORAL SEQUELAE
Calcium	Skeletal osteoporosis and osteopenia, including the lower jaw, (particularly lower jaw with total tooth loss)
Vitamin B	Tongue, gingival, lip, and mucous membrane changes. Niacin deficiency may cause the tongue to become swollen
Vitamin C	Ulcerated, edematous, and bleeding gingival tissues with halitosis
Vitamin D	Complication of calcium metabolism (skeletal osteopenia and osteoporosis)
Zinc	Taste changes

7. List oral symptoms caused by systemic conditions.

Oral Manifestations Due to Systemic Conditions

SYSTEMIC CONDITION	CAUSE	ORAL MANIFESTATION
Coagulation disorders	Anticoagulation therapy Chemotherapy Liver cirrhosis Renal disease	Increased bleeding risk

(Cont'd.)

Oral Manifestations Due to Systemic Conditions (Continued)

SYSTEMIC CONDITION	CAUSE	ORAL MANIFESTATION
Immunosuppression	Alcoholic cirrhosis Chemotherapy Diabetes Medications (steroids, immunosuppressive agents) Organ transplant therapy Renal disease	Microbial infections
Radiation sequelae	Head and neck radiation	Salivary dysfunction Mucositis Increased caries risk Dysphagia Dysguesia Difficulty with mastication Microbial infections Impaired denture retention

From Ghezzi EM, Ship JA: Systemic diseases and their treatments in the elderly: Impact on oral health. J Public Health Dent 60:289–296, 2000.

8. What are some of the oral sequelae of medication intake for systemic diseases?

Oral Sequelae of Medications for Systemic Diseases

DRUG CATEGORY	DRUG	ORAL PROBLEM
Analgesics	Aspirin NSAIDs Barbiturates, codeine	Hemorrhage, erythema multiforme Hemorrhage Erythema multiforme
Antibiotics	All Erythromycin Penicillin	Oral candidiasis Hypersensitivity reaction, vesiculoulcerative stomatitis
Anticoagulants	All	Hemorrhage
Antihypertensives	All Calcium channel blockers ACE inhibitors Thiazide diuretics Captopril, diazoxide	Salivary dysfunction Gingival enlargement Vesiculoulcerative stomatitis, pemphigus vulgaris Lichenoid mucosal reaction Taste disorders
Antiparkinsonian	All	Salivary dysfunction
Anxiolytics	Benzodiazepines	Salivary dysfunction
Vasodilators	Nitroglycerine patch	Taste disorders
Psychotherapeutics	All Glutethimide, meprobamate Phenothiazines	Salivary dysfunction Erythema multiforme Oral pigmentation, tardive dyskinesia
Corticosteroids	All	Oral candidiasis, recurrent oral viral infections
Ophthalmics	Pilocarpine	Xerostomia

NSAIDs = nonsteroidal anti-inflammatory drugs, ACE = angiotensin-converting enzyme.
From Ship JA: Geriatric oral medicine. Alpha Omegan 94:44–51, 2001.

9. What oral hygiene procedures are beneficial to nursing home elders?

The oral health of elders residing in nursing homes is very poor, and inadequate plaque removal plays a key role in the poor oral health outcomes evident in this population. Consistent daily removal of plaque and cleansing of dentures dramatically improve the oral health status of such patients. Unfortunately, the oral health care of institutionalized elders is frequently given a low priority. Interdisciplinary cooperation implemented by hospital administrators, nursing staff, dentist, and dental hygienist can reduce the risk of dental caries, gingival disease, and tooth loss among nursing home elders. The following procedures are suggested to improve the oral health of nursing home elders:

Residents with teeth. Teeth should be brushed in the morning and before going to bed at night. A regular manual toothbrush may not be helpful for residents with disabilities that affect manual dexterity or for a caregiver to provide oral hygiene care. Manual toothbrushes can be adapted to accommodate the needs of the patient. The handle can be built up with a wash cloth, aluminum foil, or a sponge hair roller or inserted in a tennis ball. Electric toothbrushes may also be considered.

Residents with partial tooth loss or total tooth loss. Dentures and partial dentures should be thoroughly cleansed daily with a denture brush or toothbrush. To reduce the risk of breaking, a washcloth should be placed in the sink before cleaning under running water. Dentures should be removed at night and soaked in a denture cleanser. All prosthesis should be labeled with the resident's name.

Therapeutic agents. Fluoride gels or the antiseptic chlorexidine gel may be applied to teeth using a foam brush (Toothette). This procedure may be used for patients in which tooth brushing is not possible. Foam brushes are not as effective as tooth brushing, but do provide a mechanism for controlling plaque in difficult patients.

Health care practitioner training. Nursing home staff should request in-service training by a dentist or dental hygienist regarding the identification of common signs of oral problems and the mechanisms of daily oral and denture hygiene for residents.

10. What recommendations for oral care can medical providers give caregivers for patients with Alzheimer's disease?

Medical providers should refer patients to a dentist as soon as possible after diagnosis of Alzheimer's disease. Oral self-care skills increasingly decline, as does the ability to cooperate, as Alzheimer's disease progresses. Patients who are in the severe stages may not be aware of oral problems or capable of expressing the presence of oral pain. Such patients should be referred to the dentist for assessment and may require more frequent recall visits to ensure that there are no acute problems and that oral hygiene care is adequate. The caregiver should be trained by the dental care team to provide daily oral hygiene for the patient, with the expectation of eventually assuming this role completely as the patient's condition deteriorates. In addition, caregivers of all patients with Alzheimer's disease should be trained by the dental care team to perform an oral screening examination to note any changes in the following oral-facial regions: face and neck, lips, inside cheeks and lips, roof of mouth, floor of mouth, gums, teeth, or ill-fitting prosthesis. The medical provider can assist the oral care provider in increasing oral and general health awareness among caregivers with the following recommendations:

• Establish a regular time each day for mouth care.
• Break up the steps for cleaning into small simple steps for the patient, reminding the person one step at a time.
• Explain what you are doing in a gentle, calm manner.
• Place a small list of step-by-step instructions on a piece of paper and post it in the bathroom, if the person can still read.
• Keep labeled mouth care supplies in the same place all the time.
• Do not assume that the person will remember the next day what he or she did today.
• Maintain professional dental care visits as recommended by the dentist .
• Perform monthly oral screening examinations and seek professional dental care immediately if any changes are noted in the oral-facial region.

11. What can oral and medical providers do to promote the oral and general health of older adults?

• Health care providers can successfully deliver tobacco cessation and other health promotion programs in their offices, contributing to both overall health and oral health.

- Community-based programs for oral and general health care provide opportunities for collaborations between medical practitioners and dental practitioners at the local and state level.
- Nursing staff and medical providers should be trained to recognize common signs and symptoms of oral conditions that require a referral to the dentist.
- Medical and oral healthcare providers should form partnerships to spread awareness to policymakers of the importance of oral health to overall health and support extended federal and state assistance programs for oral health services

BIBLIOGRAPHY

1. Erikson L: Oral health promotion and prevention for older adults. Dent Clin North Am 41:727-750, 1997.
2. Ghezzi EM, Ship JA: Systemic diseases and their treatments in the elderly: Impact on oral health. J Public Health Dent 60:289–296, 2000.
3. Henry RG, Wekstein DR: Providing dental care for patients with Alzheimer's disease. Dent Clin North Am 41:915–942, 1997.
4. MacEntee MI: Oral care for successful aging in long-term care. J Public Health Dent 60:326–329, 2000.
5. Saunders MJ: Nutrition and oral health in the elderly. Dent Clin North Am 41:681–698, 1997.
6. Ship JA: Geriatric oral medicine. Alpha Omegan 94:44–51, 2001.
7. Ship JA: Improving oral health in older people. J Am Geriatr Soc 50:1454–1455, 2002.
8. U.S. Department of Health and Human Services: Oral Health in America: A Report of the Surgeon General—Executive Summary. Rockville, MD, U.S. Department of Health and Human Services, National Institute of Dental and Craniofacial Research, National Institutes of Health, 2000.
9. U.S. Department of Health and Human Services: Healthy People 2010 (conference edition in two volumes). Washington, DC, U.S. Department of Health and Human Services, 2001.

24. HEARING LOSS OF AGING: PRESBYCUSIS

Michael C. Jung and Douglas C. Bigelow, MD

1. What is presbycusis?

Hearing loss is classified as **sensorineural** (inner ear or neural etiology), **conductive** (due to the inability of sound to reach the inner ear from an external ear, tympanic membrane or middle ear problem), or **mixed** (a combination of sensorineural and conductive hearing loss). Presbycusis is defined in general terms as sensorineural hearing loss associated with advanced chronological age. Some discrepancy exists in the medical literature regarding the use of this term. Most clinicians define presbycusis as age-related hearing loss that is due to the effects of aging in addition to the combined effects of lifelong noise exposure, trauma, ototoxic agents, and other factors. Other clinicians have used a more restrictive definition of the term to indicate that portion of hearing loss that is attributable solely to advanced age. In general, however, presbycusis refers to hearing loss associated with advancing age but of multifactorial etiology where no specific cause can be identified.

2. How common is presbycusis?

Presbycusis is a very common problem. It is the most common type of sensorineural hearing loss in industrialized countries. Approximately 40% of the population of the United States over age 65 is affected. This loss increases with advancing age. Presbycusis is generally more common and more severe in men, whose hearing diminishes at a rate about twice that of women.

3. What are the clinical characteristics of presbycusis?

Presbycusis presents as a bilateral, symmetric, sensorineural hearing loss of insidious onset. Often conversation, especially in a quiet environment, remains unaffected because the frequencies involved in hearing loss are higher than those encountered in normal speech (500–2000 Hz). This high-frequency hearing loss, however, can make it more difficult to hear clearly in the presence of background sound because the high-frequency consonant sounds are most affected. One subtype of presbycusis presents with very poor speech discrimination at a relatively early stage of the disease. There tends to be a progressive loss in hearing with advancing age. The ear examination is normal, and no other otologic diseases can account for the hearing deficits observed.

4. How does presbycusis present?

Presbycusis does not present in a uniform manner. Most patients experience a slowly progressive hearing loss at high frequencies (above 2 kHz) with a relatively preserved ability to understand speech. Other patients, however, may have a markedly impaired ability to understand speech but demonstrate adequate pure tone thresholds. Some patients present early with a minor hearing loss; others can present much later or even deny having a hearing problem despite marked deterioration in hearing ability. As hearing ability declines, communication becomes more difficult, especially in noisy environments. Many patients with presbycusis withdraw socially as their ability to converse with friends and family members deteriorates. This social withdrawal can result in isolation, depression, loneliness, and curtailment of physical and mental activity. Studies have shown an association between depression in the elderly and presbycusis. In the mentally retarded or demented elderly patient, presbycusis can contribute significantly to disability.

5. What are the different types of presbycusis?

A classification system of presbycusis was developed by Schuknecht. Four types of presbycusis (sensory, neural, strial, and cochlear conductive) comprise the classic categories of presbycusis. Although many patients with presbycusis do not fit precisely into a given category, the classification system is useful for correlating pathologic and clinical findings. Two other types of presbycusis, mixed and indeterminate, have been used to describe cases of presbycusis that do not fit into one of the four classic descriptions of the disease.

Classification of Presbycusis

TYPE	SITE OF LESION	CHARACTERISTICS
Sensory	Degeneration of organ of Corti at basal end of cochlea	High-frequency hearing loss in range above 2 kHz. Speech discrimination, which involves lower frequencies, is preserved early in course of disease. Hearing loss is bilaterally symmetric and slowly progressive. Eventually middle frequencies are involved and speech discrimination diminishes.
Neural	Loss of spiral ganglion cells	Pathologically requires loss of at least 50% of spiral ganglion cells. Rapid hearing loss with very poor speech discrimination early in course of disease and preservation of pure tone thresholds until loss of greater than 90% of spiral ganglion cells. This disproportionate loss in speech discrimination relative to the degree of hearing loss is known as phonemic regression. Patients may manifest symptoms of other CNS degenerative changes (memory loss, motor weakness, loss of coordination).
Strial (metabolic)	Atrophy of stria vascularis	Pathologically defined as loss of more than 30% of strial tissue, which is important in endolymph production and the generation of the endocochlear potential. Audiometric testing shows flat hearing loss across all tested frequencies with relatively preserved speech discrimination. Slowly progressive with onset in 3rd to 6th decade of life. Good candidates for treatment with amplification.
Cochlear conductive (mechanical)	No definite histologic correlate; possibly due to thickening of basilar membrane	Presents in middle age with symmetric sensorineural hearing loss. Audiometric testing shows straight-line-sloping hearing loss increasing in severity from low to high frequencies. Speech discrimination relatively well preserved.
Mixed	Any combination of above	Any combination of above
Indeterminate	No distinct pathologic lesions seen	About 25% of patients cannot be classified into the categories above.

6. What causes presbycusis?

The precise mechanism of age-related hearing loss is unknown. However, many factors appear to contribute to the development of presbycusis. Studies have shown an association between noise exposure and presbycusis. In addition to accumulated noise trauma, other postulated etiologies of presbycusis include cardiovascular disease, hypertension, hyperlipidemia, metabolic disorders, mutations of mitochondrial DNA, and imbalances in levels of neurotransmitters such as GABA and glutamate. Heredity also appears to play a large role in the development of presbycusis.

7. Do all elderly patients with hearing loss require a complete evaluation?

It is important to remember that hearing loss, even in the elderly, is not considered to be a "normal" process. Elderly patients who manifest symptoms of hearing loss deserve a thorough medical and otologic evaluation. Hearing loss is a significant source of disability for many elderly individuals. A complete evaluation is necessary to look for correctable or reversible types of hearing loss, to rule out more serious etiologies, to help patients cope with their disability, and to plan a proper course of treatment.

8. What aspects of the history are most important?

The first step in the evaluation of presbycusis is a detailed medical and otologic history, with particular emphasis on any history of occupational or recreational noise exposure. Occupations or activities associated with chronic exposure to loud noises include working with power tools, hunting or target practice with firearms, and listening to loud music. Eliciting a family history of hearing loss can reveal a hereditary hearing disorder. The medical history should include factors that can contribute to sensorineural hearing loss later in life: a history of otitis media, exposure to ototoxic medications (especially aminoglycoside antibiotics and certain chemotherapy agents, such as cis-platinum), head trauma, radiation to the temporal bone, and metabolic disorders such as vitamin D deficiency. Vascular disease may be important in the development of presbycusis. A history of transient attacks and brainstem ischemia may necessitate an MRI or carotid Doppler study. If there is a history of asymmetric hearing loss, an MRI should be performed to rule out an acoustic neuroma.

9. Besides presbycusis, what are some other causes of sensorineural hearing loss?

- Ménière's disease. Vertigo, tinnitus, and sensorineural hearing loss that is usually unilateral but can be bilateral in about 25% of cases. History of intermittent attacks with intervening latent periods. Low tones most involved initially.
- Syphilis can cause progressive sensorineural hearing loss with no characteristic audiometric pattern. It is important to rule out this condition with an FTA-ABS test because the hearing loss can be helped or at least stabilized with treatment. It can sometimes mimic Ménière's disease and is often associated with vestibular symptoms.
- Hereditary progressive sensorineural hearing loss: hearing loss manifested at ages much earlier than those expected in presbycusis; positive family history.
- Noise-induced hearing loss: often not distinguishable from presbycusis; in fact, is a contributing factor to presbycusis, which is considered to be of multifactorial etiology. History of chronic noise exposure or of brief exposure to intense noise stimulus.
- Infections. Chronic ear infections can lead to progressive sensorineural hearing loss. This is usually unilateral but can be bilateral if the chronic infections are bilateral.
- Autoimmune disorders can present with rapidly progressive unilateral or bilateral sensorineural hearing loss. Autoimmune screening tests should be performed in cases of rapidly progressive hearing loss. May be steroid responsive if treatment started quickly. A sudden loss of hearing can be instantaneous or progress rapidly over hours to days. Usually unilateral but on rare occasions can be bilateral. Autoimmune process often implicated, especially in bilateral cases. May be steroid responsive if treatment started shortly after the onset of hearing loss.
- Head trauma. Sensorineural hearing loss, which is usually unilateral, can occur with or without temporal bone fractures.
- Otosclerosis. Advanced otosclerosis or cochlear otosclerosis can cause a progressive sensorineural hearing loss. In most cases conductive hearing loss is also present. A reddish hue over the base of the middle ear (promontory) can occasionally be seen through the tympanic membrane on physical exam known as Schwartze's sign. A CT scan of the temporal bone can occasionally show bony changes around the cochlea. Surgical exploration of stapes footplate is both diagnostic and therapeutic when conductive hearing loss is present.

10. What elements are involved in a complete hearing test (audiogram)?

The following elements are included in comprehensive audiometric testing.

Audiometric Testing

TEST	CHARACTERISTICS
Pure-tone audiometry	Measures hearing sensitivity using pure tones at octave frequencies from 250 Hz to 8000 Hz and two interoctave frequencies (3000 and 6000 Hz). Hearing thresholds for each ear are measured separately using earphones (air-conduction stimulation). Pure tones are also presented through a bone-conduction oscillator placed on the mastoid bone. A comparison of the hearing thresholds for air and bone conduction is useful for classifying hearing loss as sensorineural (no bone-air gap), conductive (loss in air conduction relative to bone conduction) or mixed (combination of sensorineural and conductive).
Speech audiometry (speech reception threshold and speech discrimination)	This test determines how well a person can decipher speech stimuli. Threshold for words and word recognition scores are measured. The speech threshold, defined as the softest intensity level at which the test subject can correctly repeat at a rate of 50% a series of equally balanced two syllable words presented to each ear. Word recognition is scored as a percent correct of a monosyllabic word list at a specific presentation (intensity level).
Acoustic immittance battery	These tests indirectly measure stiffness of the tympanic membrane and associated middle ear structures and include tympanometry and acoustic reflex assessment.
Tympanometry	Quantifies the mobility of the tympanic membrane. Can help to differentiate various causes of conductive hearing loss such as disruption of the ossicular chain, middle ear effusion, or otosclerosis.
Otoacoustic emissions	A measure of outer hair-cell function. This specialized test is not part of the typical audiogram but can be useful in mild hearing loss to help determine if the hearing loss is cochlear or neural in origin. No response will be obtained if there is a 35-dB or greater hearing loss that is cochlear (inner ear) in origin or if middle-ear pathology causes conductive hearing loss.
Auditory brainstem response (not part of a typical hearing test)	Measures the electrical response to sound stimuli as the neural action potential travels from the auditory nerve at the level of the cochlea through the brainstem auditory pathways. While not a "hearing" test per se, the test can be used to measure objectively the threshold of presented sound stimuli. Test results also can be used to help identify retrocochlear lesions such as acoustic neuromas.

11. How is presbycusis diagnosed?

A detailed history, physical exam, and diagnostic work-up that includes an audiogram are completed. Elderly patients who present with a bilaterally symmetric, high-frequency sensorineural hearing loss are diagnosed with presbycusis once other causes of sensorineural hearing loss have been ruled out and if no other specific etiologic factor can be identified.

12. What are the treatment options for presbycusis?

The sensorineural hearing loss of presbycusis is not in itself reversible; however, the ability to function with hearing loss can be greatly enhanced by technological advances made in the hearing sciences. Current treatment regimens include:

- Hearing aids. Many patients with presbycusis benefit from the use of hearing aids. The recent advances made in hearing aid technology, including the use of digital hearing aids, has improved the sound quality and functional usefulness of hearing aids. The current hearing aids can function better in the presence of background sound than older models, although unfortunately the interference from background sound amplification has not been eliminated totally. Some patients with severe-to-profound hearing loss, complex audiometric configurations, or neural presbycusis with very poor speech discrimination, however, may receive limited benefit from even the current hearing aid technology.

- Assistive listening devices can help the patient with activities of daily living. Such devices as telephone earphone amplifiers, loud door buzzers, and television and radio amplifiers can be of great use for the elderly patient with hearing loss.
- Implantable sound conduction devices, also known as implantable hearing aids, have just been approved by the FDA for use in the United States. These devices can provide increased gain and sound clarity compared to conventional hearing aids but require surgery to be implanted and at this point generally are not covered by insurance. They work by surgically attaching a magnet to move the ossicles, which amplifies the sound.
- Cochlear implants are used for patients with severe-to-profound bilateral sensorineural hearing loss who no longer obtain significant benefit from hearing aids. Multichannel electrodes are surgically implanted into the cochlea. When these electrodes are stimulated by the externally worn sound processor and transmitter, the remaining auditory nerve is electrically stimulated in a coded pattern bringing sound to the brain. In the proper candidate the hearing results can be quite dramatic.
- Counseling and emotional support. It is vitally important that health care professionals and family members provide support to the elderly patient with presbycusis. Those close to the patient must understand the social aspects involved in presbycusis. Hearing loss is a significant source of disability, and any support that can be provided to the patient with presbycusis helps the patient to cope with this problem.

13. How do hearing aids function?

A hearing aid consists of three basic components: a microphone, an amplifier, and a receiver. The microphone receives an acoustic signal and transduces this signal to a mechanical and then an electrical signal. The amplifier boosts the electrical signal received from the microphone. The receiver takes the magnified electrical signal from the amplifier and reconverts the signal to an acoustic signal. The end result is to take an acoustic signal and convert it to a boosted acoustic signal that is output to the external auditory canal. The mechanism by which incoming acoustic signals are processed has evolved over the years from analog to digitally programmable and digital signal-processing systems.

14. What different types of hearing aids are available?

Proper selection and fitting of hearing aids are extremely important to ensure a successful result. Many facilities will allow for a month-long trial period with a new hearing aid. Close follow-up is vital to ensure optimal management.

Types of Hearing Aids

TYPES	ADVANTAGES	DISADVANTAGES
Behind-the-ear	Suitable for treating mild-to-severe hearing loss due to the wide range of power available. Larger size allows adequate space for amplification apparatus.	It is a larger hearing aid and may not be acceptable cosmetically.
In-the-ear	More discreet location, making it more cosmetically appealing. Improved localization of sound stimuli with head movement. Microphone placement also enhances high-frequency amplification.	Short distance between microphone and receiver minimizes degree of amplification; therefore, not very effective for patients with severe hearing loss.
In-the-canal	More cosmetically appealing due to its increasingly discreet placement. Improved high-frequency amplification and sound localization with head movement.	Insufficient amplification for a more than moderate hearing loss. Directional microphones cannot be used due to the small size of the faceplate.

(Cont'd.)

Types of Hearing Aids (Continued)

TYPES	ADVANTAGES	DISADVANTAGES
Completely-in-the-canal	Most cosmetically appealing due to least visible placement. Very good amplification in high frequencies.	Insufficient amplification for a more than moderate hearing loss. Directional microphones cannot be used due to the small size of the faceplate. Deep placement necessitates snug fit; some patients ineligible due to ear dimensions. Chance of occlusion effect increased and more potential problems with feedback.

BIBLIOGRAPHY

1. Babin RW: Effects of aging on the auditory and vestibular systems. In Cummings CW (ed): Otolaryngology Head and Neck Surgery, 2nd ed. St. Louis, Mosby, 1993, p 3020.
2. Cohn ES: Hearing loss with aging: Presbycusis. Clin Geriatr Med 15:1, 1999.
3. Hall JW, Antonelli PJ: Assessment of peripheral and central auditory function. In Bailey BJ, Calhoun KH, Healy GB, et al (eds): Head and Neck Surgery—Otolaryngology, 3rd ed. Philadelphia, Lippincott, 2001, p 1659.
4. Jennings CR, Jones NS: Presbycusis. J Laryngol Otol 115:3, 2001.
5. Mills JH, Lambert PR: Presbycusis. In Snow JB, Ballenger JJ (eds): Ballenger's Otorhinolaryngology Head and Neck Surgery, 16th ed. Ontario, B.C. Decker, 2003, p 443.
6. Ricketts TA, DeChicchis AR, Bess FH: Hearing aids and assistive listening devices. In Bailey BJ, Calhoun KH, Healy GB, et al (eds): Head and Neck Surgery—Otolaryngology, 3rd ed. Philadelphia, Lippincott, 2001, p 1961.
7. Roland PS, Eaton D, Meyerhoff WL: Aging in the auditory and vestibular system. In Bailey BJ, Calhoun KH, Healy GB, et al (eds): Head and Neck Surgery—Otolaryngology, 3rd ed. Philadelphia, Lippincott, 2001, p 1941.
8. Sajjadi H, Paparella MM, Canalis RF: Presbycusis. In Canalis RF, Lambert PR (eds): The Ear: Comprehensive Otology. Philadelphia, Lippincott, 2000, p 545.
9. Schuknecht HF: Further observations on the pathology of presbycusis. Arch Otolaryngol 80:369, 1964.
10. Schuknecht HF: Pathology of the Ear. Cambridge, MA, Harvard University Press, 1974.

25. PODOGERIATRIC ASSESSMENT

Arthur E. Helfand, DPM, DABPPH, and Daniel F. Motter, MPT

1. What is podogeriatrics?

Podogeriatrics is a special area of podiatric medicine focusing on foot-related problems in older adults. Care of the feet is a key component of general health care of the elderly, involving health promotion and prevention as well as treatment of foot-related problems. As with any other body system, foot conditions that present in the elderly require special consideration. Health care providers must first take into account the local foot changes associated with the aging process itself as well as the residual effects of repetitive injury over the course of an individual's lifetime. In addition, older adults tend to suffer from multiple chronic diseases, many of which affect the feet. To deliver proper care, the foot specialist must understand the specific syndromes that older patients experience and be aware that he or she is one member of a team managing multiple complex diseases.

Podiatric care must also consider the relationship between foot problems and senior social issues. For example, is the patient at risk for falls? Is the patient suffering from confusion or dementia? Can the patient perform simple activities of daily living and instrumental activities of daily living? The ability to remain pain-free and mobile is a key element in maintaining an independent quality of life—something of paramount importance to most elderly people. If proper foot care can keep a patient living at home rather than in a nursing home, the podiatrist will have done that patient a great service.

The podiatric practitioner must not miss the opportunity to point the elderly patient in the direction of other needed services. In many cases, because foot-related problems are the primary complaint, the patient may seek podiatric care initially. The initial contact with a health care provider and the health care system may become a starting point for total geriatric care through appropriate referrals to the patient's primary care physician and other specialists.

2. Who is at increased risk for foot problems in the older population?

Elders with foot-related chronic diseases are at the highest risk. Examples include diabetes mellitus, arterial insufficiency, and arthritis as well as other conditions that diminish sensation or blood flow to the feet. Pain is also a significant risk factor, because it limits mobility. These issues should be concerns not only for the foot specialists but also for primary care providers. Patients with high-risk conditions should have a foot exam at each primary care visit. Routine foot exams are especially important for diabetics, who can develop significant ulceration without being aware of it. A simple exam can avoid hospitalization, disability, and limb loss.

3. What are the primary dermatologic changes that may be present in the older foot?

- Discoloration (pigmentary changes)
- Verruca (wart)
- Xerosis (excessively dry skin)
- Hyperkeratosis (e.g., callus, corn)
- Ecchymosis
- Petechiae
- Fissure (cracks)
- Swelling
- Trophic changes
- Preulcerative changes (hematoma, blister, pretibial lesion, maceration, temperature)
- Bacterial infection with or without cellulitis
- Tinea pedis

4. What are the common onychial (toenail) changes associated with the geriatric foot?
- Dystrophy: trophic changes such as ridges (onychorrhexis) and involution (onychodysplasia)
- Subungal hematoma: hemorrhage under the toenail either as a collection of blood or splinter-type
- Mycosis: fungal infection (onychomycosis)
- Onychauxis: thickening of the toenails with some deformity
- Onychogryphosis: significant thickening with marked deformity; sometimes referred to as "ram's horn nails."

5. What are the primary clinical findings related to onychomycosis?
- Discoloration
- Hypertrophy
- Subungal debris
- Onycholysis (loosening of the nail from the free edge)
- Onychomadesis (loosening of the nail from the base)
- Secondary infection (bacterial or tinea)

6. What are the primary clinical changes noted in the initial vascular assessment of the foot?
- Coldness
- Capillary filling time
- Texture
- Turgor
- Rubor/pallor with dependency and elevation
- Trophic changes (loss of hair; dry, scaly, shiny, thin)
- Dorsalis pedis absent
- Posterior tibial absent
- Edema
- Symptoms of night cramps or intermittent claudication
- Varicosities
- Atrophy of muscles
- Ulceration
- Amputation (e.g., above knee, below knee, forefoot, toe)

7. What are the primary assessment procedures performed during the initial neurologic assessment of the foot?
- Light touch
- Sharp/dull
- Temperature
- Proprioception (joint position)
- Romberg sign (test for balance)
- Loss of vibratory sense (pallesthesia): tested with a C-128 tuning fork
- Achilles reflex
- Superficial plantar reflex
- Burning, numbness, tingling, hyperesthesia
- Loss of protective sensation (LOPS): tested with a 5.07 monofilament
- Percussion hammer (reflex changes)
- Biothesiometer (measures vibratory sense)
- Coordination, balance

8. What is included in the initial musculoskeletal evaluation of the foot in geriatric patients?
1. Muscle strength, range of motion, posture, leg length discrepancy
2. Gait analysis and relationship to risk for falls

3. Foot deformities
- **Hallux valgus**: outward deviation of the tip of the great toe or longitudinal deviation of the great toe toward the lateral side of the foot. Varus splaying of the first metatarsal with valgus rotation of the great toe and hypertrophy of the first metatarsal phalangeal joint can usually be demonstrated.
- **Anterior imbalance**: inappropriate and distorted distribution of weight to the forefoot.
- **Digitus flexus**: Claw toes, hammer toes; fixed or flexible contractures of the toes on the metatarsal or interphalangeal joints.
- **Pes planus**: flattening of the medial longitudinal arch, in which the calcaneal pitch on a weight-bearing radiograph is usually below 15°.
- **Pes valgo planus**: represents the same clinical picture as pes planus, with an addition of pronation, as demonstrated by a lateral deviation of the Achilles tendon and an outward rotational deformity of the foot; distortion of the normal calcaneal pitch represents a compensatory deformity due to complex biomechanical imbalance.
- **Pes cavus**: a higher than normal arch is commonly associated with neurologic change; in older patients, associated with atrophy of the plantar fat pad, prolapsed metatarsal heads, and plantar fat-pad displacement.
- **Hallux rigidus-limitus**: a degenerative joint change involving the first metatarsal phalangeal joint, resulting from dorsal and lateral spurs. Hallux limitus is characterized by marked limitation of range of motion; hallux rigidus, by absence of range of motion. The difference is determined by radiographic interpretation and functional range of motion.
- **Morton's syndrome**: congenital shortening of the first metatarsal, which creates a distorted or abnormal metatarsal arc. Excessive stress is placed on the second and lateral metatarsal segments, modifying the dynamics, pathomechanics, and biomechanics of the foot; may enhance the development of foot deformity.
- **Bursitis**: inflammation of soft tissue joint bursa.
- **Prominent metatarsal heads**: metatarsal prolapse, or marked prominence of the metatarsal heads associated with posterior displacement of the plantar fat pad, pes cavus, and digital contracture; modifies force and stress.
- **Charcot joints**: neuropathic arthropathy, commonly associated with diabetes mellitus.
- **Exostosis**: hypertrophy of bone with cortical and medullary changes associated with arthritis changes.
- **Heel spur (calcaneal spur)**: a calcification at the insertion of the plantar fascia to the calcaneus (enthesopathy) at its attachment. The spur is usually at the medial plantar tuberosity of the calcaneus and projects anteriorly. Repetitive trauma or stress is a significant etiologic factor; associated with plantar fasciitis or heel spur syndrome.
- **Plantar fasciitis**: inflammation and pain of the plantar fascia, associated with pathomechanical and biomechanical changes and stress, calcaneal spurs, ligamentous calcification, tissue atrophy, and rotational deformities.

4. Foot changes related to gait and footwear
- Friction
- Pressure (vertical or lateral force)
- Shear (movement against the shoe)
- Weight distribution (use of material to cushion pressure or force)
- Weight dispersion (use of Plastazote, PPT, felt, foam, cork ,or other material to transfer or redistribute pressure or force)

9. What are the components and requirements for foot wear for older patients?
1. Shoes that usually provide increased depth to accommodate deformities related to biomechanical, pathomechanical and arthritic changes
2. Rounded toe and high toe box
3. Appropriate, sufficient sizing to accommodate modifications and orthotics, if indicated

4. Special considerations to meet Medicare's criteria for therapeutic shoes for at-risk diabetics, such as:
- History of partial or complete amputation of the foot
- History of previous foot ulceration
- History of preulcerative callus
- Peripheral neuropathy with evidence of callus formation
- Foot deformity
- Poor circulation

10. Discuss common orthotic considerations for the geriatric foot.

Treatment goals must be formulated for the use of orthotics in older patients. For the most part, orthotics are used to accommodate existing deformities and to provide some redistribution of weight or pressure. Adding pressure reduction is also related to soft tissue atrophy. In addition, digital silicone molds, silicone pads, and metatarsal pads can help in the management of digital deformities. Some of the materials used include leather, cork, Korex, carbon filament, plastics, open- and closed-cell foams (Plastazote and/or PPT), and other materials that provide support and optimize weight dispersion and diffusion.

11. What should be completed as part of the initial assessment of the older diabetic foot?

The podogeriatric assessment (Helfand Index) includes a history of present complaints; past history with particular emphasis on related risk diseases; systems review; review of current medications; identification of other providers; and evaluation of the dermatologic, orthopedic, neurologic, and vascular systems. The protocol also includes the stratification of risks for neurologic, vascular, ulcer, onychial, and hyperkeratotic considerations; hyperkeratotic classification; ulcer classification; and footwear assessment, including shoes and stockings. Patient education should be included as part of the initial assessment program. *Feet First* and *If the Shoe Fits*, as published by the Pennsylvania Diabetes Academy for the Pennsylvania Department of Health, are examples of appropriate educational foot health programs.

BIBLIOGRAPHY

1. Birrer RB, Dellacorte MP, Grisafi PJ: Common Foot Problems in Primary Care, 2nd ed. Philadelphia, Hanley & Belfus, 1998.
2. Bower JH, Pfeifer MA: Levin's and Oneal's The Diabetic Foot, 6th ed. St. Louis, Mosby, 2001.
3. Helfand AE (ed): The geriatric patient and considerations of aging. In Clinics in Podiatric Medicine and Surgery, vols. I and II. Philadelphia, W. B. Saunders, 1993.
4. Helfand AE (ed): Clinical geriatrics: Assessment, education and prevention. In Clinics in Podiatric Medicine and Surgery, vol. 20. Philadelphia, W. B. Saunders, 2003.
5. Helfand AE, Jessett DF: Foot problems. In Pathy MSJ (ed): Principles and Practice of Geriatric Medicine, 3rd ed. Edinburgh, John Wiley & Sons, 1998.
6. Helfand AE: Assessing the Older Diabetic Foot, Including Health Care Strategies to Access the Older "At Risk" Patient with Foot Complications Related to Diabetes Mellitus and Podogeriatric Assessment Protocol. Harrisburg, PA, Pennsylvania Diabetes Academy, Pennsylvania Department of Health, Temple University School of Medicine, Department of Continuing Medical Education, 2001.
7. Helfand AE: Diseases and disorders of the foot. In Cobbs EL, Duthie ED, Murphy JB (eds): Geriatric Review Syllabus: A Core Curriculum in Geriatric Medicine, 5th ed. Malden MA, Blackwell Publishing for the American Geriatrics Society; 2002, pp 287–294.
8. Lorimer D, French G, West S: Neale's Common Foot Disorders: Diagnosis and Management, 6th ed. New York, Churchill Livingstone, 2002.

Website
www.apma.org

26. PARKINSON'S DISEASE

Howard Hurtig, MD

1. Who is Parkinson's disease named after?

In 1817 James Parkinson wrote *Essay on the Shaking Palsy*. Because of its seminal and lasting impact, his name was affixed to the disease later in the 19th century.

2. How is Parkinson's disease different from parkinsonian syndrome?

Parkinsonian syndrome, or parkinsonism, is an umbrella term that applies to a recognizable cluster of neurologic symptoms (fatigue, tremor, slowed mobility, difficulty walking) and signs (bradykinesia, stooped posture, shuffling gait, cogwheel rigidity, rest tremor, and postural instability). Symptoms usually appear in middle-aged adults and increase in frequency with advancing age. Approximately 1% of people over age 60 in developed countries have some form of parkinsonism, although it is prevalent everywhere in the world.

Any combination of signs and symptoms of parkinsonism can occur, most often emerging gradually or even imperceptibly. Not all components of the symptom complex are present in every patient. Unilateral rest tremor is the most common early symptom, but because it is distinctively different from other types of tremors (i.e., action or intention tremors), it is usually recognizable to the trained eye as distinctly parkinsonian. Rarely, self-recognition of signs of parkinsonism is abrupt; for example, in the form of tremor starting in the aftermath of physical or psychological trauma. There is no evidence that either type of trauma actually causes parkinsonism or accelerates the naturally progressive course.

Eighty to 90% of people who develop the cardinal symptoms and signs of parkinsonism will have *idiopathic* parkinsonism or **Parkinson's disease** (PD). A diagnosis of PD can be made confidently if at least three major signs are identified. PD is a *clinical* diagnosis, reached after other causes of parkinsonism have been excluded by a careful history, thorough physical examination, and a few specific laboratory tests. Brain imaging studies, such as magnetic resonance imaging (MRI), are rarely helpful except to rule out specific structural disorders.

Criteria for Diagnosis of Parkinson's Disease*

Unilateral onset and persistent asymmetry	Levodopa-induced dyskinesias
Rest tremor	Levodopa response for ≥ 5 yr
Progressive disability	Clinical course of ≥ 10 yr
Excellent response to levodopa	

* Three or more required for diagnosis of definite Parkinson's disease.
From United Kingdom Parkinson's Disease Society Brain Bank.

3. Describe the pathology of Parkinson's disease.

The disease is primarily confined to the upper brainstem, (midbrain) in a region known as the substantia nigra, where melanin-containing neurons undergo progressive degeneration. The cause and the reasons that this particular part of the brain is vulnerable to selective cell death are unknown. The **Lewy body** (LB), an intracytoplasmic inclusion body found at autopsy in the few nigral neurons that survive the process of progressive nigral degeneration, is the histologic signature of PD. LBs are also found at postmortem examination in the cerebral cortex, especially among patients who have significant cognitive dysfunction, the prevalence of which increases with advancing motor disability. Approximately one-third of patients with PD become demented late in late stages of the disease. Cortical LBs are found in most demented parkinsonian patients, but some will have the pathology of Alzheimer's disease.

Nigral neurons, when healthy, are the main source of the brain's supply of the neurotransmitter **dopamine**. Dopamine is transported from the midbrain via the **nigrostriatal** anatomic pathway to the caudate putamen in the **basal ganglia,** which lie adjacent to the lateral and third ventricles. Dopamine is one of several important neurotransmitters that are active in the physiologic circuitry connecting the basal ganglia to the cerebral cortex and that contribute to or are responsible for the execution of normal motor programs of the brain. Dopamine replacement therapy with the dopamine precursor **levodopa** often alleviates many of PD's most disabling symptoms, but it does not stop the relentless but protracted natural progression of the disease.

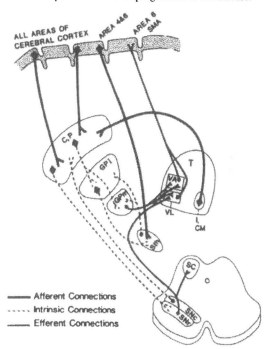

Major afferent, efferent, and internuclear pathways of the basal ganglia. C,P = caudate nucleus and putamen (striatum), GP = globus pallidus (l = lateral, m = medial), SN = substantia nigra (c = compacta, r = reticulata), Sth = subthalamic nucleus, T = thalamus (nuclei: VA = ventral anterior, VL = ventrolateral, CM = centromedian, I = other intralaminar nuclei), SMA = supplementary motor area of cortex, SC = superior colliculus. (From Riley DE, Lang AE: Movement disorders. In Bradley WG, et al (eds): Neurology in Clinical Practice. Boston, Butterworth-Heinemann, 1996, with permission.)

4. What are the major and minor signs and symptoms of parkinsonism?

Signs of Parkinsonism

MAJOR OR CARDINAL SIGNS	MINOR SIGNS	
Rest tremor (4–6 Hz)	Masked facies	Urinary frequency
Bradykinesia	Micrographia	Constipation
Muscular rigidity	Fatigue	Depression
Postural instability	Drooling	Cognitive slowing
	Hypophonia	

5. Which other neurologic disorders have parkinsonism as a major clinical feature?

Parkinson-plus syndrome. Approximately 10% of people with parkinsonism have pathology in anatomic sites in addition to the pigmented neurons of the substantia nigra. Degenerative disorders such as progressive supranuclear palsy (PSP), striatonigral degeneration, and parkinsonism with autonomic failure (Shy-Drager syndrome) often resemble PD early in their course, except that patients with Parkinson-plus syndromes are less likely to have tremor and more likely to have postural instability with significant gait problems at the beginning of the illness. The generic term **multisystemic atrophy** (MSA) has become a popular label for a parkinsonian syndrome that is characterized by increasing bradykinesia, rigidity and postural instability, and findings on neurologic exam that reflect multiple anatomic sites of degeneration (basal ganglia, brainstem, cerebellum, pyramidal tract). MSA is another umbrella term that encompasses the older names, such as Shy-Drager syndrome, olivopontocerebellar atrophy, and striatonigral degeneration. PSP is a separate, pathologically distinct disease and is not a part of the MSA complex. Levodopa usually gives little or no benefit to patients with Parkinson-plus syndrome, and as a result, the rate of progression is often faster. Autopsy of patients with MSA shows widespread neurodegeneration but no LBs.

Cerebrovascular disease. In the elderly with vascular risk factors, especially hypertension, parkinsonism can evolve as a result of multifocal ischemia and be almost indistinguishable from PD. History of stroke, early onset of gait instability, presence of frontal release signs, prominent cognitive loss, little or no tremor, and an MRI scan showing multiple infarcts are a few features that help to separate vascular parkinsonism from the other parkinsonian syndromes.

6. Can medications cause parkinsonism?

Any drug classified as a neuroleptic (antipsychotic) that is used for any length of time can produce signs of parkinsonism (also known as extrapyramidal signs) and other movement disorders (e.g., tardive dyskinesia) in older patients. It is important to remember that metoclopramide (Reglan) is a neuroleptic with the same potential for causing parkinsonism as the more potent drugs, such as chlorpromazine and haloperidol. Neuroleptics cause parkinsonism by the same mechanism that they relieve the symptoms of psychosis; they block postsynaptic dopamine receptors in the basal ganglia and mesolimbic cerebral cortex. The newer "atypical" neuroleptics, such as clozapine (Clozaril), olanzapine (Zyprexa), risperidone (Risperdal), and quetiapine (Seroquel), produce parkinsonian side effects less often. Reserpine, once a standard antihypertensive, is still used occasionally, often in a combination drug. Reserpine causes parkinsonism by depleting the presynaptic stores of catecholamines, including dopamine. It has no effect on dopamine receptors.

7. What disorders of the nervous system are often confused with parkinsonism?

1. **"Senile gait"** is a disorder of locomotion among older people that resembles the shuffle of parkinsonism, and it can be so severe that walking is impossible due to the inability to initiate or sustain the rhythmic sequence of movements basic to normal walking. This condition has been called **lower-body parkinsonism** because the other usual symptoms of parkinsonism found above the waist are missing or relatively mild. Senile gait overlaps with the mincing steps of older persons who have a background of multiple small strokes and with "gait ignition failure," transient freezing that occurs with initiation of walking. The pathophysiology of these nonparkinsonian gait disorders is obscure.

2. **Essential tremor** (ET) is another common cause of tremor in the elderly. It is familial (autosomal dominant) in at least half of cases and increases in frequency and severity with aging. It is the mirror image of parkinsonian rest tremor; i.e., it is activated by voluntary movement and subsides at rest. A careful neurologic exam is the key to separating ET from PD. Handwriting is often a clue: micrographic and tight in PD (usually not shaky), shaky and large in ET. The other differentiating factor is a normal gait in patients with ET.

3. **Stroke** is sometimes diagnosed in patients with unilateral parkinsonism. Since parkinsonism often starts on one side, especially in PD, a flexed and rigid arm or leg can look as if it were caused by stroke (especially if tremor is absent). Yet examination shows the tell-tale signs of parkinsonism (cogwheel rigidity, bradykinesia of fingers and toes) and the absence of findings typically seen in stroke-related neurologic deficits—that is, strength and sensation are normal, reflexes symmetrical, and Babinski signs absent. On the other hand, multiple small strokes can cause a parkinsonian syndrome that highly resembles PD. A neurologic exam with pyramidal findings, an abnormal MRI scan showing strokes in the basal ganglia, and a poor response to levodopa usually delineate the two disorders.

8. Describe the relationship between Alzheimer's disease and PD.

Alzheimer's dementia (AD) is by far the most common neurologic disorder of aging in the Western world. Mild parkinsonism occurs in 20–30% of patients with AD, a reflection of the frequent autopsy finding of a moderate decrease in the number of neurons in the substantia nigra of Alzheimer-affected brains. This interesting overlap between AD and PD is also evident in the higher-than-chance occurrence (20–30%) of dementia in a cross-section of elderly patients with PD, a significant number of whom have Alzheimer's pathology and cortical LBs at autopsy.

A clinical diagnosis dementia with parkinsonism vs. PD with dementia is a common chicken-and-egg dilemma in this setting. It is often unscrambled by identifying the symptom complex that came first as a primary disorder. Under such circumstances, dementia followed by or coterminus with signs of parkinsonism is now called dementia with Lewy bodies or diffuse Lewy body disease. The patient with typical parkinsonism followed by onset of dementia after an interval of at least 2–3 years is classified as having PD with dementia. In most cases, autopsy shows similar pathology despite these clinical distinctions, namely LBs in the substantia nigra and cortex with or without AD pathology.

9. Describe an appropriate diagnostic work-up for someone with parkinsonism.

In reality, the diagnosis of classic PD is purely clinical and no tests are needed. However, when diagnostic criteria are not met confidently, many doctors choose to do a **brain imaging study**, especially an MRI scan. MRI or computed tomography (CT) scans show no definitive abnormalities in PD and only occasionally are helpful in patients with the atypical forms of parkinsonism. Rarely, **severe hydrocephalus** can cause parkinsonism, and only a CT or MRI can show the large ventricles. A ventriculoperitoneal shunt will improve neurologic function in these cases. In parkinsonian patients with longstanding uncontrolled hypertension and a history of stroke, a scan might show signs of widespread ischemic injury to the brain. Such patients are likely to have a mixture of pyramidal and extrapyramidal findings on neurologic examination.

Blood and urine tests for **copper** are mandatory in the work-up of parkinsonism in anyone under 40 years of age to exclude **Wilson's disease**, an inherited (autosomal recessive) disorder of copper metabolism. Parkinsonism in children and young adults also can be part of the phenotype in certain other hereditary conditions, such as the autosomal dominant **Machado-Joseph disease** (MJD), now classified as spinocerebellar atrophy type III. The gene for this disorder has been cloned, and DNA testing is available in specialized diagnostic laboratories.

A strongly positive response to an adequate trial of **levodopa** is usually the best indicator that classic PD is the right diagnosis. As a rule, a weak or absent response suggests one of the atypical parkinsonian states, although a significant response to levodopa may occur early but transiently in the course of any form of parkinsonism.

10. What organ systems does parkinsonism affect?

Gastrointestinal tract
  Dysphagia
  Slowed gastric and intestinal motility
  Constipation
  Pseudo-obstruction or megacolon (rare)
Urinary tract
  Increased frequency and urgency
  Urge incontinence

Respiratory system
  Hypoventilation
  Laryngeal stridor in MSA
  Hypophonic speech
Visual system
  Visual blurring
  Diplopia
Olfactory system
  Anosmia

11. What causes Parkinson's disease?

This question tantalizes everyone. Although there is enough circumstantial evidence to permit experts to formulate a unified working causal hypothesis, the mystery of causation for the most part has not been deciphered. The evidence falls into three broad categories with many points of convergence and intersection:

1. Although it has been known for most of the 20th century that approximately 10–15% of patients with PD have a positive family history of parkinsonism, autosomal dominant pedigrees with autopsy proof of PD (higher cell loss with Lewy bodies) have been rare. Moreover, studies of identical twins have shown a relatively low rate of concordance when one twin has PD. Yet these autosomal dominant families and the more common, nonspecific familial aggregations of PD give some weight to the belief that one or more abnormal genes with variable penetrance and expressivity are responsible for *all* cases of PD. This conjecture was given weight in 1997 with the discovery of a gene responsible for familial parkinsonism in several large families with an autosomal dominant pattern of inheritance. The gene lies on chromosome 4 and codes for the presynaptic protein **alpha synuclein** (a-syn). Subsequent investigations have shown that immunostaining of a-syn in the brain localizes to nigral and cortical LBs. Since 1997 three other genes have been identified in other pedigrees, including the widely prevalent gene known as parkin.

2. Numerous epidemiologic studies have suggested, albeit weakly, that a host of environmental insults, including past head injury, chronic exposure to pesticides (or other toxins), and rural living, might be risk factors for later development of PD.

3. Neurons die slowly as the brain ages, and neural tissue does not regenerate. Consequently, advancing age contributes to the loss of chemical transmitters manufactured by those dying neurons, and the result in susceptible individuals (i.e., those genetically predisposed or environmentally exposed) is age-related neurologic illness, such as PD and AD. Programmed cell death, known as apoptosis, may be an important factor in neurodegeneration.

12. What is neuroprotection or neuroprotective therapy?

The basis of neuroprotection is the hypothesis that neural degeneration can be slowed or halted by using agents that stabilize cells and keep them from dying. The fundamental pathogenesis of neurodegeneration is thought to be linked to oxidative stress, which in turn is mediated by the generation of an excessive amount of toxic, oxygen-rich free radical molecules. Free radicals are highly destructive to cell membranes. The discovery that the drug **deprenyl**, an inhibitor of a subtype of the enzyme monoamine oxidase (type B), could block the formation of MPP+ from MPTP (MPP+ is a highly neurotoxic, oxidized byproduct of the recreational drug MPTP that produces severe parkinsonism) and thereby prevent its toxicity led to the hypothesis that deprenyl could slow progression of the disability of PD by preventing the formation of oxygen free radicals that result from the oxidation of dopamine. In the 1980s, a double-blind, randomized clinical trial of deprenyl in patients with early PD showed that deprenyl delayed the need for levodopa therapy by almost a year compared with placebo. Unfortunately, solid proof that deprenyl actually does protect neurons has been elusive because it also has a mild but significant potential to reduce parkinsonian symptoms by a separate mechanism. Many neurologists still prescribe deprenyl in early PD for its putative neuroprotective effect, despite absence of proof.

The search for other neuroprotective agents has intensified in recent years. Some indirect basic and clinical evidence suggests that the class of antiparkinson drugs known as **dopamine agonists** may have neuroprotective qualities, and NIH has launched a major effort to encourage investigators to conduct clinical trials of other putative neuroprotective agents in patients with early PD to see whether the rate of progression can be slowed. **Coenzyme Q_{10}**, an antioxidant and fortifier of mitochondria, was shown in a well-designed phase II clinical trial (reported in late 2002) to postpone the need for symptomatic antiparkinson therapy in early parkinsonian patients not taking antiparkinson drugs. Coenzyme Q_{10} has no known effect on Parkinson symptoms.

The recent discovery of a variety of **growth factors** in the human nervous system has created the possibility of an entirely new form of clinically viable neuroprotection. These biologically active substances naturally promote growth and membrane stability of all cells during development. Phase II clinical trials have yielded encouraging tentative results. These results, however, do not yet constitute proof of neuroprotection by coenzyme Q_{10}.

13. Which drugs are most effective in treating Parkinson's disease?

See table on following page.

Drugs for Treatment of Parkinson's Disease

DRUG	MECHANISM OF ACTION	RELATIVE POTENCY	SIDE EFFECTS
Carbidopa/levodopa (Sinemet)	Activates DA_1 and DA_2 receptors (DA = dopamine)	++++	Nausea Dyskinesia Psychosis Hypotension Constipation Sedation
Dopamine agonists (bromocriptine pergolide, pramipexole, ropinirole)	Activates DA_2 receptors	++	Nausea Hypotension Leg edema Psychosis Sedation
Entacapone	Same as tolcapone	++	Dyskinesia Orange urine Rare diarrhea
Amantadine (Symmetrel)	Releases DA from vesicles Has antiglutamate and anti-cholinergic properties	+	Psychosis Leg edema Livedo reticularis
Anticholinergics (Artane, Cogentin, Kemadrin)	Block acetylcholine receptors	+	Memory loss Blurred vision Psychosis Dry mouth
Deprenyl (Eldepryl)	Monoamine oxidase inhibitor—blocks reuptake of DA Neuroprotection (?)	+	Psychosis Hypotension
Tolcapone	Catechol O methyl transferase inhibition—blocks reuptake of DA	+	Dyskinesia Diarrhea Liver damage

Five important axioms apply to the use of any of these drugs in the treatment of PD:
1. Never start treatment with more than one drug.
2. Start with the lowest practical dose and increase slowly to avoid side effects.
3. Never make more than one change at a time when raising or lowering doses, unless the patient is in crisis.
4. Multiple drugs at the same time (rational polypharmacy) may be necessary. Many neurologists introduce second and third drugs early in the treatment if the primary one (usually levodopa or a dopamine agonist) is not giving adequate benefit.
5. Dopamine agonists are useful first-line agents drugs in younger patients (< 65) if symptoms are evolving slowly.

14. Why is levodopa given with carbidopa?

Levodopa, 35 years after its introduction, remains the best drug with the best therapeutic margin (fewest side effects in relation to benefit), despite its short half-life. A precursor of dopamine, levodopa is biochemically inert (i.e., not a neurotransmitter), but it crosses the blood-brain barrier (BBB) to get into the brain, where it is converted to dopamine by the enzyme dopa-decarboxylase (DD). The active transmitter dopamine, on the other hand, is excluded from the brain because its molecular structure does not permit it to cross the BBB from the systemic circulation. The problem is that levodopa is rapidly decarboxylated to dopamine peripherally by DD in the gut and liver before it reaches the brain; thus it is useless for clinical purposes unless given in large amounts to saturate the converting enzyme, in which case intolerable nausea usually occurs.

The solution to this therapeutic "catch 22" came in the early 1970s with the development of the DD inhibitor, **carbidopa**. When carbidopa is given in combination with levodopa (Sinemet), it prevents peripheral decarboxylation and reduces by 80% the amount of levodopa required to have a clinical effect. Therefore, through reduced frequency of side effects associated with the use of pure levodopa, levodopa becomes accessible to a much larger population of patients.

15. Do all patients with parkinsonism and all symptoms of parkinsonism respond to treatment?

Unfortunately, no. The cardinal symptoms of early disease—rest tremor, rigidity, and bradykinesia—usually respond well but not necessarily at the same time. Tremor tends to lag behind the other two. Approximately 50–60% of responders will grade the response as very good or excellent. A completely negative response to levodopa-carbidopa usually portends an unfavorable prognosis and the diagnosis of one of the Parkinson-plus disorders.

The most vexing of all symptoms of parkinsonism is loss of balance or postural instability (PI). Most drugs, including Sinemet, have little or no effect on PI, although occasional significant improvements in balance make the effort of trying the various available dopaminergic medications worthwhile in every parkinsonian patient. The relatively poor response of PI to dopamine replacement therapy compared with many of the other symptoms of parkinsonism suggests a nondopaminergic pathophysiology for this most disabling symptom.

16. What are the important adjunctive drugs used in treating secondary problems in PD?

Adjunctive Drugs Used in Parkinson's Disease

DRUG	INDICATION	DRUG	INDICATION
1. Antidepressants Tricyclics SSRIs	Depression	5. Lactulose Laxatives Stool softeners	Constipation
2. Anxiolytics Benzodiazepines	Anxiety, panic	6. Atypical neuroleptics Clozapine Quetiapine	Drug-induced psychosis
3. Carbidopa	Sinemet-induced nausea	7. Fludrocortisone Midodrine	Orthostatic hypotension
4. Oxybutynin Tolterodine	Urinary urgency	8. Hypnotics Benzodiazepines Diphenhydramine	Insomnia

17. What drugs can interfere with the anti-Parkinson drugs (APDs)?

Drugs That Can Aggravate Parkinsonism

DRUG	HOW USED	ADVERSE PHARMACOLOGIC EFFECT
Alpha-methyldopa	Antihypertensive	Depletes presynaptic catecholamines
Amiodarone	Antiarrhythmic	Unknown
Amoxapine	Antidepressant	Blocks DA receptors
Lithium	Antipsychotic, bipolar disease	Unknown
MAO inhibitors*	Antidepressants	Blocks reuptake of DA and NE
Meperidine	Analgesic	Drug-drug interaction
Metoclopramide	GI promotility	Blocks DA receptors
Neuroleptics (except clozapine and certain other atypical neuroleptics)	Antipsychotic	Blocks DA receptors

(Cont'd.)

Drugs That Can Aggravate Parkinsonism (Continued)

DRUG	HOW USED	ADVERSE PHARMACOLOGIC EFFECT
Papaverine	Vasodilator	Blocks DA receptors (?)
Reserpine	Antihypertensive	Depletes presynaptic catecholamines

MAO = monoamine oxidase, DA = dopamine, NE = norepinephrine.
* MAO inhibitors of subtypes A and B—to be distinguished from deprenyl, which inhibits only subtype B. But MAO inhibitors can cause severe hypertension when used in combination with Sinemet and are contraindicated.

The above table lists the drugs that anyone with PD should avoid or at least be aware of when using APDs. Neuroleptics (antipsychotics and metoclopramide) head the list because they block dopamine receptors in the striatum and can produce severe "extrapyramidal" (parkinsonian) side effects in patients with or without PD. The introduction of clozapine, an atypical neuroleptic that does not produce extrapyramidal side effects, has facilitated control of drug-induced hallucinations and delusions in patients with advanced PD and cognitive impairment. Other atypical neuroleptics are useful as antipsychotics in PD, but some may aggravate the symptoms of PD.

Recently a warning was issued against the simultaneous use of deprenyl and antidepressants that inhibit serotonin uptake (selective serotonin reuptake inhibitors and tricyclics) because of the rare occurrence of an acute serotonin crisis (hypertension, sweating, agitation, psychosis).

18. Can nonpharmacologic treatments help?

The most important are physical, occupational, and speech therapy. Each has a place and a time and may be repeated without fear of overdosing. **Physical exercise** is good for conditioning, strengthening, and stretching stiff, underutilized muscles. Working with a good therapist can restore confidence and stability to a deteriorating patient, especially when drug options are limited in the more advanced stages of disease.

Good **nutrition** also keeps the body strong. Most patients are aware that large protein meals may block or truncate the response to a dose of Sinemet taken near mealtime. Transport of the large neutral amino acids in the blood following breakdown of ingested protein uses the same carrier system that delivers absorbed levodopa to the brain. Competition for delivery to the brain via an overloaded transport system in effect reduces access of drugs to the brain and aggravates symptoms.

Acupuncture may relieve pain and even depression associated with parkinsonism. Despite centuries of use, its mechanism of action in the nervous system remains unknown.

Psychotherapy and **counseling** of patient and family can be vitally helpful when depression is a chronic handicap or in times of crisis.

19. What surgical procedures are available for the treatment of PD?

Neurosurgical treatment of PD falls into three broad categories:

1. **Ablative procedures** permanently destroy small, precisely targeted groups of cells in strategic locations within the basal ganglia. The medial globus pallidus and the ventral-lateral thalamus are specific anatomic targets in the two most common operations, because pathologically hyperactive neurons in these regions contribute to the severity of bradykinesia, rigidity, and rest tremors. **Pallidotomy** was popular in the 1950s but disappeared after the introduction of levodopa in the late 1960s. It began a comeback in the early 1990s when it was shown to relieve some of the more serious motor problems related to chronic levodopa usage, particularly on-off fluctuations and dyskinesias. Sophisticated computerized imaging (not available in the 1950s) has allowed stereotactic localization of anatomic targets to become more precise. **Thalamotomy** has been used specifically to control medically intractable parkinsonian tremor. The other symptoms of PD are alleviated much less by thalamotomy than by pallidotomy.

2. **Deep brain electrical stimulation** (DBS) has emerged in the past five years as a safer and more effective procedure than surgical ablation. Approved by the Food and Drug Administration in early 2002, DBS has supplanted all of the –otomy procedures because of the

lower risk of perioperative complications and its reversibility in patients who may not tolerate its effect on neurologic function. DBS works by suppressing abnormal neural outputs from critical anatomic sites in the basal ganglia with high-frequency stimulation, powered by a portable battery implanted much like a cardiac pacemaker. DBS, like the ablative procedures, is appropriate for only a select minority of patients with PD—mainly young, levodopa-responsive patients with on-off fluctuations, dyskinesias, and preserved cognitive function.

3. **Restorative procedures** include transplantation with fetal dopamine-producing neurons of various genetically engineered cell lines or devices that deliver dopamine directly into neuron-rich striatal tissue. **Fetal tissue transplantation** is done in only a few places in the world. Its usefulness is still uncertain after almost two decades of experimental application to humans and primates. Ethical and logistical concerns probably will restrict its use in the future. Furthermore, the results of two clinical trials of fetal cell implants were published in 2002 and 2003. Neither showed consistent efficacy. Other implantation techniques, using genetically altered viral vectors or cultured cells that deliver dopamine and growth factors, are under development in experimental animals. Human trials are also planned.

20. Can pain and altered sensation be part of the symptom complex of PD?

Yes, fairly often. It is not uncommon for patients to report stiff, achy joints or numbness and tingling at an early stage before the diagnosis is made. Since PD usually presents as a unilateral or asymmetric clinical disorder, pain and sensory symptoms tend to occur on the side of greater motor involvement. A stiff or painful frozen shoulder is a common precursor to the onset of more recognizable signs of unilateral parkinsonism. Effective pharmacotherapy alleviates pain in parallel with the relief of rigidity and improved joint mobility. Physical therapy is often a valuable adjunct to the loosening effect of drugs.

Pain also can occur as a side effect from APD therapy. Levodopa sometimes induces painful dystonic contractions of limb muscles, either at peak dose effect or as the drug is wearing off. Painful dystonia of the foot on awakening from sleep in the morning is a common symptom of overnight depletion of dopamine stores and usually clears after the first dose of Sinemet of the day.

21. How common is depression in PD?

Very common. Depression occurs throughout the course of PD, and although antidepressants or psychotherapy helps, depression tends to recur. Serious and unexplained depression, often sudden in onset, may herald or precede the onset of the motor symptoms by months or years.

Dopamine deficiency in the basal ganglia is the major biochemical abnormality responsible for the motor disorder in PD. Norepinephrine and serotonin also are depleted, but to a lesser extent than dopamine. Virtually all of the current antidepressants work in the brain by blocking reuptake of serotonin, norepinephrine, or both at the synapse so that more of these transmitters are available to stimulate noradrenergic or serotonergic receptors. The major and minor biochemical losses in PD, therefore, predispose every patient to a combination of motor and mental changes that include depression as a natural expression of the underlying pathology.

22. What cognitive problems occur in PD?

Most patients with PD, even early in the course of illness, have abnormalities of memory and mental processing. These subtle changes are usually mild or even clinically insignificant. Many patients, however, complain of mental sluggishness and difficulty with the highest levels of cognition, especially if occupational demands are both physically and intellectually taxing. The term **bradyphrenia** has been applied to this state of slowed thinking. Abnormalities of executive function (decision-making) are well-documented in the intermediate stages of disease progression and may force patients in high-pressure jobs to take early retirement, even when they are still independent in every respect outside the office.

Mental and motor deterioration tend to occur in parallel as PD progresses. Serious mental disturbances, such as periodic confusion, visual hallucinations, delusions, and agitation with insomnia at night occur later in the course and are frequently caused or aggravated by the various

APDs. Drug-induced delirium is more likely to occur in patients whose cognitive function is already compromised by the underlying illness. Dementia, which affects 20–30% of patients, occurs late in the course in most cases, when motor function is severely impaired, but not always. The dementia of PD has a more complicated effect on social and personal functions than does Alzheimer's disease because of the additive impact of the motor disabilities. Unlike Alzheimer's dementia, which is classified neuropsychologically as a **cortical dementia** because of the high frequency of language dysfunction (aphasia) in late stages, Parkinson dementia is designated a **subcortical dementia**. Nonlanguage functions, such as memory retrieval, visual-spatial orientation, and frontal lobe executive functions are the most seriously impaired areas of performance.

Sleep is commonly disturbed in patients with PD. Most patients report sleep interruption, often due to urinary frequency, and nocturnal restlessness. Sleep deprivation at night can lead to excessive daytime sleeping, which is further aggravated by the daytime sedating effect of most antiparkinson drugs. **Rapid-eye-movement (REM) behavior disorder** (RBD) is extremely common in PD. It is characterized by active dreaming, dream enactment behavior (talking, thrashing movements, pugilistic encounters with a frightened bed partner, and other bizarre actions) and no awareness of the altered behavior. RBD can also precede the onset of classic symptoms of PD by years. About half of all people with RBD without signs of parkinsonism eventually develop PD.

23. Describe the natural history of PD.

Variability is the single most remarkable feature of the natural history of PD. All patients tend to get worse over many years, but the pace of progression differs. Few if any features are reliable indicators of prognosis.

Most patients notice a very gradual increase in disability, sometimes over a period of 25 or more years. The timing of the onset of PI during the course of illness is also unpredictable, but it usually appears several years after the other symptoms have been treated successfully. When and if it occurs, postural instability signals a major increase in disability, although steady deterioration does not necessarily follow. Many patients, again unpredictably, remain on the new plateau for variable amounts of time until the next sign of progression occurs. Onset of PI early in the course of progressive illness is an ominous marker for a Parkinson-plus disorder, and it usually heralds a more rapid rate of deterioration.

24. Is chronic levodopa usage harmful?

The possibility that chronic levodopa usage might accelerate progression has been hotly debated without resolution for over three decades. Levodopa, with its potential to generate oxygen free radicals and to downregulate dopamine receptors, reaches a point of diminishing returns with prolonged usage, according to the skeptics. Therefore, the treating physician should delay starting it for as long as possible and use the other APDs first. Levodopa promoters, on the other hand, point to the normalization of life span for patients with PD, compared with shortened life spans in the era before levodopa, and to the vastly improved quality of life in most users, regardless of the complications that may eventually occur. Therefore, they argue, why not start it as soon as the patient's disability dictates a need for effective treatment?

Irreconcilable positions notwithstanding, one fact is indisputable: Everyone with PD at some point requires levodopa to achieve maximal functional ability, usually around 3 years into the disease. Postponing the use of the best drug for a year or two when the disease often runs a 20- or 25-year course does not buy much time. Besides, there is essentially no hard clinical evidence that withholding levodopa improves long-term outcome, and there are no data in humans proving that levodopa is toxic.

25. How do people with PD die?

Patients with PD live a relatively normal life span now compared with expectations 35 years ago before levodopa was introduced. Many die in old age or earlier of other diseases before they progress to the point of extreme immobility. The general rate of deterioration is usually slow enough that most patients learn to accommodate, although none too happily, as the next level of compromise is reached.

In some instances, deterioration and progression to end-stage disability are unpredictably precipitous after years of stability. The cause of this rare abrupt decline is unknown, but rapid worsening sometimes follows hospitalizations (e.g., for surgery, a broken hip, or heart attack) or some other period of forced immobilization associated with an intercurrent illness. Nigral cell loss at postmortem exam is usually directly proportional to the degree of clinical disability at the time of death. It is likely that an accelerated increase in disability at the end of life reflects the death of the substantia nigra's last few cells. The conversion of levodopa to dopamine in the brain can no longer take place because there are no cells with enough dopa decarboxylase to promote the conversion. The patient's clinical response to Sinemet ceases, and voluntary movement becomes impossible. A parallel decline in cognitive function is a common end-stage occurrence. Dementia, especially in very old patients, affects as many as 50% at the end of life. Pneumonia, urinary tract infections, and pulmonary emboli are often the direct antecedents of death from cardiac arrhythmia or myocardial infarction.

BIBLIOGRAPHY

1. DBS for PD Study Group: DBS of the subthalamic nucleus or globus pallidum interna in PD. N Engl J Med 345:956–963, 2001.
2. Hoehn MM, Yahr MD: Parkinsonism: Onset, progression and mortality. Neurology 17:427–442, 1967.
3. Hurtig HI, Trojanowski JQ, Galvin J, et al: Alpha-synuclein cortical Lewy bodies correlate with dementia in PD. Neurology 54:1916–1921, 2000.
4. Jankovic J, Tolosa E (eds): Parkinson's Disease and Movement Disorders, 2nd ed. Baltimore, Williams & Wilkins, 1993.
5. Lang AE, Lozano AM: Parkinson's disease. N Engl J Med 339:1044–1053 (Part I) and 1130–1143 (Part II), 1998.
6. Marsden CD, Fahn S: Akinetic rigid syndromes. In Marsden CD, Fahn S (eds): Movement Disorders, 3rd ed. Oxford, Butterworth-Heinemann, 1994.
7. Miyasak JM, Martin W, Sucherowsky O, et al: Practice parameter: Initiation of treatment for PD: An evidence-based review. Neurology 58:11–17, 2002.
8. Olanow CW, Watts RL, Koller WC: An algorithm (decision tree) for management of PD: Treatment guidelines. Neurology 56(Suppl 5):1–88, 2001.
9. Parkinson Study Group: Pramipexole vs. Levodopa as initial treatment for PD. JAMA 284:1931–1938, 2000.
10. Schapira AHV (ed): Progress in Parkinson's disease. Neurology 61(Suppl 3):1–63, 2003.
11. Siderowf A, Stern M: Update on Parkinson's disease. Ann Intern Med 138:651–658, 2003.
12. Stern MB: The early treatment of PD: Levodopa, dopamine agonist or both. Parkins Rel Disord 7:27–33, 2001.

27. ORAL ANTICOAGULATION IN THE ELDERLY

Angela C. Cafiero, PharmD, CGP, and Dina H. Salman, PharmD

1. What is warfarin (Coumadin)?

Warfarin, a vitamin K antagonist, is an oral anticoagulant that produces its effect by inhibiting the enzymes responsible for the synthesis of the vitamin K-dependent clotting factors. The vitamin K-dependent clotting factors are protein C, protein S, and factors II, VII, IX, and X.

2. What laboratory monitoring parameters are needed during warfarin therapy?

Warfarin requires frequent monitoring to ensure optimal therapeutic benefit to minimize adverse effects. The prothrombin time (PT) or protime has been used to measure anticoagulant effects. The PT measures the biologic activity of factors II, VII, and IX, which correlate to warfarin's anticoagulant effect. The PT measures the time required for clot formation in the citrated plasma after calcium and a thromboplastin have been added. Thromboplastins are rich in tissue factor, which is extracted from mammalian tissue (lung, brain, placenta) or from recombinant human tissue factor.

Although the PT is the best test available for anticoagulation, it has a wide variability in the sensitivity of the thromboplastin reagents. Thus, the same blood sample can produce different results with different thromboplastins. The standardization of the PT involves using the international normalized ratio (INR), which corrects for differences in the thromboplastin reagents. The equation to convert PT to INR takes into consideration the patient's PT in comparison with the control PT, as shown in the following equation:

$$INR = (PT^{patient}/PT^{control})^{ISI}$$

The international sensitivity index (ISI) measures the thromboplastin's responsiveness compared with standard thromboplastin. The INR is the best standardized system available to monitor anticoagulation. The goal INR range depends on the therapeutic indication. A baseline complete blood count (CBC) and PT/INR should be taken before initiation of therapy. INR monitoring is recommended every 2–6 weeks, depending on the previous recorded value and individual patient risk factors for warfarin-associated bleeding. In the elderly, monitoring of the PT/INR may be more frequent, approximately every 2–4 weeks, especially if the patient has a history of nonadherence with warfarin directions. Any changes in the patient's condition or medications require closer monitoring of the INR.

3. What are the FDA-approved indications and therapeutic ranges for warfarin?

INDICATIONS	INTERNATIONAL NORMALIZED RATIO (INR) RANGE
Prophylaxis for venous thromboembolism	2.0–3.0
Treatment of venous thromboembolism	2.0–3.0
Arterial thrombosis and stroke prevention	
Atrial fibrillation	2.0–3.0
Mechanical prosthetic valve in aortic position	2.0–3.0
Acute myocardial infarction	2.0–3.0
Mechanical prosthetic valve in mitral position	2.5–3.5

Indications listed above are FDA-approved for warfarin therapy. There are no differences in the INR goals based on increased age.

4. What adverse effects are associated with warfarin?

The main adverse effect associated with warfarin is the increased risk of bleeding, which depends on the intensity and duration of anticoagulation therapy. Hemorrhaging can occur in any part of the body and can range from mild to severe. The most common site for hemorrhage is the gastrointestinal (GI) tract. In patients older than 65 years with comorbid conditions or a history of GI bleeding or taking concomitant antiplatelet therapy, the risk of GI hemorrhage increased significantly.

Other bleeding effects commonly associated with warfarin include enhanced bruising, increased bleeding of gums when brushing teeth and epistaxis. Most bleeds are mild, but any bleed has the potential to become life-threatening on warfarin therapy. One of the more common life-threatening bleeds includes intracranial hemorrhage. The risk of intracranial hemorrhage increases in patients older than 65, a history of stroke, or other comorbid conditions and in patients with a history of falls or at a high risk for falls.

Other rare adverse reactions associated with warfarin therapy include purple toe syndrome and skin necrosis. Purple toe syndrome is a purplish discoloration of the toes as a result of cholesterol microembolization into the arterial circulation of the toe. This syndrome is not associated with pain, tenderness, or sensory changes. Skin necrosis within the subcutaneous fat is due to an imbalance between the procoagulant and anticoagulant proteins early in the course of warfarin therapy, resulting in capillary thrombosis and secondary hemorrhages. The incidence of skin necrosis is < 0.1%; it is more common in persons with protein C deficiency and, to a lesser extent, protein S deficiency. To off-set the transient procoagulant state associated with warfarin's inactivation of protein C and protein S, heparin or low-molecular-weight heparin is simultaneously initiated with warfarin and continued until the INR has reached the therapeutic range in two separate measurements.

5. How is warfarin dosed?

Warfarin dosing may be separated into initial and maintenance phases. The initial dose of warfarin therapy is determined by approximating the average maintenance dose. A loading dose of warfarin is not recommended because of the increased risk of hemorrhage without a decrease in time to achieve a therapeutic INR. For most patients under 65 years old, the starting dose of warfarin is 5 mg once daily. However, elderly patients have an increased sensitivity to warfarin because of their increased pharmacodynamic response to warfarin, potential drug interactions, decreased protein binding, or concomitant disease states (e.g., hepatic disease, thyroid disease, malnutrition, GI hemorrhage). Therefore, the dose initiated in the geriatric population is lower, approximately 2.5 mg once daily.

The half-life of the vitamin K-dependent coagulation factors ranges from 4 to 6 hours for factor VII and from 3 to 5 days for factor II. As a result, a complete therapeutic response to the initial warfarin dose is not observed until all the vitamin K-dependent coagulation factors have been fully inhibited. Initially the INR should be monitored every 3–5 days, and dose adjustments should be made no sooner than 3–5 days after a change in the warfarin dose to allow sufficient time for changes in the INR. If a dose adjustment is needed, it should be limited to an increase or decrease of 5–20% of the total weekly dose due to the nonlinear pharmacokinetics of warfarin.

6. How do you manage a supratherapeutic vs. subtherapeutic INR?

Warfarin therapy is individualized to account for interpatient and intrapatient variability in response. In evaluating a subtherapeutic or supratherapeutic INR, it is important to check for factors contributing to the decreased or increased INR. Factors that influence the development of a subtherapeutic or supratherapeutic INR include patient nonadherence with warfarin therapy, initiation of a new medication, changes in dietary consumption of vitamin K_1 foods, alcohol consumption, changes in vitamin K_1 or warfarin absorption, and changes in warfarin metabolism.

Evaluating a warfarin regimen is based on the total weekly dose. When the INR is not at goal, the dose should be increased or decreased by approximately 5–20% of the total weekly dose. The effect of this small dose change may not become apparent for up to 1 week later.

For a subtherapeutic INR, the dose of warfarin should be increased based on the same principle of a 5–20% increase. Allow approximately 2 days after the dosing change for the clotting factors to equilibrate. A complete blockade of the coagulation factors may take up to 1 week.

There are several approaches to the management of a supratherapeutic INR. The first option is to holding 1 or 2 doses (days) of warfarin. When a rapid decrease in INR is needed, the administration of vitamin K_1 (phytonadione) will replete the vitamin K_1-dependent clotting factors. Vitamin K_1 can be administered orally, intravenously, subcutaneously, and intramuscularly. The oral route is preferred because of the risks associated with the other routes. The intravenous route produces a quicker decline in the INR compared with the oral route but is associated with the risk of anaphylaxis. The subcutaneous route is associated with erratic absorption and significant bruising. The intramuscular route is not recommended due to poor absorption and risk of hematoma. Oral vitamin K produces a substantial decrease in the INR within 24 hours with minimal side effects and risk to the patient.

The goal of vitamin K is to decrease the INR to within therapeutic range. High doses of vitamin K can lower the INR to subtherapeutic range and lead to warfarin resistance for up to 5–7 days, depending on the dose of vitamin K. If the event is life-threatening, infusion of fresh frozen plasma or prothrombin concentrate repletes the clotting factors and produces the most dramatic decrease in the INR. Low-dose vitamin K is warranted in the elderly population more frequently than in younger adults due to an increased risk of a hemorrhagic event.

In general, dose adjustments in the elderly should be made no sooner than every 3 days to fully deplete the clotting factors. Sufficient amount of time is necessary for changes in the INR to occur.

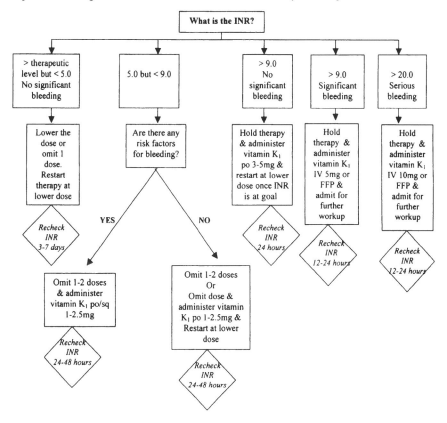

Management of supratherapeutic INRs.

7. What are the potential mechanisms for pharmacokinetic interactions with warfarin therapy in the elderly?

Elderly patients are at an increased risk of pharmacokinetic interactions with warfarin. A potential mechanism for interaction results from alterations in plasma proteins. Warfarin is approximately 98% protein-bound. Frail, malnourished elderly patients can have a reduction in plasma proteins, which can result in an increase of the unbound, active form of warfarin.

Another potential mechanism for interaction results from an age-related decrease in hepatic phase I metabolism. This decrease in metabolism can result in decreased clearance of medications, including warfarin. Warfarin is a racemic mixture of two optically active isomers, the R-isomer and the S-isomer. The S-isomer is 5 times more potent than the R-isomer and is metabolized by cytochrome P450 2C9 and 2C19 enzymes. The R-isomer is metabolized by the cytochrome P450 1A2 and 3A4 enzymes. Interactions with the S-isomer are more clinically significant; however, when both isoenzymes of the R-isomer are inhibited, an interaction can be significant. Drugs and herbs that either induce, inhibit, or are metabolized by any of the enzymes that metabolize warfarin can result in a drug–drug or drug–herb interaction.

Drugs That May Increase Warfarin Response

Alcohol (acute)	Danazol	Flutamide	Metronidazole
Allopurinol	Diflunisal	Fluvastatin	Methylthiouracil
Amiodarone	Disulfiram	Fluvoxamine	Miconazole
Anabolic steroids	Erythromycin	Gemfibrozil	NSAIDs
Capecitabine	Fenofibrate	Indomethacin	Pentoxyfylline
Celecoxib	Fluconazole	Influenza vaccine	Omeprazole
Chloral hydrate	Fluoroquinolones	Isoniazid	Rofecoxib
Cimetidine	Fluorouracil	Itraconazole	Quinidine
Clarithromycin	Fluoxetine	Lovastatin	Sulfamethoxazole
			Tamoxifen

Drugs That May Decrease Warfarin Response

Alcohol (chronic)	Cholestyramine	Estrogens	Vitamin K
Barbiturates	Clozapine	Griseofulvin	Raloxifene
Carbamazepine	Dicloxacillin	Nafcillin	Rifampin
		Trazodone	Rifabutnin

Herbal Supplements That May Increase Warfarin Response

Alfalfa	Celery	Ginger	Parsley
Aloe gel	Chamomile	Ginkgo biloba	Passion flower
Aniseed	Clove	Ginseng (Panax)	Quassia
Arnica	Dandelion	Horse chestnut	Red clover
Aspen	Dong quai	Horseradish	Sweet clover
Black cohosh	(Angelica)	Inositol nicotinate	Sweet woodruff
Black haw	Fenugreek	Licorice	Tamarind
Bladder wrack	Feverfew	Meadowsweet	Tonka beans
Buchu	Garlic	Nettle	Willow
Capsicum	German sarparilla	Onion	Wintergreen

Herbal Supplements That May Decrease Warfarin Response

Coenzyme Q10	Mistletoe	Yarrow
Goldenseal	St. John's wort	

8. What dietary restrictions should be observed during warfarin use?

Maintaining a consistent diet is important with the use of warfarin. Foods rich in vitamin K_1 replete the vitamin K-dependent clotting factors and thus reverse the action of warfarin. Large changes in the amount of vitamin K_1 foods can affect the anticoagulant properties of warfarin. These foods should be consumed in small portions and limited in their consumption. In general, patients on warfarin should maintain a diet consistently low in vitamin K_1. An exception to this dietary restriction is in the frail elderly, in whom oral intake is more important than enforced dietary restrictions. Such patients require close monitoring of the INR due to the fluctuation of their diet.

The consumption of alcohol has mixed effect on warfarin and can influence the INR. Acute consumption can slightly increase the INR, whereas patients with a history of chronic alcohol use can have a lower INR. Maintaining a consistent diet and avoiding alcohol assist in stabilizing the INR.

Vitamin K_1 Content of Foods

HIGH	MEDIUM	LOW
Basil	Apple, green	Apple, red
Broccoli	Asparagus	Avocado
Brussels sprouts	Dill pickle	Breads
Butterhead lettuce	Green peas	Carrot
Cabbage	Iceberg lettuce	Cauliflower
Canola oil	Margarine	Celery
Chick pea	Pistachio nuts	Coffee
Coleslaw	Red cabbage	Cola
Collard greens	Summer squash	Corn
Green onion		Dairy products
Green tea		Eggs
Kale		Fish
Liver		Green beans
Mayonnaise		Meats
Mustard greens		Pasta
Parsley		Peanuts
Red leaf lettuce		Potato
Spinach		Poultry
Turnip greens		Rice
Watercress		Tomato

9. What information should elderly patients be aware of while taking warfarin?

Patient and caregiver education is of utmost importance. It is necessary for patients to understand the indication for the use of warfarin, the duration of warfarin therapy, and the consequences of missing a dose or taking extra doses. Warfarin is an important medication that needs to be taken around the same time every day to keep consistent drug levels. If the patient forgets to take the dose, he or she should be instructed to take it as soon as possible on the same day. If the patient completely forgets a dose, he or she should be instructed to skip the dose and not to double the dose of warfarin the next day to make up for the missed dose.

Many medications interact with warfarin. In general, it is best to assume that every medication, including over-the-counter and herbal products, can interact with warfarin unless otherwise noted. Patients should advise health care professionals of their warfarin therapy before they start any new medication. Patients should be counseled to maintain a diet consistently low in vitamin K_1-containing foods and to limit the use of alcohol.

Any signs or symptoms of bleeding should be reported immediately. If bleeding persists, patients should present to the emergency department. Avoidance of heavy bodily contact assists in decreasing the risk of bleeding.

10. What are the risks vs. benefits of warfarin therapy?

Balancing the risks of hemorrhage vs. the benefit of prevention of a thromboembolic event is essential in any patient population but assumes increased importance in the geriatric population. The most common complications associated with warfarin therapy involve upper gastrointestinal bleeding (GI) and, to a lesser extent, intracranial hemorrhage. On average, the risk of a bleeding complication associated with warfarin therapy is 3% per year; the annual risk of death due to hemorrhage is approximately 0.6%. The risk is related to the intensity of anticoagulation and concomitant administration of aspirin, nonsteroidal anti-inflammatory drugs, and other drugs that impair platelet function and produce gastric erosions. In addition, age > 65, a history of stroke or GI bleeding, history of falls, and other comorbid conditions have been shown to increase the risk of major bleeding.

Despite potential bleeding complications, long-term anticoagulation with warfarin reduces the risk of a stroke associated with atrial fibrillation by 65%, whereas aspirin decreases that risk by only 20%. Treatment of venous thrombosis with warfarin decreases the rate of a recurrent event by greater than 90%. Given the benefits of warfarin therapy in prevention of stroke and venous thrombosis, individual patient risk factors should be assessed and the threshold for warfarin initiation should be lower.

11. How does warfarin differ from other anticoagulants?

CLASS	AGENT	CONSIDERATIONS	DOSAGE FORM
Antiplatelet	Aspirin Clopidogrel (Plavix) Extended-release dipyridamole-aspirin combination (Aggrenox) Ticlopidine (Ticlid)	Inhibits platelet function Not as effective in the prevention of thromboembolism	Tablet Capsule
Heparin	Heparin	Variable patient response Must monitor aPTT Coadministered with warfarin until INR in therapeutic range	Intravenous injection Subcutaneous injection
Low-molecular-weight heparin	Enoxaparin (Lovenox) Tinzaparin (Innohep) Dalteparin (Fragmin)	Similar mechanism and indications as heparin More predictable response than heparin Does not require aPTT monitoring Coadministered with warfarin until INR in therapeutic range	Subcutaneous injection
Direct thrombin inhibitors	Lepirudin (Refludan) Bivalirudin (Angiomax) Argatroban	Indicated for use in patients with history of heparin-induced thrombocytopenia	Intravenous infusion
Factor Xa inhibitors	Fondaparinux (Arixtra)	Indicated only for the prevention of venous thromboembolism after lower extremity orthopedic procedures	Subcutaneous injection

aPTT = activated partial thromboplastin time.

12. How is warfarin managed during the perioperative period?

Perioperative management of patients requiring warfarin therapy is a challenge because it often requires discontinuation of warfarin and normalization of the PT/INR to prevent excessive bleeding during the procedure. To determine which patients are candidates for discontinuation of warfarin, the risk of bleeding during a specific procedure vs. the risk of a thromboembolic event must be carefully assessed. No specific recommendations exist for perioperative management in the elderly; however, because the elderly are at an increased risk of adverse events related to warfarin, one may be more inclined to withhold warfarin therapy through the procedure.

A recently published systematic review by Dunn and Turpie examined the literature involving the perioperative management of patients on oral anticoagulation. Overall, the available literature was poor, with no randomized controlled trials, and the duration of follow-up was rarely stated. However, based on the available literature the authors concluded that patients undergoing dental procedures, arthrocentesis, cataract surgery, and diagnostic endoscopy or colonoscopy with or without biopsy do not require discontinuation of oral anticoagulation therapy. This recommendation to continue warfarin through the perioperative period is based on a relatively low risk of uncontrolled bleeding compared with developing a thromboembolic event. For more invasive procedures and surgery requiring discontinuation of warfarin, individual patient characteristics should be assessed to determine whether heparin or low-molecular-weight heparins bridging should be used for anticoagulation while the PT/INR normalizes. The table below lists recommendations for perioperative management of warfarin for procedures requiring discontinuation of warfarin.

INDICATIONS FOR WARFARIN THERAPY	RECOMMENDATION
Atrial fibrillation without history of thromboembolic stroke	Hold warfarin
Mechanical aortic valve	Hold warfarin Optional use of treatment dose heparin or LMWH while PT/INR is subtherapeutic
Mechanical mitral valve Atrial fibrillation with history of thromboembolic stroke	Hold warfarin Use treatment dose heparin or LMWH while INR is subtherapeutic
Venous thromboembolism	Hold warfarin Assess need for bridging with heparin or LMWH on an individual basis

Modified from Dunn A, Turpie A: Perioperative management of patients receiving oral anticoagulation. Arch Intern Med 163:901–908, 2003.

13. What are some considerations for managing an elderly patient on warfarin?

Managing an elderly patient on warfarin is a complex task, especially if the patient has cognitive impairment, diminished eyesight, decreased dexterity, or no assistance at home. In such patients, adherence with clinic appointments and warfarin therapy becomes an issue. Involving another person in the patient's care—for example, a nursing assistant or neighbor—can assist in managing the warfarin. Medication calendars and pillboxes are useful tools to assist in ensuring adherence. Medication calendars include a list of the daily dosage of warfarin. Assistance in filling a weekly pillbox with the correct daily dosage of warfarin can be beneficial, especially in patients with cognitive impairment and impaired vision.

The best recommendation for managing warfarin therapy in an elderly patient is to keep the regimen simple. Having the patient take the same dosage every day assists with adherence. For example, if a patient needs to take a weekly dosage of 16 mg, a simple regimen would be 2 mg 6 days per week and 4 mg 1 day per week.

Patients in a structured nursing facility are more likely to be a candidate for warfarin therapy. However, it is still important to assess risks, especially if the patient is mobile. Medication adherence is more reliable in a controlled environment. Dietary intake also is more predictable in a nursing home, where meals are prepared for the patient. Besides these advantages, nursing home patients have the same issues as the community dwelling elderly.

Evaluation of the risks and benefits of warfarin therapy is important in an elderly patient. Warfarin therapy may not be appropriate in a patient with risk factors for falls, history of bleeding, or adherence problems. Aggressiveness of utilization of warfarin therapy is assessed on an individual basis.

BIBLIOGRAPHY

1. Ansell J, Hirsh J, Dalen J, et al: Managing oral anticoagulant therapy. Chest 119:22S–38S, 2001.
2. Copland M, Walker I, Tait R, et al: Oral anticoagulation and hemorrhagic complications in an elderly population with atrial fibrillation. Arch Intern Med 16:2125–2128, 2001.
3. Coumarin and indandione derivatives: General statement. In McEnvoy GK (ed): AHFS Drug Information. Bethesda, MD, American Society of Health System Pharmacists, 2002, pp 1410–1421.
4. Current guidelines for practice: Oral Anticoagulation for Older Adults. American Geriatrics Society, 2002. Available at <www.americangeriatrics.org>.
5. Dunn A, Turpie A: Perioperative management of patients receiving oral anticoagulation. Arch Intern Med 163:901–908, 2003.
6. Haines S, Racine E, Zeolla M: Venous thromboembolism. In Dipiro J, Talbert R, Yee G, et al (eds): Pharmacotherapy: A Pathophysiologic Approach, 5th ed. New York, McGraw-Hill, 2002, pp 337–373.
7. Hirsh J, Dalen JE, Anderson DR, et al: Oral anticoagulants: Mechanism of action, clinical effectiveness, and optimal therapeutic range. Chest 119:8S0–21S, 2001.
8. Hirsh J, Fuster V, Ansell J, et al: American Heart Association/American College of Cardiology Foundation Guide to Warfarin Therapy. Circulation 107:1692–1711, 2003.
9. Jacobs L: The use of oral anticoagulants (warfarin) in older people: American Geriatrics Society guideline abstracted from Chest 2001;S119. J Am Geriatr Soc 50:1439–1445, 2002.
10. Man-Son-Hing M, Laupacis A: Balancing the risks of stroke and upper gastrointestinal tract bleeding in older patients with atrial fibrillation. Arch Intern Med 162:541–550, 2002.
11. Warfarin sodium. In Kastrup EK (ed): Drug Facts and Comparisons, 57th ed. St. Louis, Facts and Comparisons, 2002, pp 177–181.

28. CARDIOVASCULAR DISEASE: PRIMARY AND SECONDARY PREVENTION

Marjorie Marenberg, MD, PhD

1. Describe the epidemiology of coronary artery disease in the elderly.

The incidence of coronary artery disease (CAD) increases with age. Over 50% of all coronary events and 85% of all deaths from coronary artery disease occur after the age of 65.

2. Are risk factors for coronary artery disease similar in elderly and younger populations?

Yes. Several major epidemiologic studies in the elderly have shown that the traditional risk factors of hypertension, diabetes, lack of exercise, and ratio of high total cholesterol to high-density lipoprotein continue to predict coronary events and cardiovascular disease mortality even after the age of 75. The prevalence of some of these risk factors also increases with age. Although the magnitude of the relative risk associated with these risk factors is attenuated at older ages, the *attributable risk* of hypertension, diabetes, and hypercholesterolemia to the likelihood of a future coronary event actually *increases* with age.

3. What is the difference between primary and secondary prevention of CAD?

Traditionally, primary prevention refers to interventions that reduce the incidence of CAD and secondary prevention to modalities that prevent a recurrent event in people with established CAD. However, since atherosclerosis progressively increases with age, it is difficult to distinguish fully between these two prevention measures in the elderly. A large number of people may be at high risk for CAD that has not yet clinically manifested. This situation is known as subclinical cardiovascular disease.

4. How can subclinical cardiovascular disease be measured?

Several measures of subclinical cardiovascular disease have been developed to determine subclinical atherosclerotic disease. Electron-beam computerized tomography (EBCT) measures the amount of calcification in the coronary arteries. Carotid ultrasound can measure the degree of plaque in the carotid arteries, which has been shown to predict risk of stroke. Ankle-brachial index (ABI) measures the ratio of blood pressure in the brachial, posterior tibial, and dorsalis pedis arteries. The highest of four measurements in the arm, divided by the highest of four measurements in the ankle, is used to determine the ABI. A ratio of less than 1 is suggestive of peripheral arterial disease. Although these subclinical measurements target different vascular beds, they may be suggestive of the burden of atherosclerotic disease in the vascular beds of other organs.

Not all older adults have significant plaque burden. In fact, there is quite a large degree of heterogeneity in the degree of atherosclerosis among the elderly.

5. HMG co-A reductase inhibitors (statins) reduce risk of primary and secondary disease in middle-aged people. Is there evidence that treating older persons with statins reduces the risk of cardiovascular disease in the elderly?

Yes. Two recent landmark studies have proved the efficacy of statin use in older persons. The Heart Protection Study was a double-blind, randomized clinical trial of 20,536 people aged 40–80 years at high risk for cardiovascular disease. Included were persons with known coronary disease (such as a history of a prior myocardial infarction, unstable angina, angioplasty) or a history of a nondisabling stroke, transient ischemic attack, carotid artery disease, or diabetes. After 5 years of follow-up, treatment with simvastatin significantly reduced the risk of a future nonfatal or fatal coronary event, even in people over the age of 70. Interestingly, statins reduced the risk of CAD even in people with normal cholesterol levels. Finally, the Heart Protection Study demonstrated for the first time in an older population that use of a statin can be protective for ischemic strokes.

The Prospective Study of Pravastatin in the Elderly (PROSPER) is the only clinical trial that has exclusively examined reducing cardiovascular risk in elderly persons. This randomized, double-blinded, controlled clinical trial of 5804 people aged 70–82, after 3 years of follow-up, demonstrated a significantly reduced risk of nonfatal and fatal cardiovascular disease (by almost 20%). However, in contrast to the HPS, PROSPER did not demonstrate a reduction in stroke risk. The authors attribute this difference in results to an insufficient follow-up period; it may take 5 years, as it does in HPS, to demonstrate a benefit from pravastatin use.

Both these important secondary prevention studies demonstrate the clinical relevance of treating older persons at high risk for cardiovascular disease with a statin. Based on these, and earlier studies, the ATPIII guidelines state that "no hard and fast age restrictions appear necessary when selecting persons with established CHD for LDL cholesterol-lowering therapy."

6. The HPS and PROSPER study were secondary prevention studies. Are there any primary prevention studies of statins in older people?

There have been two primary prevention studies of statin therapy: the West of Scotland Coronary Prevention Group (WOSCOPs) and the Air Force/Texas Coronary Atherosclerosis Prevention Study (AFCAPS/TexCAPS). In both studies, roughly 20% of the cohort was over 65. In these subgroups, use of the statin significantly lowered the risk of developing CAD (fatal and nonfatal combined). Based on these findings, the ATPIII guidelines recommend treating older adults on a case-by-case basis. However, in addition to these trials, a recent prospective epidemiologic study showed that statin use reduced new-onset CAD events even in adults over the age of 75. The results of this study offer more compelling evidence that treating older persons with statins can reduce the incidence of coronary artery events.

7. What are the current recommendations for cholesterol management?

The National Cholesterol Education Program established the Adult Treatment Guidelines (ATPIII) for lipid management in 2001:

1. Establish the presence or absence of clinical atherosclerotic disease, defined as clinical coronary heart disease(CHD), symptomatic carotid artery disease, peripheral arterial disease, or abdominal aortic aneurysm. Diabetes is considered a CHD risk equivalent.

2. Determine the major risk factors for CHD that modify LDL goals:
   • Cigarette smoking
   • Hypertension (blood pressure greater than or equal to 140/90 mmHg) or taking antihypertensive medication
   • Low high-density lipoprotein (HDL) cholesterol (< 40 mg/dl)
   • Family history of premature CHD (first-degree relative less than 55 in males, 65 in females)
   • Age (men greater than or equal to 45, women greater than or equal to 55)

3. If there are more than two risk factors, assess the 10-year CHD risk (using Framingham tables). If the 10-year risk is greater than 20%, the risk should be considered as a CHD-equivalent.

4. Through the table below, establish the low-density lipoprotein (LDL) goal of therapy, and determine the need for therapeutic lifestyle changes or drug therapy.

RISK CATEGORY	LDL GOAL	LDL LEVEL AT WHICH TO INITIATE TLC	LDL LEVEL AT WHICH TO CONSIDER DRUG THERAPY
CHD or CHD risk equivalents	≤ 100 mg/dl	≥ 100 mg/dl	≥ 130 mg/dl
2+ risk factors	< 130 mg/dl	≥ 130 mg/dl	≥ 130 mg/dl (if 10-year risk 10–20%; otherwise, 160 mg/dl)
0–1 risk factors	≤ 160 mg/dl	≥ 160 mg/dl	≥ 190 mg/dl

TLC = therapeutic lifestyle changes.

8. What are the recommendations by ATPIII for therapeutic lifestyle changes?

The therapeutic changes outlined by the National Cholesterol Education Program in ATPIII include the following:

1. Diet
   - Saturated fat < 7% of calories
   - Increased fiber (10–25 gm/day)
2. Weight management (optimal body mass index ≤ 24)
3. Increased physical activity

In addition to the dietary recommendations above, other essential ingredients for weight loss include a balanced diet consisting of fruits, vegetables, and no more than 55% carbohydrates, complex carbohydrates with restriction of refined carbohydrates (e.g., sugar, candy, white flour), and portion control. At this time, there is no clear evidence that high-protein, low-carbohydrate diets are beneficial in the long term for prevention of CAD.

9. What is the metabolic syndrome?

The metabolic syndrome is thought to stem from the interrelationship between obesity and the development of insulin resistance, which can then lead to hypertension and an abnormal lipid profile. Specifically, the ATPIII defines the metabolic syndrome as any three of the following: (1) abnormal obesity (waist circumference > 40 inches in men, > 35 inches in women); (2) triglycerides greater than 150 mg/dl; (3) HDL < 40 mg/dl for men, < 50 mg/dl for women; (4) blood pressure > 130/85 mmHg; and (5) fasting glucose ≥ 100 mg/dl. A recent study from the Third National Health and Nutrition Survey estimated the population prevalence of the metabolic syndrome as 22%. The study also found that this prevalence increased with age; over age 70, the prevalence was 42%! This is clearly a growing epidemic among the aging population.

10. Does evidence suggest that treating people with the metabolic syndrome reduces cardiovascular risk?

Although no clinical trials have addressed the primary prevention of CAD among people with the metabolic syndrome, the VA-HIT trial randomized men with CAD who had normal LDL, low HDL, and elevated triglycerides to either gemfibrozil or placebo. After 5 years, men in the gemfibrozil group had a reduced risk of cardiovascular events, which has attributed to this medication's effect on raising HDL levels.

11. What are the ATPIII recommendations for treating metabolic syndrome?

The first recommendations include lifestyle modification by intensifying weight loss and increasing physical activity. Lowering triglycerides can be achieved by carbohydrate restriction, specifically targeting processed sugars and refined bread products.

For pharmacologic treatment of triglycerides, treatment of elevated LDL is the primary goal. However, if the triglycerides are greater than 500 mg/dl, treating triglycerides becomes the primary goal to prevent pancreatitis.

12. What therapeutic agents should be used to treat LDL and the dyslipidemias of the metabolic syndrome? What are the relative lipid-lowering effects of these classes of medications?

	LDL	HDL	TRIGLYCERIDES
First-line agents			
HMG coreductase inhibitors	↓↓	↔↑	↔↓
Fibrates	↔	↑	↓↓
Second-line agents			
Bile acid resins	↓	↔	↑
Nicotinic acid	↓	↑↑	↓
Fish oils			↓↓

In general, statins can lower LDL by 15–20% at the starting dose. Raising the dose increases the lowering effect usually by only another 5%. Side effects and toxicity increase with increasing dose. Using both statins and fibrates can increase the risk of adverse events; thus, statins should generally be used at lower doses in combination with low doses of fibrates, if both triglycerides and LDL need to be targeted.

A recently approved medication, ezetimibe, reduces LDL by inhibiting cholesterol absorption and has been marketed for use in combination with statins without increasing the risk of myopathy because it is generally not systemically absorbed. However, given the increase in gastrointestinal transit time in older adults, systemic absorption may occur, and further postmarketing data in older subjects are needed to characterize the side effects of ezetimibe.

13. What are the side effects from statins? What are the risk factors for statin-induced adverse events in the elderly?

Statins are generally well tolerated, but elevated hepatic transaminases and myopathy are the most common side effects. Increased transaminases occur among 0.5–2.0% of people taking statins and are reversible after stopping the medication.

The most common clinical manifestation of myopathy is muscle aches with no associated increase in creatinine kinase. This effect occurs in roughly 1.6–5% of people taking statins. Despite the fact that in several placebo-controlled trials, the incidence of myalgias between the treatment and control group have been similar, it is possible to have creatinine kinase (CK) elevation without complaints of myalgias. Statin use cannot be excluded as a cause of these side effects.

The most concerning side effects of statins are myositis and rhabdomyolysis, defined as muscle pain associated with CK levels 10 times greater than normal. Cerivastatin was withdrawn from the market in August 2001 because it was associated with 31 deaths due to rhabdomyolysis in the U.S. Data from the FDA and National Prescription Audit Plus revealed that the death rate for cerivastatin was 16–80 times higher than for other statins. The following factors can increase risk for statin-associated myopathy:

- Advanced age (> 80 years)
- Impaired drug metabolism
- Frequent surgical procedures
- Polypharmacy
- Comorbidity
- Weight loss or decreased nutritional state
- Small body frame and frailty
- Presence of diabetes with chronic renal insufficiency
- Specific medications including fibrates (especially gemfibrozil), nicotinic acid (rarely), cyclosporine, azole antifungals, macrolide antibiotics, HIV protease inhibitors, verapamil, amiodarone, digoxin, warfarin, and grapefruit juice
- Alcohol abuse

14. How does one choose whether or not to start an older person on a statin for CAD prevention?

It is important to weigh the risk and benefits. Clearly, poor functional status and multiple comorbidities may place a person at a high risk of adverse events in the setting of a limited life expectancy. However, a person age 85 with known diabetes and CAD who is functionally independent still would benefit from the reduced risk for further coronary events with a statin. In addition, according to the Heart Protection Study, treatment with a statin may reduce risk for stroke in such people. Therefore, age alone should not be a criterion for initiating treatment with a statin, but functional status, active life expectancy, and risk for a vascular even should be considered in the decision.

15. What is the significance of the newer risk factors for CAD, such as C-reactive protein, lipoprotein a, and homocysteine?

C-reactive protein (CRP) is a marker of chronic inflammation that has been shown to be predictive of CAD. A recent prospective study demonstrated that CRP is a stronger risk than LDL cholesterol. However, although no randomized clinical trials have shown that lowering CRP reduces cardiovascular risk, studies are clearly under way. Current recommendations are to measure

CRP at the time of cholesterol screening. CRP levels < 1, 1–3, and > 3 mg/L represent low-, medium-, and high-risk groups. For people with cholesterol levels requiring pharmacologic therapy, elevated CRP should encourage strict compliance. In people with LDL levels between 130 and 160, an elevated CRP should lead to better compliance with ATPIII guidelines and perhaps initiate a switch from lifestyle to therapeutic modification. In people at low risk for CAD by LDL level, an elevated CRP should lead to greater compliance initially with lifestyle modification.

Lipoprotein a [Lp(a)] is a lipoprotein with an attached glycoprotein (aopA) that is structurally similar to plasminogen and is thought to cause impairment in fibrinolysis. Studies of the normal distribution of Lp(a) have shown that levels appear to be higher in African-Americans than whites. Lp(a) is also strongly genetically determined. It is generally not recommended to screen for Lp(a) unless there is a strong family history of CAD. The primary goal of Lp(a) therapy is LDL reduction.

Homocysteine is a protein that has been associated with low vitamin B12 and folic acid levels and has been found in epidemiologic studies to be a weak independent risk factor for CAD. Although no clinical trials have shown that reducing homocysteine reduces CAD risk, treatment with folic acid and vitamins B5 and B12 does not appear to have adverse effects and may be useful in people with elevated homocysteine and normal LDL levels who are otherwise at risk for CAD.

16. Have antihypertensive medications also been shown to reduce cardiovascular risk in both primary and secondary prevention in the elderly?

Yes. Hypertension has repeatedly been shown to be a risk factor for CAD, and this risk doubles with each 20/10 mmHg increment in blood pressure. Therefore, the recent Joint National Committee on Prevention, Detection, Evaluation and Treatment of High Blood Pressure (JNC7) has recommended that people with a systolic blood pressure of 120–139 mmHg and a diastolic blood pressure of 80–89 mmHg be considered as "prehypertensive." JNC7 recommended thiazide diuretics as first-line therapy for hypertension. However, given the risk of orthostasis in thiazide use, this recommendation must be used cautiously in elderly persons, and screening for orthostasis both before and after the administration of a diuretic is advised.

Beta blockers have long been the mainstay for treatment after myocardial infarction and recently for congestive heart failure and should be used for hypertension in such patients. ACE inhibitors and angiotensin II antagonists have also recently been shown to prevent CAD and stroke in high-risk people and are also recommended in patients with congestive heart failure, prior CAD, prior stroke, or TIA.

BIBLIOGRAPHY

1. Chobanaian AV, Bakris GI, Black HR, Cushman WC: The Seventh Report of the Joint National Committee on Prevention, Detection, Evaluation, and Treatment of High Blood Pressure. JAMA 389:2560–2572, 2003.
2. Ford ES, Giles WH, Dietz WH: Prevalence of the metabolic syndrome among US adults: Findings from the third National Health and Nutrition Examination Survey. JAMA 287:356–359, 2002.
3. Grundy SM: The National Cholesterol Education Program (NCEP)—The National Cholesterol Guidelines in 2001, Adult Treatment Panel (ATP III). Approach to lipoprotein management in 2001 National Cholesterol Guidelines. Am J Cardiol 90:(8A):11i–21i, 2001.
4. Heart Protective Study Collaborative Group: MRC/BHF Heart Protection Study of cholesterol lowering with simvastatin in 20,536 high risk individuals: A randomized placebo-controlled trial. Lancet 360:7–22, 2002.
5. LIPID Study Group: Long term effectiveness and safety of pravastatin in 9014 patients with coronary heart disease and average cholesterol concentrations: The LIPID trial follow-up. Lancet 359:1379–1387, 2002.
6. Pasternak RC, Smith SC, Bairey-Merz CN, Grundy SC: ACC/AHA/NHLBI Clinical Advisory on the Use and Safety of Statins. J Am Coll Cardiol 40:568–573, 2002.
7. Ridker PM: Clinical application of C-reactive protein for cardiovascular disease detection and prevention. Circulation 107:363–369, 2003.
8. Shepherd J, Blauw GJ, Murphy MB, Bollen ELEM: Pravastatin in elderly individuals at risk of vascular disease (PROSPER): A randomized controlled trial. Lancet 360:1623–1630, 2002.
9. Thompson PD, Clarkson P, Karas RH: Statin-associated myopathy. JAMA 289:1681–1690, 2003.

29. HEART FAILURE

Ross R. Zimmer, MD, and Brian M. Drachman, MD

1. Define heart failure.

Heart failure has been classically defined as a condition in which heart function is unable to meet the needs of the body. However, this definition is inadequate. Recently we have begun to define heart failure as a clinical syndrome of functional limitations and physical examination findings due to cardiac pathology. Furthermore, and of no less importance, heart failure is a progressive disorder, often accompanied by decreased survival, in part due to neurohormonal activation and unpredictable cardiac arrhythmias. However, patients with cardiac dysfunction can also be asymptomatic, and the disease process can be abated in part by a combination of education, lifestyle modification, medical therapies, and appropriate percutaneous or surgical interventions as needed.

2. Is heart failure more common in the elderly?

Heart failure is predominantly a disease of the elderly; 6–10% of people older than 65 years old have heart failure. Approximately 80% of the patients hospitalized with heart failure are older than 65 years, and more Medicare dollars are spent for its diagnosis and treatment than any other. This is predominantly due to the number of cardiovascular risk factors, such as hypertension, diabetes mellitus, and hypercholesterolemia, that develop over many years to create progressive end-organ effects. Furthermore, hospitalizations due to heart failure exacerbations become more frequent over time as older patients potentially have more trouble taking their increasingly complex medical regimens and often lack the support that is needed to be compliant with the accompanying dietary restrictions.

3. What causes heart failure?

The causes of heart failure must be broken down into systolic or diastolic dysfunction. Systolic dysfunction is present when the ejection fraction is less than 40% (normal ejection fraction: 55–60%). Common causes of **systolic dysfunction** in the elderly include:
- Coronary artery disease (most common)
- Idiopathic (diagnosis of exclusion)
- Hypertension
- Valvular heart disease
- Alcohol abuse
- Thyroid disease
- Myocarditis
- Systemic causes such as lupus or hemachromatosis

Diastolic dysfunction, which accounts for about 20–30% of patients with heart failure, is defined as heart failure with an ejection fraction greater than 40% and no significant valvular or pericardial disease. The bulk of patients with this disorder have no identified underlying cardiac disease. Many have had longstanding hypertension, and echocardiography may reveal concentric left ventricular hypertrophy. Diastolic dysfunction is more common in elderly women, due in part to increased myocardial stiffness related to fibrosis as well as accompanying neurohormonal abnormalities that further exacerbate this problem.

Other causes of heart failure in the elderly include valvular disease, especially aortic stenosis. Occasionally, patients with restrictive cardiomyopathy present at a later age, such as those with multiple myeloma and accompanying cardiac amyloid.

4. How do patients with heart failure present?

The presentation of heart failure, whether due to systolic or diastolic dysfunction, pericardial or restrictive disease, is quite varied. Many patients can have structural heart disease and no symptoms at all. Abnormalities of cardiac function may be found on a screening echocardiogram done for unrelated reasons, such as preoperative cardiac evaluation. A typical presentation often includes some degree of shortness of breath, sometimes with exertion or at rest if the patient is less compensated. Orthopnea may also be present as well as paroxysmal nocturnal dyspnea. Other typical presenting complaints include fatigue and lower extremity swelling. In the elderly population, the presentation may be less specific and may include a change in mental status or decreased appetite.

Physical examination findings include elevated neck veins, rales, and edema. Typically, the cardiac examination in patients with systolic dysfunction reveals an S3, whereas an S4 is present in patients with diastolic dysfunction. It should be noted, however, that the physical examination often underrepresents the degree of cardiac pathology over time in patients with marked left ventricular systolic dysfunction. The venous capacitance vessels (veins/lymphatics) adapt to the longstanding heart failure, and often minimal edema and clear lungs may be seen at the time of presentation. Elevation of jugular venous pressure greater than 8 cmH$_2$O may be the most reliable physical finding.

Other presentations include new onset of palpitations and arrhythmias such as atrial fibrillation or even sudden cardiac death. Finally, patients may present with an exacerbation of an underlying cardiac problem, such as angina or infarct with coronary artery disease, or hair loss and fatigue with thyroid disease, more common in the older population.

5. Outline a diagnostic approach to heart failure.

Key questions in history

- Dyspnea
- Orthopnea
- Paroxysmal nocturnal dyspnea
- Chest pain
- Palpitations
- Lightheadedness
- Near syncope or syncope
- Cardiac risk factors

Key components of physical examination

- Vital signs
- Jugular venous pressure
- Presence of rales or pleural effusion
- Cardiac examination for S3, S4, murmurs, and rubs
- Hepatomegaly or pulsatile liver
- Edema
- Bruits

Select diagnostic studies are essential to the work-up and treatment of patients with heart failure. An electrocardiogram may be helpful, especially if it reveals an infarct pattern. A chest radiograph may be of limited value but may confirm the diagnosis of heart failure or reveal a noncardiac source of dyspnea. The best diagnostic study remains echocardiography, which reveals evidence of systolic left ventricular dysfunction or preserved left ventricular function with associated findings that may be consistent with diastolic dysfunction. However, the diagnosis of diastolic dysfunction by an echocardiogram is a difficult one, especially in the elderly, in whom certain parameters to make this diagnosis lose their specificity. Echocardiography can also reveal significant valvular disease. An echocardiogram is also helpful for evaluation of the pericardium (e.g., constrictive pericarditis leading to heart failure).

Consideration should be given to an ischemic evaluation if the patient complains of anginal chest pain. An exercise or pharmacologic nuclear or echocardiographic stress test is a safe and simple screening test for the presence and degree of coronary artery disease. Unfortunately, stress tests are often unreliable in patients with marked left ventricular dysfunction. In patients with abnormal stress tests, marked left ventricular dysfunction or a high probability of ischemic heart disease, cardiac catheterization should be performed. Many of these patients have multivessel disease and thus should be considered for surgery. Their functional status and other comorbidities must be assessed before embarking on this more invasive and aggressive approach. Other basic testing that should be considered, especially in the elderly, includes a thyroid-stimulating hormone level as well as studies ordered based on the clinical presentation, such as a serum ferritin if there is a suspicion for hemochromatosis given accompanying hepatic or dermatologic findings.

6. How do you treat patients with heart failure?
- Correction of conditions that cause or exacerbate heart failure
- Lifestyle modifications
- Pharmacologic therapy (systolic and diastolic function)
- Device therapy
- Surgical options

7. Discuss correction of conditions that cause or exacerbate heart failure.
This important factor is often overlooked in the treatment of heart failure. Ischemic heart disease, for example, remains the most common cause of heart failure; thus, it is crucial that patients with left ventricular systolic dysfunction be evaluated for ischemia, and that revascularization, if indicated, be performed. Similarly, hypertension can both cause and exacerbate heart failure due to other conditions. Aggressive blood pressure control is essential. Other factors include:
- Correction of underlying valvular disease (e.g., aortic stenosis, mitral regurgitation)
- Alcohol restriction/cessation
- Treatment of systemic factors, including thyroid disease, infection, anemia
- Removal of drugs that can contribute to heart failure (e.g., nonsteroidal anti-inflammatory agents, certain calcium channel blockers)
- Treatment of supraventricular arrhythmias (most commonly atrial fibrillation) and sustained ventricular arrhythmias
- Treatment of certain systemic disorders (e.g., hemochromatosis, sarcoidosis)

8. What lifestyle modifications are advised?
Changes in diet and lifestyle play an important part in the management of heart failure, whether due to systolic or diastolic dysfunction. Examples include:
- Sodium restriction to 2–3 gm/day. Patients should be instructed to avoid table salt, to minimize cooking with salt, and to evaluate the sodium content of purchased foods.
- Concomitant fluid/water restriction to 64 ounces/day.
- Daily weight monitoring to evaluate for early changes in fluid accumulation.
- Participation in cardiac rehabilitation/regular structured exercise. Although most patients should not participate in heavy labor or exhaustive activities, randomized trials have shown that exercise training can improve quality of life, lessen symptoms, and improve exercise intolerance.
- Weight loss in overweight patients.
- Smoking cessation and avoidance of illicit drugs; occasional and limited alcohol consumption is acceptable.
- Patient education to better understand the early symptoms of decompensated heart failure.

9. Discuss pharmacologic therapy for systolic dysfunction.
1. **Diuretics.** Diuretics improve symptoms by decreasing preload and relieving vascular congestion. However, some patients can avoid the need for these agents by practicing careful sodium and fluid restriction. Overzealous use of diuretics, especially in the elderly, may lead to metabolic disturbances, such as hypokalemia, as well as a fall in cardiac output and blood pressure often associated with orthostatic hypotension and progressive renal insufficiency.

2. **Angiotensin-converting enzyme (ACE) inhibitors.** ACE inhibitors improve outcomes in all patients with systolic dysfunction, ranging from those with asymptomatic LV dysfunction to those with severe symptomatic disease (NYHA Class I–IV). Studies confirming these findings include SOLVD and CONSENSUS. All patients should be started on ACE inhibitors, although it should be noted that the elderly are often underrepresented in clinical trials.

- Therapy should be started with low doses, particularly in the elderly, to minimize symptomatic hypotension and other side effects.
- If tolerated, drugs should then be uptitrated to the doses used in clinical trials (e.g., captopril 50 mg tid, enalapril 10 mg bid, lisinopril 20 mg bid). However, there is some debate as to whether these high doses are substantially more effective than modest dose therapy.
- African Americans may experience less benefit from ACE inhibitors than Caucasians.
- Side effects include cough, hyperkalemia and renal insufficiency.

3. **Angiotensin II receptor blockers (ARBs)**. ARBs appear to be as effective or slightly less effective than ACE inhibitors in systolic dysfunction. They have not been studied in as diverse a patient population as has been done with ACE inhibitors and should not be used in place of ACE inhibitors as first-line therapy. However, one of the few studies to look predominantly at an older population was ELITE II, which suggested that ARBs were safe to use in the elderly and, given similar outcomes, may be a reasonable alternative to patients who do not tolerate ACE inhibitors. Despite initial concerns that combination therapy with ACE inhibitors, ARBs, and beta blockers may be detrimental, more recent data suggest that the addition of an ARB to an ACE inhibitor may be useful in selected patients with CHF.

4. **Hydralazine and nitrates**. The combination of nitrates and hydralazine has been shown to improve mortality compared with placebo in systolic dysfunction (VHeFT I). However, this regimen is less effective than ACE inhibitors, and the increased dosing frequency and the higher incidence of adverse reactions makes it poorly tolerated.

- The main indication is for patients who do not tolerate ACE inhibitors and ARBs secondary to azotemia, hyperkalemia, or symptomatic hypotension.
- Consider an alternative in African Americans, who may respond less favorably to ACE inhibitors.
- Titrate hydralazine to a maximum of 100 mg tid and nitrates to 120–160 mg qd (doses used in trials).

5. **Beta blockers**. Most beta blockers studied (carvedilol in the U.S. Carvedilol Trials, metoprolol extended release in MERIT-HF, and bisoprolol in CIBIS II) were found to improve outcomes, including survival, in symptomatic systolic dysfunction (NYHA class II–IV) to a degree that rivals that seen with ACE inhibitors.

- Most other beta blockers have not been studied. Drugs with intrinsic sympathomimetic activity (e.g., pindolol and acebutolol) should be avoided.
- Patients should be clinically euvolemic and on stable doses of ACE inhibitors, diuretics, and other heart failure medications before therapy is initiated.
- Beta blockers should be started in all symptomatic patients unless contraindicated (class IV patients under consultative guidance of experienced cardiologist).
- Symptoms may worsen over first several weeks. Careful monitoring is necessary.
- Start at low doses (3.125 mg 2 times/day of carvedilol, 12.5 to 25 mg/day of metoprolol XL, 1.25 mg/day of bisoprolol).
- Improvement appears to be dose-dependent. Drugs should be uptitrated as possible (25–50 mg 2 times/day of carvedilol, 150 mg/day of metoprolol XL, 5–10 mg/day of bisoprolol).

6. **Digoxin**. Digoxin improves symptoms in patients with systolic dysfunction. It did not appear to affect total mortality in the large NIH-sponsored DIG trial. It is, therefore, indicated only in patients with symptomatic heart failure (NYHA class II–IV). It can also be useful for rate control in patients with atrial fibrillation.

- The usual maintenance dose of digoxin is 0.125–0.25 mg qd. However, digoxin is renally cleared and the dosage must be reduced in patients with renal dysfunction and in elderly patients.
- No evidence indicates that higher serum levels are more efficacious, and higher levels may increase risk of toxicity. We recommend maintaining levels between 0.7 to 1.2 ng/ml.
- Some evidence suggests digoxin may increase mortality in women and thus one should have a higher threshold for starting it in this population.

7. **Spironolactone**. The RALES trial demonstrated improved survival in patients randomized to spironolactone on top of standard medical therapy. However, only a small percentage of the patients in this trial were receiving beta blockers.

- Spironolactone is indicated in patients with advanced heart failure (NYHA class III–IV). Patients with less severe disease have not been studied.
- Patients must be monitored carefully for hyperkalemia, especially elderly patients and those with renal insufficiency. Spironolactone should be avoided in patients with a creatinine greater than 2.5 mg/dl.
- Male patients may experience gynecomastia/breast tenderness. Recently, more selective aldosterone blockers have been studied that limit this side effect.
- The usual maintenance dose is 25 mg/day. There is minimal diuretic effect at this dosage.

8. **Calcium channel blockers**. There is no direct role for calcium channel blockers in the management of systolic dysfunction. Verapamil and cardizem should be avoided given their negative inotropic effects with accompanying neurohormonal activation, especially of catecholamines. Second-generation dihydropyridines such as amlodipine and felodipine can be safely used in patients with systolic dysfunction if indicated for other conditions (e.g., angina or hypertension) based on the PRAISE and V-HeFT III trials, respectively.

9. **Warfarin**. Patients with systolic dysfunction are at increased risk of thromboembolic events, presumably due to stasis of blood in the dysfunctional left atrium and left ventricle.

- Warfarin is indicated in patients who have experienced a previous embolic event or who have paroxysmal or chronic atrial fibrillation.
- There are no published randomized trials of warfarin (or other antithrombotic agents) in heart failure. Nonetheless, some physicians recommend warfarin in selected patients with severely depressed systolic function (ejection fraction [EF] < 30%). The benefit of this practice is unclear. A trial is currently underway to evaluate this question.

10. Discuss pharmacologic therapy for diastolic dysfunction.

Unlike with systolic dysfunction, no large randomized trials have assessed the effect of drug therapy in patients with diastolic dysfunction. The treatment remains empirical with little data available. That said, the following guidelines have been recommended:

- Diuretics should be used to reduce vascular congestion and improve symptoms. However, patients are often very sensitive to preload reduction with a fall in cardiac output and blood pressure. This scenario can lead to dizziness or syncope.
- Beta blockers and nondihydropyridine calcium channel blockers (particularly verapamil) may be beneficial by slowing heart rate. This increases the time available for LV filling and coronary blood flow, particularly during exercise. Calcium blockers may also have a direct lusitropic effect, leading to enhanced relaxation during diastole.
- ACE inhibitors and ARBs may be more effective than other antihypertensive agents in causing regression of left ventricular hypertrophy, which often contributes to diastolic dysfunction. These agents may also directly diminish myocardial stiffness.
- Digoxin is generally not recommended in these patients. However, in the DIG trial, digoxin appeared to reduce hospitalization in patients with preserved systolic function, suggesting a possible benefit in this population.

11. Discuss the role of device therapy.

A detailed review of pacemaker and implantable cardioverter defibrillator (ICD) therapy in heart failure is beyond the scope of this chapter. However, the following guidelines apply.

- An ICD is indicated for secondary prevention in patients with a history of sudden death or hemodynamically unstable ventricular arrhythmia.
- The role of an ICD for primary prevention is less clear. Data for ICD use in patients with coronary disease and severely depressed LV function are increasing. In contrast, data in patients with nonischemic cardiomyopathy are limited. Although the risk of ICD implantation

is not high, procedures that simply affect survival and not quality of life must be embarked upon in an older population with caution.

• Biventricular pacing improves symptoms in selected patients with systolic dysfunction who have a bundle-branch block. It should be considered in patients with prolonged QRS duration who remain severely symptomatic despite optimal medical therapy.

12. What are the surgical options for heart failure?

Elderly patients often can be reasonable candidates for surgical interventions. Surgery should be more strongly considered for patients with marked symptoms or limited prognosis due to cardiac condition. Furthermore, they should have a reasonable functional status along with no other major comorbidities that would limit their recovery.

Surgical options include coronary artery bypass grafting for symptomatic coronary artery disease with left ventricular dysfunction. Surgical risk, including death, stroke, and infection, is higher in patients over 80 years of age and may be as high as 20%. Valve replacement surgery can also be performed. Patients greater than 80 years old have done quite well, especially with aortic valve replacement surgery for aortic stenosis. Cardiac transplantation in even the most aggressive centers is typically limited to patients who are under 70 years old, especially given the lack of organs available. However, a growing body of data potentially support the use of ventricular assist devices for patients who are older than 70 years of age with class IV heart failure but with a limited number of other medical issues.

13. Is there a best approach to end-of-life issues in an elderly patient with heart failure?

Heart failure is a progressive disease, and patients have variable but progressive decline of quality of life. The mortality associated with heart failure is also significant; patients with class IV heart failure due to systolic dysfunction have as high as a 50% 1-year mortality rate. In patients whose quality of life is markedly limited despite aggressive medical and surgical interventions, early discussions of potential end-of-life issues must be initiated. This is obviously even more important in the elderly population, in which there are fewer options to improve quality of life and survival.

The approach to end-of-life care will always be, in part, based on patient and family beliefs, but the treating physician should take an active role in this process to educate them about the symptomatic and progressive nature of heart failure to allow an educated decision regarding issues such as code status and even hospice care.

BIBLIOGRAPHY

1. Digitalis Investigation Group: The effect of digoxin on morbidity and mortality in heart failure. N Engl J Med 336:525, 1997.
2. Hunt SA, et al: ACC/AHA Guidelines for the evaluation and management of chronic heart failure in the adult. J Am Coll Cardiol 38:2101–2113, 2001.
3. Packer M, Bristow MR, Cohn JN, et al: The effect of carvedilol on morbidity and mortality in patients with chronic heart failure. US Carvedilol Heart Failure Study Group. N Engl J Med 334:1349–1355, 1996.
4. Pitt B, Segal R, Martinez FA, et al: Randomised trial of losartan versus captopril in patients over 65 with heart failure (Evaluation of Losartan in the Elderly Study, ELITE). Lancet 349:747–752, 1997.
5. SOLVD Investigators: Effect of enalapril on survival in patients with reduced left ventricular ejection fractions and congestive heart failure. N Engl J Med 325:293–302, 1991.

30. PERIPHERAL VASCULAR DISEASE

William Kavesh, MD, MPH

1. What is peripheral vascular disease?

Peripheral vascular disease (PVD) generally refers to arterial and venous disorders of the arms and legs. Lymphedema (swelling of an extremity caused by damage or obstruction to the lymphatic system) also falls within the broad category of PVD, but this chapter focuses on arterial and venous disorders.

2. Why is peripheral vascular disease important?

- **PVD is common.** Venous insufficiency affects up to 20% of adults and is especially common in the elderly. Complications include deep vein thrombosis and venous leg ulcers. Arterial disease of the lower extremities, known as peripheral arterial disease (PAD), generally affects the elderly and is about equally distributed between men and women in the elderly population. Among persons under age 70, however, the prevalence is higher in men. About 10–16% of adults over the age of 55 have evidence of PAD, and about two-thirds of these patients are asymptomatic.

- **PVD, especially PAD, is insidious.** Neither asymptomatic patients nor their physicians are usually aware that they have the disease, even though asymptomatic patients are at much higher risk for cardiovascular death than the general population. Progression of symptomatic disease is slow. After 5–10 years, more than 70% of patients report either no change or improvement in their symptoms, 20–30% have progressive symptoms requiring intervention, and less than 5% need amputation . Much less frequently, occlusive symptoms can have an abrupt onset, most often as the result of an embolism from the heart or other vessels.

- **PVD is a major source of morbidity.** Pain, impairment of the ability to walk, and chronic leg ulceration associated with either arterial or venous insufficiency can impair independence, radically alter the personal and work life of the afflicted person, and have life-threatening complications. The concurrent presence of both conditions can be particularly problematic to treat.

- **PAD is a harbinger of serious vascular disease elsewhere in the body.** At least 10% of patients with lower extremity arterial disease have cerebrovascular disease, and 28% have coronary heart disease. The 5-year mortality rate for patients with symptomatic arterial insufficiency is 30%; 75% of this mortality is due to coronary or cerebrovascular events. Asymptomatic patients with evidence of PAD also have up to a fourfold increase in risk of all-cause mortality.

3. Who gets PVD?

PVD is a disease of elderly people, patients with hypertension or hyperlipidemia, smokers, and diabetics. Combinations of these risk factors are common and increase the chance that arterial insufficiency will develop. Reduction of risk factors is associated with improvement of symptoms or decrease in the progression of disease.

Frequency of Peripheral Vascular Disease Manifestations in Various Risk Groups

POPULATION AT RISK	CONDITION	RISK OF CONDITION
Elderly people	Varicose veins	50% prevalence > 65 yr 10% prevalence < 35 yr
	Claudication	1–2%prevalence < 50 yr 5% prevalence > 50 yr

(Cont'd.)

Frequency of Peripheral Vascular Disease Manifestations in Various Risk Groups (Continued)

POPULATION AT RISK	CONDITION	RISK OF CONDITION
Hypertensives	Claudication	Risk doubles in men Risk quadruples in women
Hyperlipidemia	Claudication	Risk doubles for cholesterol > 270 Present in almost half of PAD patients.
Smokers	PAD	Risk increases up to 8-fold Smoking plays a role in up to two-thirds of cases
Diabetics.	PAD Leg amputation	Up to 4-fold increase in risk Up to 7-fold increase in risk

4. How can you determine if someone has PVD?

Venous and arterial insufficiency present quite differently, although some manifestations, such as pain or ulceration, may occur in both diseases. History and physical examination are augmented by laboratory studies, particularly ultrasound, which provides detailed information about the degree of disease. Ultrasound can provide both anatomic data about the degree of obstruction and the rate of flow through a blood vessel. In the case of arterial disease, the most useful measurement for general screening is a measurement of flow known as the ankle-brachial index (ABI). This index is a measurement of the ratio of systolic blood pressure in the lower legs to systolic blood pressure in the arms. An ABI less than 0.90–0.95 indicates the presence of atherosclerotic disease. Symptoms do not usually appear until the ABI is less than 0.70.

5. What are the manifestations of venous disease?

- **Varicose veins.** Varicose veins may occur as a primary phenomenon related to obesity, prolonged standing (a professional hazard of surgeons, for example), or pregnancy. Familial predisposition also seems to play a significant role. Once the venous walls have separated from each other, the delicate valves that control blood flow do not fully close. Backward flow then can occur, increasing pressure on vessel walls and causing leakage of blood cells and other plasma components.
- **Venous insufficiency.** Once leakage of plasma components has occurred, the condition is known as venous insufficiency. It results in a cascade of findings that reflect progressive deterioration:
  1. **Rusty brown discoloration of the skin.** Discoloration is patchy at first, then confluent.
  2. **Leathery skin.** This condition may occur over time and skin ulcers may develop, either spontaneously or after minor trauma. Discoloration and ulceration typically develop in a region from the mid-calf to the ankles, known (primarily by the British) as the gaiter area. Ulceration can be chronic and debilitating. This manifestation is discussed in detail below.
  3. **Cellulitis** (either spontaneous or due to local trauma).
  4. **Discomfort, particularly in the dependent position.** Varicosities without other complications may simply produce an aching or burning sensation on standing. Once venous insufficiency develops, especially when considerable edema has accumulated, the patient may complain of heavy limbs and aching during ambulation. This symptom is usually relieved promptly on elevating the legs.
  5. **Deep vein thrombosis** (the most serious complication of venous insufficiency).
- **Abnormalities on laboratory assessment by ultrasound and other techniques.**

6. What laboratory tests aid in the diagnosis of venous diseases?

1. **Venogram**

Description: injection of radioopaque material into a vein in the foot, demonstrating the proximal veins sequentially for the presence of filling defects.

Advantage: gold standard for diagnosis of deep vein thrombosis

Disadvantage: extremely uncomfortable and cumbersome procedure

Frequency of use: rare; alternative may be magnetic resonance venography.

2. Ultrasound

Description: utilization of reflected high-frequency sound waves to visualize and measure blood flow in arteries or veins (duplex ultrasound)

Advantages

- Highly accurate in the diagnosis of venous blockage between the knee and the inguinal ligament. The sensitivity and specificity of duplex ultrasound for the diagnosis of thrombosis approach 95%.
- It is also a good modality for diagnosing chronic damage to the venous system, which may show abnormal flow patterns and anatomic changes even in the absence of acute thrombosis.

Disadvantages

- Less accurate in detecting disease below the knee. However, since pulmonary emboli are much less likely to occur from thrombosis below the knee, this shortcoming has not been considered major.
- Misleading results may occur in the presence of marked edema, severe congestive heart failure, or ascites.
- Duplex ultrasound requires imaging machinery and is therefore found mainly in radiology departments and vascular labs.

Frequency of use: currently the primary approach to the diagnosis of deep vein thrombosis.

3. Continuous-wave Doppler

Description: measures blood flow, which is occluded in deep vein thrombosis.

Advantage: devices are portable and less expensive.

Disadvantage: devices are not as accurate as duplex ultrasound.

Frequency of use: relatively infrequent. Continuous-wave Doppler should be used in locations distant from a radiology suite or vascular lab, and the patient should be moved to a facility with duplex ultrasound as soon as possible for a more accurate diagnosis.

7. What disorders may be confused with venous insufficiency?

The aching of venous insufficiency is a nonspecific discomfort when the legs are in the dependent position. In advanced cases with massive edema, pain on walking may occur. However, other conditions may also present with discomfort and should be considered.

Key guideline: Elderly patients often present with more than one condition simultaneously. The final explanation for a particular symptom and its variations may involve the interaction of two or more of these conditions.

Differential Diagnosis of the Findings in Venous Insufficiency

CONDITION	DIFFERENTIATING FEATURES
Arthritis in legs	Arthritic pain usually localizes in joints and reproduces during physical examination.
	Improves with rest but not with elevation, as does the typical pain of venous insufficiency.
Lymphedema	Massive, nonpitting edema.
	Does not disappear overnight, as edema of venous insufficiency often does.
	Long-standing venous insufficiency may result in development of a brawny edema that may be hard to differentiate from lymphedema.
Muscular tears and other muscular conditions	Muscular conditions worsen with walking and do not improve with elevation.
Arterial insufficiency	Pain of arterial insufficiency improves with dependency.
	Ultrasound distinguishes the two conditions.

(Cont'd.)

Differential Diagnosis of the Findings in Venous Insufficiency (Continued)

CONDITION	DIFFERENTIATING FEATURES
Spinal stenosis	Arthritic condition of the lumbosacral spine; may present with pain in the legs on standing, but this pain typically starts in the back and radiates to the buttocks and then possibly the lower legs, whereas venous insufficiency presents with discomfort primarily in the lower legs. There should be no back pain with venous insufficiency unless two separate conditions are present.

8. What is deep vein thrombosis?

Deep vein thrombosis is an obstructive disorder of the veins, most often occurring in the lower extremities, although it may also occur in pelvic vessels. More superficial thrombophletis is increasingly seen as a complication of intravenous lines. Deep vein thrombosis can occur in legs already affected by venous insufficiency but can also be a cause of venous insufficiency. Damage to veins by an initial episode of deep vein thrombosis may predispose to recurrent episodes.

9. What factors predispose to deep vein thrombosis?

- Familial predisposition
- Occult or overt cancers
- Immobility
- Primary or medication related disorders of clotting factors
- Traumatic injuries
- Previous deep vein thrombosis

10. How do you diagnose deep vein thrombosis?

1. **Location:** commonly in the calf, thigh, or both.
2. **Manifestations**
   - Swelling and edema, usually unilateral, not always painful, in the lower leg; often exacerbated by walking.
   - Tenderness over veins; positive Homan's sign (pain on flexion of the calf muscles) common but imprecise.
   - *Key guideline:* always examine the area behind and proximal to the knee as well as the femoral triangle in the upper thigh, looking for spread.
3. **Complications:** deep vein thrombosis below the knee is much less likely to result in pulmonary embolization than deep vein thrombosis above the knee.
4. **Key diagnostic issues**

   Clinical diagnosis: Unreliable; confirmed by ultrasound in less than half of cases.

   Other diagnoses: Baker's cyst (posterior knee pain and swelling)

   Torn calf muscle (pain and swelling)

   Intra-abdominal obstruction (decreased venous outflow)

   Unilateral edema due to previous strokes, vein harvesting for bypass surgery (look for tell-tale leg scars), vein stripping for other reasons

   Key guideline: Unilateral edema due to previous stroke or vein harvesting may occur for many years or mainfest as new unilateral edema at the onset of congestive heart failure or other condition that eventually will produce bilateral edema as the condition worsens.

   Be aware of the many medications that can produce edema (e.g., NSAIDs, antihypertensive agents). The first manifestation may be unilateral edema in a patient already predisposed by a stroke or bypass surgery.

11. What are the stages of arterial insufficiency?

1. **Asymptomatic stage.** PAD may be asymptomatic for many years until a critical level of vessel occlusion develops. The degree of obstruction necessary to produce symptoms varies from person to person, and the ABI in symptomatic patients may vary from 0.40–0.70,

2. **Symptomatic stage**
   - *Intermittent claudication.* The classic symptom of peripheral arterial insufficiency is intermittent claudication. Patients describe a sensation of muscle tightness or aching, predictably brought on by exercise. The distance or time to the onset of pain is usually predictable. It is shortened on hills or stairs—and pain on walking uphill may be the first symptom. With progression of the disease, the time or distance to onset of pain may gradually shorten. An abrupt decrease in time or distance to onset of pain may suggest thrombosis or embolus, and prompt evaluation is indicated. Typically, the pain starts in the calf and may progress proximally. Pain starting initially in the buttocks or knee should prompt a search for other diagnoses such as spinal stenosis or arthritis in other joints; the differential diagnosis is described in more detail below. The pain ceases after a few minutes of rest but recurs when walking is resumed.
   - *Rest pain.* As the disease progresses, pain occurs at rest, at first when the leg is elevated; this pain typically is relieved by hanging the leg down—as opposed to the pain of venous insufficiency, which improves with elevation. In this situation, the person may also develop coexisting edema due to sleeping in a chair in an effort to prevent or reduce the pain. Eventually the pain occurs no matter what the patient tries to relieve it.
   - *Leg ulceration and gangrene.* Eventually, at the most advanced stages, skin breakdown may occur. At this point, diagnosis and treatment may be urgent.

12. What are the physical findings in arterial insufficiency?

1. **Asymptomatic phase.** Physical examination of the patient with PAD may show nothing abnormal prior to the onset of symptoms—even when laboratory studies may show evidence of 50–70% arterial occlusion.

2. **Symptomatic phase:** changes in pulse, temperature, and skin.
   - *Diminished or absent pulses.* Typically, by the time that symptoms begin, foot pulses are no longer palpable. The absence of pulses on physical examination is not necessarily a sign of critical occlusion. The opposite finding, however, can be helpful (i.e., the presence of foot pulses predicts the absence of significant occlusive disease). Examination of pulses proximal to the foot can also be useful. The popliteal pulse, located behind the knee and slightly laterally, can often be felt if the knee is flexed slightly by the examiner while the fingers are placed firmly into the popliteal space. Femoral pulses can be found about halfway along and slightly distal to the inguinal ligament. In the presence of PAD, bruits are often readily heard over a femoral artery, even when the pulse is difficult to appreciate. When severe narrowing occurs, the bruit may disappear—a significant sign in a patient who is known to have a prior bruit.
   - *Temperature.* The temperature of the feet is useful in certain circumstances. Cool feet may simply represent a benign condition of excessive vasomotor tone. In this situation, both feet are usually cool. If one foot is cool or significantly cooler distally, the likelihood of significant PAD increases.
   - *Skin color and character.* Dependent rubor is a condition of intense vasodilation that is the response of the superficial circulatory system to inadequate flow. In this situation, the toes, or typically the toes and a portion of the distal foot, become reddened with dependency. The skin may also become atrophied and shiny in the chronically ischemic foot. In advanced stages, ulceration may develop, which may be quite painful. Ischemic ulcers are discussed further in the section on foot ulceration.

3. **Maneuvers to assist examination.** Timed pallor and venous refilling are useful at the bedside, although they have been superceded to some extent by laboratory flow studies that are described later in more detail.

- *Timed pallor.* Examination for pallor is carried out by elevating both feet above the level of the heart. The foot is then held up for 1 minute. The absence of pallor indicates normal foot circulation. Pallor appearing within 30 seconds of elevation suggests significant occlusive disease. Pallor without elevation suggests severe PAD.
- *Venous refill time.* Once measurements of the feet are made in the elevated position, the feet are lowered and the time to venous refilling is measured. Refilling within 15 seconds indicates normal arterial circulation; at up to 30 seconds, moderate disease; and more than 40 seconds, severe disease.

13. What laboratory tests aid in the diagnosis of arterial insufficiency?

1. **Ankle-brachial index (ABI)**

Description: A continuous-wave Doppler device is used to measure pressures in both arms and legs. These devices are portable and inexpensive and can be carried in a coat pocket. The blood pressure cuff is placed sequentially on both upper arms and above the ankle; the Doppler recorder is positioned over an artery just distal to the cuff. The highest brachial arm pressure is chosen. The ratio of the ankle to arm pressure is measured. Because pressures in the legs are slightly higher than those in the arms, an ABI of 1.0–1.2 is normal. An ABI greater than 1.2 can occur in the presence of calcified vessels, which do not compress unless high pressures are applied. The calcifications can sometimes be felt on examination or seen on an x-ray. In such cases, the pressure should be measured in the toe, which is less likely to have calcification. The normal toe:brachial index is above 0.60. An ABI less than 0.95 is abnormal. Symptoms and signs associated with lower ABIs are summarized in the table below. There is no absolute cutoff, and the ABI that correlates with the onset of particular symptoms may vary from person to person.

Clinical Correlates of the Ankle-brachial Index

SIGNIFICANCE	ABI
Normal	> 0.90–0.95
Claudication	0.40–0.70
Rest pain	0.30–0.50
Tissue at risk of necrosis	< 0.30

Advantage: ABI is a simple concept that has become the standard test for detecting and following arterial insufficiency over time.

Disadvantage: ABI requires a skilled person to perform the test and avoid errors caused by calcified vessels.

Frequency of use: standard test for arterial insufficiency.

2. **Segmental pressure**

Description: Pressure measurements in the thigh and calf by using a blood pressure cuff and Doppler device in the same way that the ABI is measured. Thigh, calf, and ankle indices are known as segmental pressures.

Advantage: can be followed over time and correlated with symptoms.

Disadvantage: same as ABI.

Frequency of use: common.

3. **Color ultrasound and magnetic resonance angiography (MRA)**

Description: Color ultrasound has become a standard method of measuring the anatomic features of an artery. Flow patterns detected on ultrasound also provide important information. MRA is increasingly used to provide a detailed picture of the vascular system.

Advantage: noninvasive.

Disadvantage: If bypass surgery is being considered, arteriography is usually required to define the anatomy most precisely.

4. **Exercise testing.** This approach may be helpful when more than one cause of exercise-induced leg pain is considered (e.g., spinal stenosis and PAD). If the onset of symptoms correlates with a striking drop in systolic pressure at the ankle, the diagnosis of PAD is confirmed.

5. **Transcutaneous oximetry.** This test measures oxygen diffusion from the skin. Transcutaneous oxygen values reflect the patency of small vessels and may be helpful in diabetes and in predicting tissue viability.

14. What conditions may mimic arterial intermittent claudication?

Conditions That Mimic Arterial Claudication

CONDITION	DIFFERENTIATING FEATURES
Spinal stenosis	Back pain and buttock pain on standing relieved by lumbar flexion
Arthritis of the hips	Hip and buttock pain on passive hip motions
Trochanteric bursitis	Tenderness over the greater trochanter
Arthritis of the knees	Knee pain on standing
Baker's cyst	Popliteal mass on exam and ultrasound
Polymyositis	Proximal muscle pain and weakness
Venous claudication	Relief with elevation of the leg; venous dilatation, cyanotic hue, and edema
Painful peripheral neuropathy	Pain persists even when activity ceases

In elderly people, the major differential consideration is lumbar spinal stenosis. This disorder, due to bony encroachment on the cauda equina or spinal nerve roots, causes pain and paresthesias in the back, buttocks, and further down the leg in the distribution of the involved nerves. Pain typically begins when the patient is standing, is exacerbated by walking and lumbar extension, and is relieved by leaning forward (which reduces pressure on spinal outflow)—the "supermarket cart" sign. Bilateral leg pain is common. About 75% of patients report numbness or paresthesia, and 80% or more may report weakness. Relief of neurogenic claudication is said to take up to 10 minutes as compared with the pain of PAD, which resolves after a few minutes of rest. Reproduction of symptoms on extension and positive findings on MRI usually confirm the diagnosis.

15. What do leg ulcers have to do with peripheral vascular disease?

Leg ulcers complicate both venous and arterial disease, usually at an advanced stage. They also may occur in a number of other conditions, including neuropathic conditions such as diabetes, pressure over bony prominences, hypertension, vasculitis, hemolytic anemias, dermatologic conditions, warfarin necrosis, and neoplasms. Certain features may aid in diagnosing the cause of a leg ulcer, including location, presence or absence of pain, rate of development, and appearance of the ulcer.

Atypical presentations are not uncommon. Treatment of venous and arterial ulcers is discussed in the next section. Treatment of other types of ulcers is also mentioned briefly in the next section.

Characteristics of Leg Ulcers

TYPE	LOCATION	PAIN	PROGRESSION	APPEARANCE
Arterial	Lateral ankle/distal	+	Slow	Sharp, necrotic, dryer
Venous	Medial ankle	–	Fast	Irregular, shallow, moist
Neuropathic	Distal	–	Slow	Deep, infected, rim of callous skin
Pressure	Feet, ankles, knees	–	Slow	Shallow to deep
Hypertensive	Posterolateral legs	+	Fast	Similar to arterial
Vasculitic	Distal legs	+	Fast	Similar to arterial, blue/red rim
Hemolytic	Ankles	+	Slow	Similar to arterial, multiple

(Cont'd.)

Characteristics of Leg Ulcers (Continued)

TYPE	LOCATION	PAIN	PROGRESSION	APPEARANCE
Dermatologic	Shins/calves	±	Slow	Blistering(pemphigoid) Necrotic (diabetic necrobiosis) Papular (pyoderma)
Warfarin	Shins/calves	+	Fast	Purpuric
Neoplastic	Shins/calves	±	Slower	Irregular(squamous cell, lymphoma) Alligatored (Kaposi's sarcoma, non-HIV)

16. What treatments are helpful for venous insufficiency?

1. **Prevention.** The keys to prevention are weight loss, position change, and moisturizing creams and steroid creams to reduce scratching and risk of skin ulceration and infection.

2. **Elastic stockings.** Standard stocking pressures for various conditions are described in the table below. For patients whose legs do not fit standard sizes, custom compression stockings are available. Stockings should be replaced at about 6 months because most stockings lose much of their elasticity by then.

Pressures of Elastic Stockings for Various Conditions

CONDITION	PRESSURE OF STOCKING
Standing with little movement (e.g., surgeons, guards)	20 mmHg
Varicose veins	20–30 mmHg at ankles, gradual reduction toward knees
Previous ulcerations	40–50 mmHg at ankles

Difficulties with elastic stockings include putting them on, especially for older patients with arthritis or a previous stroke that limits movement and strength. Solutions include rubber globes to improve grip and frames on which the stockings can be stretched, with the leg inserted as if putting on a boot and the frame removed. Zippered stockings and Velcro wraps have their advocates.

3. **Pneumatic compression devices.** These devices can be quite effective in reducing edema, especially when some component of lymphedema is present. They also may be combined with elevation of the affected leg.

17. Outline the principles of treatment for venous ulcers.

Treatment of leg ulcers approaches an art form. New agents become available on a regular basis.

Treatment of Venous Ulcers

TREATMENT	COMMENT
Elevation	Reduces edema. Lie in bed several times a day with legs on pillow above heart. Elevation of legs on a stool is not helpful.
External compression	Determine first that arterial circulation is intact by exam or arterial Doppler. Apply Unna boot (see description below)
Absorption of exudate	Unna boot is generally adequate. For exuberant exudate, treat for a short period with absorptive dressing such as calcium alginate.
Antibiotic treatment of secondary cellulitis	Treat when spreading redness and tenderness appear. Oral antibiotics are usually sufficient. Cover for skin pathogens.
Prevention of recurrence	Elastic stockings, fitted if necessary (e.g., Jobst) for atypical leg shapes; treat medical problems that produce edema; antipruritic, moisturizing agents.

Unna boots (named for the physician who invented them) are external compression bandages impregnated with zinc oxide and other elements to absorb exudate. They are applied like a cast from the foot to just below the knee and then covered with an Ace bandage to hold the bandages firmly in place. If the ulcer has a great deal of exudate or debris, it may be treated with absorptive dressings such as calcium alginate for a short period before starting Unna boot treatment. The Unna boot is usually changed on a weekly basis until the ulcer is healed, then replaced with an elastic compression stocking. When conscientiously applied and monitored, Unna boots can heal over 90% of venous ulcers, but full healing often takes months. Other modalities have been tried, but Unna boots seem to have the best record of success. For very large venous ulcers, some surgeons have had success with skin grafting to hasten the healing process.

18. What treatments are effective for deep vein thrombosis?

1. **Immediate anticoagulation.** Unfractionated heparin remains the treatment of choice and should be started immediately on diagnosis or prior to diagnosis if definitive diagnosis will be delayed. In patients at high risk for bleeding, a vena caval filter may be placed to prevent pulmonary embolization. Leg elevation and warm soaks often make the patient feel more comfortable. Low-molecular-weight heparin is a safe and effective alternative for selected patients and may be especially helpful for home-bound patients. Low-molecular-weight heparin requires less monitoring, but present formulations must be administered twice daily by injection; therefore, it is suitable only when trained personnel are available.

2. **Chronic anticoagulation.** As soon as the heparin dose is stabilized or at the outset of treatment with low-molecular-weight heparin, patients should be started on warfarin (Coumadin) unless there is a contraindication to long-term anticoagulation. Laboratory services are usually available in most urban and suburban areas to draw blood at home for monitoring of home-bound patients. Demented patients who live alone or have poor support systems may be unable to manage a medication with such a narrow therapeutic index as warfarin. Chronic fallers who injure their heads may be at risk of subdural hematoma. In such situations, a vena caval filter may be the best choice. Patients should be advised that over-the-counter GI-irritant drugs such as NSAIDs should be avoided, although low-dose enteric-coated aspirin can be prescribed for cardiac prevention. The international normalized ratio (INR) is traditionally maintained at about 2.0–3.0. Controversy exists as to whether a lower target INR of 1.5–2.0 may also provide effective coagulation. The length of time that a person must remain on warfarin after deep vein thrombosis remains somewhat unclear. However, longer treatment times have become commonplace. Current treatment recommendations are summarized in the table below.

Duration of Therapy for Deep Vein Thrombosis

TIME INTERVAL	INDICATION
3–6 mo	First DVT with reversible or time-limited risk factor: surgery, trauma, transient immobilization or estrogen use
6 mo–2 yr, possibly longer	Idiopathic DVT, first event
12 mo to lifetime	Recurrent event, idiopathic or with thrombophilia First event with cancer until resolved, anticardiolipin antibody, antithrombin deficiency

DVT = deep vein thrombosis.
Adapted from Hyers TM, et al: Antithrombotic therapy for venous thromboembolic disease. Chest 119: 176S–193S, 2001.

3. **Treatment of precipitants.** Discontinuation of drugs, treatment of cancer, and changes in lifestyle may be necessary to reduce the likelihood of recurrence.

19. Outine the five elements in the treatment of PAD.

1. **Reduction of risk factors.** Treatment of hyperlipidemia with statins improves pain-free walking time and may have other beneficial effects. Poor control of diabetes and hypertension are associated with progression, as is continued smoking.

2. **Protection and care of the feet.** Small injuries, maceration of tissue between the toes due to poor hygiene, and pressure from poorly fitting shoes can predispose to the development of foot ulcers that may take months to heal (if they heal at all). If concurrent peripheral neuropathy due to diabetes, alcohol, or another cause complicates the picture, patients may not recognize significant injuries. Daily foot checks, regular podiatry care, and protection of pressure sites are mandatory, especially in bedbound or chairbound patients. Air mattresses for prophylaxis, alternating pressure mattresses or special beds for active ulcers, and aggressive debridement of necrotic tissue surgically or enzymatically also may be needed to promote healing. Hydrocolloid dressings may then be applied to keep the wound moist and to provide protection against further pressure. Ulcers with a neuropathic component are often deep and painless. They may be particularly resistant to treatment, especially in the setting of PAD. The same principles apply as for ulcers due to vascular insufficiency.

3. **Exercise.** Walking programs consisting of as little as 20–30 minutes four or five days per week have been shown to significantly increase walking distance. Every patient who can walk should participate in a structured walking program. Use of a treadmill is recommended, but even walking outside is better than nothing.

4. **Medical therapy.** Antiplatelet agents are the mainstay of medical therapy for PAD. Clopidogrel was demonstrated to be more effective than aspirin in one large study, but aspirin was almost as good. Combining the two appears to confer additional benefit. Cilostazol, a recently released and highly expensive drug, also has been shown to improve walking distance. Dipyridamole has no demonstrable effect, according to a number of studies. Pentoxifylline has trace if any effect on improving claudication symptoms compared with placebo.

5. **Revascularization.** Revascularization is indicated for rest pain, nonhealing ulcers, or patients who must walk to earn a living or find the limitations of their situation intolerable. Angioplasty and stenting can be done with low morbidity. Bypass techniques continue to improve, although distal vessels still have a high rate of restenosis due to low flow.

CONCLUSION

Peripheral vascular disease is a source of major, and unnecessary, morbidity and mortality. Prudent screening and attention to the early manifestations of both venous and arterial disease could improve the lives of many persons who now suffer the complications of these disorders.

BIBLIOGRAPHY

1. Criqui MH, et al: Mortality over a period of 10 years in patients with peripheral arterial Ddsease. N Engl J Med 326:381–385, 1992.
2. Hyers TM, et al: Antithrombotic therapy for venous thromboembolic disease. Chest 19:176S–193S, 2001.
3. Weitz JI, et al: Diagnosis and treatment of chronic arterial insufficiency of the lower extremities: A critical review. Circulation 94:3026–3049, 1996.
4. Wennberg PW, Rooke TW: Diagnosis and management of diseases of the peripheral arteries and veins. In Fuster V, Alexander RW, O'Rourke RA, et al (eds): Hurst's The Heart. New York, McGraw-Hill, 2001.
5. Young, JR, Olin JW, Bartholomew JR: Peripheral Vascular Diseases. St. Louis, Mosby, 1996.

31. RHEUMATOLOGIC CONDITIONS IN THE ELDERLY

Edna P. Schwab, MD

1. What are the characteristic features of polymyalgia rheumatica?

Polymyalgia rheumatica is a common cause of musculoskeletal pain in older individuals. The etiology is unknown. In a survey of Olmsted County, Minnesota, conducted by the Mayo Clinic, its prevalence was found to be 700/100,000 persons over age 50. Most patients are at least 50 years old. Female sex predominates by a ratio of 2.5:1.

Bilateral aching and stiffness of the shoulder girdle and upper arms, neck and torso, hip girdle, and thigh muscles in association with constitutional symptoms and an elevated Westergren erythrocyte sedimentation rate (ESR) characterize polymyalgia rheumatica. These symptoms are most common in the morning and frequently are associated with malaise, weight loss, and low-grade fever. Physical examination is remarkable for tenderness and limitation of motion of the shoulders and hips. Weakness, however, is not evident. Synovitis has been demonstrated by arthroscopy and biopsy of shoulder joints. More recently, swelling and pitting edema of the distal extremities have been described in a small subset of patients similar to what is seen in remitting symmetrical seronegative synovitis with pitting edema. The diagnosis of polymyalgia rheumatica is made when symptoms of pain and morning stiffness are present for at least one month and other diagnostic possibilities have been excluded.

The onset of polymyalgia rheumatica may be gradual but more often is sudden. This condition rarely responds to nonsteroidal anti-inflammatory drugs and often requires the initiation of corticosteroids. Low doses of prednisone (10 mg/day) usually result in an excellent therapeutic response. Polymyalgia rheumatica is a self-limited disease but also may have a more prolonged course. In patients whose ESR is normal, the diagnosis is made if characteristic symptoms are present and the response to prednisone is rapid and complete. Sometimes, it may be difficult to distinguish between the diagnosis of polymyalgia rheumatica and rheumatoid arthritis because of the similarities in presentation and lack of positive serologies in older patients. A high index of suspicion should be maintained for a closely associated disease, temporal arteritis, which occurs in 15–20% of patients with polymyalgia rheumatica.

2. Which laboratory findings are characteristic of polymyalgia rheumatica?

The ESR is often elevated to > 40 mm/hr and commonly to > 100 mm/hr. Evidence of an anemia due to chronic disease along with mildly elevated liver function abnormalities is usually present. Radiographs of the joints may demonstrate soft-tissue inflammation without evidence of erosions.

3. Define giant cell arteritis and describe its features.

Giant cell arteritis is a large-vessel vasculitis that often affects the vessels of the aortic arch. It has a reported prevalence of 200/100,000 people over age 50, as surveyed by the Mayo Clinic in Olmsted County, Minnesota. Superficial vessels, such as the occipital and external carotid and its branches, including the temporal, lingual, and facial arteries, may be involved. Deeper vessels also may be affected, including the vertebral artery and internal carotid along with its branches. Vessels lacking elastic tissue, such as the intracranial arteries, are spared. Most often, however, the branches of the aorta, occipital, or temporal artery become inflamed, with patients developing symptoms associated with the involved vessels.

Common symptoms consist of occipital or temporal headaches in 90% of patients, along with jaw claudication and tenderness over the temporal artery. Diplopia may occur as a result of ischemia to the extraocular muscles. The most dreaded complication is irreversible visual loss, which occurs in 15% of patients, most commonly due to ischemic optic neuritis with involvement of the ciliary branches of the internal carotid. Stroke and TIA are rare complications of giant cell arteritis. Other neurologic manifestations may include peripheral neuropathies and mononeuropathy. As in polymyalgia rheumatica, these symptoms are often accompanied by constitutional symptoms of fever, malaise, anorexia, and weight loss. These nonspecific symptoms often prompt an evaluation for an occult malignancy. Polymyalgia rheumatica may be present in up to 60% of cases of giant cell arteritis.

4. Which laboratory and histologic features are diagnostic for giant cell arteritis?

In a patient who has characteristic findings of giant cell arteritis, laboratory evaluation usually demonstrates an elevated ESR at least > 50 mm/hr but usually > 100 mm/hr. Anemia and mildly elevated liver function tests also may be present. However, a normal ESR may be present in up to 22% of cases of giant cell arteritis, making the diagnosis more challenging. The C-reactive protein is a more sensitive test of disease activity in addition to elevated ILG levels. The latter is not used in routine clinical practice.

The diagnosis is made by a temporal artery biopsy demonstrating destruction of the internal elastic lamina associated with granulomatous inflammation. Histologic examination reveals areas of inflammation of the media and fragmentation of the elastic lamina of the artery. This pattern of involvement follows those vessels that contain internal elastic lamina. Granulomas contain lymphocytes, histiocytes, and giant cells. Inflammatory edema or thrombus may occlude the vessel, leading to ischemic symptoms typically seen in this disorder. It is important to remember that the entire vessel is generally not involved. Skip lesions, areas of inflammation interspersed with normal-appearing vessel, may be found on a temporal artery biopsy. Biopsies should include at least 1 inch of vessel. Although biopsies may still remain positive after 2 weeks of treatment, they should be obtained prior to initiating therapy.

5. How is giant cell arteritis treated?

When the diagnosis of giant cell arteritis is considered, temporal artery biopsy should be obtained. Treatment should be started promptly with high-dose corticosteroids, at least 40–60 mg/day of prednisone, and continued after the diagnosis is confirmed. Solumedrol, 1 gm/day intravenously for 3 days, is given when visual loss is a concern. Symptoms as well as ESR should determine the tapering schedule. Clinicians also should start appropriate therapies, such as calcium and vitamin D, to lessen the toxicity of corticosteroids. To date, steroid-sparing agents such as methotrexate had conflicting results but may be useful in patients who require prolonged high-dose steroids.

6. What are the characteristic features of elderly-onset rheumatoid arthritis?

Rheumatoid arthritis (RA) is a chronic inflammatory disease involving the synovium that may be accompanied by systemic manifestations of fever, malaise, fatigue, and weight loss. The etiology of the disease is unknown. Typically, it affects patients during the third to fifth decades of life with a prevalence rate of 0.3–3%. Women are affected more often than men with a ratio of 2:1 to 3:1. The prevalence of RA increases with age. The proportion of affected men also rises with age. Patients with long-standing RA often have more severe disease with extraarticular manifestations, joint deformities, and comorbidities.

Patients who develop RA after age 60 generally have been perceived to have milder arthritis, lack rheumatoid nodules, and are rheumatoid factor-positive in only 32–58%, unlike disease seen in younger patients. Patients with RA gradually develop symmetric pain, swelling, and stiffness in peripheral joints, sparing the distal interphalangeal joints. Occasionally, RA presents acutely. In hemiplegic patients, the paralyzed side is not affected by the disease. In the elderly patient, large joints, such as shoulders, are more frequently affected and may be mistaken for polymyalgia rheumatica. In general, the features of polymyalgia rheumatica and remitting seronegative symmetric synovitis with pitting edema and rheumatoid arthritis overlap. Often an immediate response to low-dose steroids help to distinguish polymyalgia rheumatica from other disorders. Studies evaluating the prognosis of elderly-onset RA have been contradictory. Most early studies describe a rapid decline, whereas more recent reports describe a more benign course. Other diagnostic considerations in the elderly patient who develops an acute symmetric polyarticular synovitis include pseudogout, polyarticular gout (especially in women on diuretics), systemic lupus erythematosus, and paraneoplastic disease.

7. How often does systemic lupus erythematosus occur in older adults?

Systemic lupus erythematosus (SLE) may present in 15–20% of elderly patients with women being more frequently affected. Unlike the female-to-male ratio of 5–8:1 that is found in the younger population, the ratio is 2:1 in the elderly. The disease in the elderly also is milder, with manifestations of serositis, joint pain, interstitial lung disease, and sicca symptoms being more common. Central nervous system (CNS) involvement and renal disease are less frequent. Laboratory tests may include a positive antinuclear antibody (ANA), low complement levels, and positive antibodies to ds-DNA, SS-A, SS-B or Sm. Healthy older adults may have a low-titer positive ANA present in their serum without evidence of any systemic disease.

Drug-induced SLE occurs more commonly in the elderly and should alert the physician to detect the causative agent. Inciting drugs include procainamide, hydralazine, and isoniazid. Antihistone antibodies, in addition to a positive ANA, are found in 70–95% of patients. Symptoms resemble those seen in older-onset SLE.

8. What are the features of primary Sjögren's syndrome?

Primary Sjögren's syndrome is a frequent diagnosis in elderly patients who present with sicca symptoms. Patients often complain of grittiness in their eyes and dryness of their mouth associated with odynophagia. Polyarthritis, arthralgias, myalgias, fever, and fatigue may be accompanying symptoms. Systemic manifestations of vasculitis, interstitial nephritis, Raynaud's phenomenon, interstitial lung disease, hypothyroidism, and central and peripheral nervous system involvement occur infrequently.

9. What is rheumatism?

Many elderly patients complain of having "rheumatism" when they describe generalized musculoskeletal pain. Rheumatism refers to painful, nondeforming, nonsystemic musculoskeletal conditions that arise from soft tissue, bursa, ligaments, and tendons rather than bone or joints. Rheumatism may be localized to a bursa or tendon or to a region such as the neck or back or may be generalized as in fibromyalgia syndrome.

10. Which conditions are associated with nonarticular or soft-tissue rheumatism?

Soft-tissue rheumatism is another entity frequently reported in the elderly. It refers to conditions such as fibromyalgia, bursitis, tendinitis, low back pain, and cervical spine pain syndromes. It is important to realize that low back pain may be due simply to back strain but also may have more serious causes, including compression fractures secondary to osteoporosis or primary or secondary malignancies such as multiple myeloma and metastatic cancer. Other common soft-tissue conditions in the elderly include rotator cuff tendinitis, which may result in severe shoulder pain that radiates to the elbow and impairs range of motion of the shoulder. Elderly men and women may develop adhesive capsulitis that results following a period of inactivity of the shoulder. The presentation is that of progressive stiffness and discomfort of the shoulder with limitation of motion. Pain often occurs with movement.

11. Describe the fibromyalgia syndrome.

Fibromyalgia syndrome (FMS) is a noninflammatory musculoskeletal disorder manifested by chronic widespread pain and dysregulation of neuroendocrine function and sleep. Associated symptoms include stiffness, fatigue, memory and concentration difficulties, subjective hand puffiness, dizziness, headaches, Raynaud's phenomenon, paresthesias, sicca symptoms, irritable bowel and bladder syndrome, and disrupted sleep. Criteria for diagnosis of FMS have been established by the American College of Rheumatology and include widespread pain present for at least three months and pain on digital palpation in 11 of 18 tender point sites. Laboratory and radiographic studies frequently are unremarkable. FMS has not been well studied in the elderly, although recent estimates have demonstrated a rising prevalence rate among the elderly. Wolfe demonstrated rates of 2% among 30- to 39-year-olds, 5.6% among 50- to 59-year-olds, and 7.4% among 70-year-olds. Fibromyalgia was found to be 6 times more prevalent among women over the age of 50 years than men. The increased frequency seen in the elderly may be due to the rising presence of other musculoskeletal pain disorders contributing to persistent nociceptive input and sustained hyperalgesia. Fibromyalgia may coexist with other rheumatologic disorders including osteoarthritis, rheumatoid arthritis, systemic lupus erythematosus, Sjögren's syndrome, and psoriatic arthritis. It also has been described in patients with chronic fatigue syndrome, hypothyroidism, and conditions associated with the administration or withdrawal of steroids.

12. How does reflex sympathetic dystrophy syndrome present?

Reflex sympathetic dystrophy occurs commonly in the elderly with diabetes or following trauma, cerebrovascular events, or peripheral nerve pathology. It presents with severe burning pain and swelling of an extremity, hand, or foot. Signs of vasomotor instability are often present, manifested by temperature changes, edema, sweating, and trophic changes of hair, skin, and nails. As the disorder progresses, skin and muscle atrophy occurs with the development of contractures and restricted motion. During the later stages of the disorder, radiographs of the extremity often reveal diffuse osteoporosis.

13. What are the common rheumatic manifestations of endocrinopathies and malignancies?

Endocrinopathies such as hypothyroidism may be associated with joint and muscle pain and stiffness. Weakness is not a prominent feature. Hyperthyroidism can present as a painless proximal myopathy or, infrequently, with soft-tissue swelling, clubbing, and periostitis called thyroid acropachy. Acromegaly frequently produces degenerative changes of cartilage. Carpal tunnel syndrome may be a manifestation of diabetes, hypothyroidism, and acromegaly. Diabetes also has been associated with diffuse idiopathic skeletal hyperostosis, Charcot joints, and limited joint mobility. Pseudogout has been associated with hypothyroidism and hyperparathyroidism.

Primary **malignancies** and metastatic tumors may present with polyarticular joint pain, and these diagnoses should be considered in patients with an abrupt onset of a rheumatologic condition. Lymphomas and leukemias may present in the elderly with synovitis that resembles rheumatoid arthritis or polymyalgia rheumatica. Hypertrophic osteoarthropathy may be seen with pulmonary malignancies and other cancers. Neoplasms have been associated with the development of polymyositis and dermatomyositis. In one series, 25% of cases were associated with neoplasia of the breast, lung, ovary, colon, stomach, and uterus.

14. What are the features of remitting seronegative symmetric synovitis with pitting edema?

This disorder primarily occurs in older men, with a male-to-female ratio of 2:1. It presents as an acute symmetric polyarthritis involving the wrists, flexor digitorum tendon sheaths, metacarpophalangeal joints, tarsal and metatarsophalangeal joints, and interphalangeal joints. Associated pitting edema of the hands, soft tissue swelling of the distal upper and lower limbs, and morning stiffness are present.

Constitutional symptoms are often absent. This disease may be closely related to seronegative rheumatoid arthritis. Synovial fluid is mildly inflammatory, and the ESR is often elevated. The disease occurs more often in autumn but can occur throughout the year. The overall prognosis is good, and response to treatment with low-dose prednisone is often immediate.

BIBLIOGRAPHY

1. Abu-Shakra M, Bukila D: Cancer and autoimmunity: Autoimmune and rheumatic features in patients with malignancies. Ann Rheum Dis 60(5):433–441, 2001.
2. Evans JM, Hunder GG: Polymyalgia rheumatica and giant cell arteritis. Clin Geriatr Med 14:455–473, 1998.

3. Goldenberg DL: Office management of fibromyalgia. Rheum Dis Clin North Am 28(2):437–446, 2002.
4. Lawrence RC, Helmick CE, Arnett FC, et al: Estimates of the prevalence of arthritis and selected musculoskeletal disorders in the United States. Arthritis Rheum 41:778–799, 1998.
5. Lockshin UD: Endocrine origins of rheumatic disease. Diagnostic clues to interrelated syndromes.
   Postgrad Med 11(4):87–88, 91–93, 2002.
6. McCarty DJ: Perspective syndrome of remitting seronegative symmetric synovitis with pitting edema. J
   Clin Rheumatol 1:203–204, 1995.
7. McGuire JL: The endocrine system and connective tissue disorders. Bull Rheum Dis 39(4):1–8, 1990.
8. Michet CJ, Evans JM, Fleming KC, et al: Common rheumatologic disease in elderly patients. Mayo Clin
   Proc 70:1205–1214, 1995.
9. Salvarani C, Cantini F, Boiardi L, Hunder GG: Polymyalgia pheumatica and giant cell arteritis. N Engl J
   Med 342:261–271, 2002.
10. Salvarani C, Gabriel S, O'Fallon WM, Hunder GG: Epidemiology of polymyalgia rheumatica in
    Olmsted County, Minnesota, 1970–1991. Arthritis Rheum 3:369–373, 1995.
11. Salvarini C, Hunder GG: Giant cell arteritis with low erythrocyte sedimentation rate: Frequency of oc-
    currence in a population-based study. Arthritis Rheum 45:140–145, 2001.
12. Van Schaardenburg D: Rheumatoid arthritis in the elderly. Prevalence and optimal management. Drugs
    Aging 7:30–37, 1995.
13. Van Schaardenburg D, Breedveld F: Elderly-onset rheumatoid arthritis. Semin Arthritis Rheum
    23:367–368, 1994.
14. Wolfe F, Ross K, Anderson J, et al: The prevalence and characteristics of fibromyalgia in the general
    population. Arthritis Rheum 38:19–28, 1995.

32. ARTHRITIS AND MUSCULOSKELETAL PAIN IN THE ELDERLY

Edna P. Schwab, MD

1. What changes occur in the aging joint and how are they related to the development of osteoarthritis?

Aging is a risk factor for the development of osteoarthritis. There are distinctions in the pathogenesis of the aging joint and the joint affected by osteoarthritis. Cartilage matrix is composed of predominantly type II collagen, proteoglycans consisting of a protein core, and side chains of the glycosaminoglycans chondroitin sulfate and keratan sulfate. Sixty percent of this tissue is composed of water. With aging one sees decreased strength and stiffness of this organized network. Tissue damage may occur secondary to the inability of cartilage to accommodate increased mechanical loading and result in increased fibrillations, erosions, and permeability to fluids. The increased water content within cartilage may predispose the joint to development of osteoarthritis. Aging also is associated with chondrocyte senescence, a state in which chondrocytes can no longer replicate. Although these cells remain metabolically active and respond to cytokines such as IL-1, as senescent cells accumulate their rate of synthesis and degradation appears to be reduced even among growth factors and cytokines. Currently, it is not clear if these changes predispose to osteoarthritis. Less is known about the aging changes found in subchondral bone and its association with osteoarthritis.

Periarticular muscles are the major shock absorbers protecting the joint. When a load occurs unexpectedly, damage can occur to the articular cartilage and subchondral bone rather than the load being absorbed by the muscle. Joint trauma has been linked to the development of osteoarthritis in this manner. As muscle mass and strength diminish with age, the joint may be predisposed to increased loads and joint injury. Quadriceps strengthening in the elderly may retard the rate of muscle loss, diminish pain, and improve gait and knee strength as well as decrease joint trauma.

In the joint affected by osteoarthritis, the dominant feature is cartilage loss. The water content of cartilage is increased, and inflammatory mediators, either derived from chondrocytes or synovial fluid, decrease proteoglycan composition and synthesis while degrading proteoglycans and collagens.

2. How prevalent are arthritic conditions in the elderly?

Arthritis and musculoskeletal disorders are two of the most prevalent chronic conditions among the elderly and are important public health problems among adults of working age. As the population ages, the prevalence of arthritis, with its negative impact on function, is expected to rise. In a study by Hughes, the most frequent musculoskeletal conditions diagnosed among a sample of elderly persons over age 60 were osteoarthritis (83%), old fractures (32%), and soft-tissue rheumatism (13%). Joint impairment was most frequently observed in the upper and lower spine (92%), hands (58%), feet (55%), knees (35%), and hips (20%). Joint impairment, pain, and psychological status all had an effect on predicting future disability.

3. What is the impact of pain?

Pain and limitation in motion from arthritis can restrict the independence of older persons by impairing their performance of activities of daily living (ADLs). Upper extremity impairment is more pronounced in men and significantly related to inability in performing ADLs, whereas lower extremity impairment is more common in women and is significantly related to impairment in instrumental ADLs. Both upper and lower extremity impairments occur in increased frequency in both sexes over the age of 80.

Data from the Longitudinal Study on Aging indicate that the extent of arthritis-related disabilities increases with time. These impairments were found to be strong risk factors for predicting adverse outcome, including nursing home care.

Prevention by the identification of risk factors preceding the development of musculoskeletal disorders, early diagnosis, and implementation of appropriate treatment will help to prevent or retard disability associated with arthritis and enhance an older person's quality of life. Symptoms in the elderly, however, may not be as apparent as in younger persons due to multiple coexisting conditions and cognitive impairment. A decline in function may not be perceived by a patient, family member, or staff members until impairment or disability is significant.

4. What are the causes of musculoskeletal symptoms in the elderly?

Symptoms of joint pain, limitation of motion, swelling, and morning stiffness are features of various arthritides. A thorough history with a review of systems and physical examination will help to differentiate the various rheumatic conditions in the elderly, such as those with articular or soft-tissue involvement (i.e., osteoarthritis, crystal arthropathies, periarthritis, tendinitis, bursitis, and entrapment neuropathies) from conditions that also have systemic manifestations. These conditions include infectious arthritides, polymyalgia rheumatica, giant cell arteritis, elderly-onset rheumatoid arthritis, and other connective tissue disorders. Appropriate radiographs and laboratory tests including synovial fluid analysis help to establish an early and accurate diagnosis.

5. Which is the most common form of chronic arthritis?

By far, the most common and disabling rheumatic condition in patients over 55 years of age is **osteoarthritis**. Radiographic changes often precede symptoms and frequently may not correlate well with symptoms until marked progression and cartilage loss occur. Approximately 65% of elderly patients have symptoms of joint pain, stiffness, and limitation in range of motion (ROM). Studies have demonstrated that 12% of elderly patients cannot perform ADLs as a result of pain and limitation from osteoarthritis. About half of these individuals end up confined to the bed or wheelchair. Predictors of disability include the severity of other coexisting diseases, visual or hearing impairment, functional capacity, social support, education level, income, and availability of social and home-care services. Anxiety, depression, and coping mechanisms also influence the development and severity of disability.

6. Describe the common symptoms and findings characteristic of osteoarthritis.

Joints that are commonly involved in osteoarthritis include areas of weight-bearing, such as the lumbar spine, hips, and knees. Hands (especially the first carpometacarpal joint), cervical spine, and feet (primarily the first metatarsophalangeal joints) are also commonly involved. Early morning stiffness, when present, characteristically lasts 10–30 minutes. Stiffness may occur following periods of inactivity, whereas pain often increases with activity and improves with rest. Patients may complain of buckling or instability as well as loss of motion. Musculoskeletal examination may reveal swelling, deformities, bony overgrowth (referred to as Heberden's and Bouchard's nodes when involving the distal and proximal interphalangeal joints of the hands, respectively), crepitus, limitation of motion, and synovial effusions. Muscle spasm, tendon contractures, and capsular contractures also may be observed depending on the site of involvement.

Cervical and lumbar pain may result from arthritis of the apophyseal joints, osteophyte formation, pressure on surrounding tissue, and muscle spasm. Radicular symptoms are caused by nerve root impingement. Cervical and lumbar stenosis develops when facet joints and the ligamentum flavum hypertrophy as a result of disc degeneration, which narrows the spinal canal causing compression of the cord. Anterior vertebral osteophytes also may contribute to cord compression. Patients may develop localized pain, extremity weakness, gait ataxia, or abnormal neurologic findings. Pseudoclaudication is a characteristic feature of lumbar stenosis and is described as pain in the buttocks or thighs occurring with ambulation and relieved by rest or lumbar flexion. Hip pain is usually felt in the groin or the lateral or medial aspects of the thigh; however, it can be referred to the knee or buttocks and may be misdiagnosed as lumbar stenosis.

7. What are the laboratory and radiographic findings in osteoarthritis?

Laboratory findings in osteoarthritis are usually normal. Radiographs classically reveal the presence of joint-space narrowing with subchondral sclerosis as an early finding. As arthritis progresses, the development of marginal osteophytes, subchondral bone cysts with sclerosis, and subluxation occurs. In advanced disease, loose bodies and subchondral bone collapse may be evident. Synovial fluid analysis reveals noninflammatory fluid (< 500 cells/ml).

8. What risk factors are associated with the development of osteoarthritis?

- Age (although not everyone develops pain and immobility)
- Genetic predisposition
- Female sex and menopausal status
- Obesity
- Ethnic/racial background
- Prior trauma
- Occupational knee bending/physical labor
- Abnormal biomechanics and physical loading (soccer players and weight lifters)
- Increased bone mineral density
- Quadriceps weakness (also implicated in the pathogenesis of the disease)
- Congenital abnormalities (Perthes' disease and congenital dislocation of the hip)
- Inflammatory conditions (crystal arthropathies, septic arthritis)
- Chondrocalcinosis
- Metabolic disorders (acromegaly and hemachromatosis)

9. How is osteoarthritis best managed?

Realistic goals need to be established with the patient. Pain often leads to deconditioning, loss of ROM and disability. The physician should educate the patient about arthritis prevention, exercise, joint protection, knee bracing, and incorporation of rest periods in order to alleviate pain and delay disease progression. Preventive techniques include identification of risk factors such as obesity and behavioral modification for weight loss, diminishing injury during exercise, and altering job demands in those who experience repetitive trauma and joint injury. The patient should be made aware of the various treatment options available for the management of osteoarthritis. The suggested course of management might include a combination of the following:

Nonpharmacologic Therapies

Exercise and Rehabilitation: Resting the joint for prolonged periods, especially in the elderly, may result in deconditioning, muscle atrophy, contractures, and osteoporosis. A supervised exercise program with a physical therapist and occupational therapist will help to strengthen weakened muscles and improve range of motion. An evaluation for appropriate assistive devices and appliances should be performed. Aerobic exercise, resistive exercise, and aquatic therapy have been demonstrated to improve function and disability in addition to decreasing pain. The application of **heat or cold packs** following exercise is often helpful. Acute inflammation responds to the application of cold, whereas chronic pain improves with heat. **Acupuncture** has been used for treatment, especially in Asian countries; however, controlled trials have not demonstrated significant improvement. **Transcutaneous electrical nerve stimulation, low-power laser therapy**, and **pulsed electric and electromagnetic fields** have not been extensively studied.

Psychological counseling: Relaxation techniques and biofeedback may be effective in diminishing the degree of pain in some affected patients. The older patient may require psychological counseling, especially if depression is evident. Persistent pain, disability, deformity, decline in function, and limited independence can often lead to depression. This depression can be exacerbated if the patient has sexual difficulties and/or is unable to work as a result of arthritis. The patient should receive psychiatric, sexual, or financial counseling if any of these situations arise.

Pharmacologic Therapy

Initiation of drug therapy should take into account the side effect profile of the drug, comorbidities of the patient, and potential drug interactions.

Analgesics

Acetaminophen is an effective analgesic agent used to treat osteoarthritis. It has fewer side effects than nonsteroidal anti-inflammatory drugs (NSAIDs) when used in therapeutic doses (4.0 gm/day) and is as effective as NSAIDs in many patients. Use in patients with liver disease or alcohol-induced cirrhosis should be monitored closely, and renal function should be assessed in chronic users of analgesics.

Opioids such as codeine, hydrocodone, and oxycodone may be used when conservative therapies are ineffective or when contraindications exist to the use of traditional NSAIDs. These are frequently used when there is bony collapse, as in avascular necrosis, or in situations involving nerve impingement.

Tramadol, a centrally acting analgesic, has also been found to be useful in controlling symptoms.

The practitioner using these agents should monitor for common adverse effects including delirium, dizziness, somnolence, and constipation, especially when used in patients who also take other centrally acting agents (i.e., antidepressants).

Analgesic/Anti-inflammatory Agents

NSAIDs are the most commonly prescribed agents to treat arthritis, but the elderly are at increased risk of adverse effects from these drugs, including acute renal failure, gastric ulceration and bleeding, cardiovascular effects, hepatotoxicity, and cognitive impairment. Patients using NSAIDs should be monitored closely for evidence of adverse reactions. Risk factors identified for the development of gastrointestinal complications include increasing age, history of peptic ulcer disease, concomitant corticosteroid or anticoagulant use, cigarette smoking or alcohol use, and ingestion of multiple NSAIDs. H_2 blockers or misoprostol, a prostaglandin E2 inhibitor, should also be prescribed in patients at high risk for gastrointestinal complications.

Cyclooxygenase-2 inhibitors (COX-2) have been promoted as safer alternatives to traditional NSAIDs in the treatment of pain due to their relative reduction in GI complications. Although controversial the enthusiasm for these agents is blunted by perceived increased risk in cardiovascular events. Further trials need to be conducted to evaluate the cardiovascular risks of these agents.

Antidepressants have been found to control chronic pain with some success when used in low doses. The blockage of serotonin reuptake augments the inhibitory pathways of the spinal tract, thereby inhibiting pain perception.

Intraarticular corticosteroid injections may be used to alleviate the pain from arthritis. These agents should not be used more than 3–4 times a year because of possible deleterious effects on cartilage. **Viscosupplementation with hyaluronic acid** derivatives also have been shown to provide superior relief when compared to intraarticular corticosteroids and NSAIDs.

Topical analgesic creams such as methylsalicylate or capsaicin, an inhibitor of the release of substance P from nerve terminals, have been helpful in alleviating joint pain. Side effects frequently encountered include burning at the site of application.

Alternative remedies have become increasingly popular among patients as a result of limited pain relief with the traditional agents available. **Glucosamine sulfate** and **chondroitin sulfate** have demonstrated improved symptom relief and limited studies have demonstrated diminished joint space narrowing. The mechanism of action for glucosamine is not yet known. Both are available in health food stores. Compared to ibuprofen, however, the effects of glucosamine were not statistically different. The role of antioxidants such as **vitamin C**, **vitamin E**, and **beta carotene** in preventing disease progression requires further investigation.

Investigational agents used to modify disease have yet to be established. These agents include enzyme inhibitors, growth factors, and cytokine inhibitors. Osteochondral grafts of chondrocytes and/or stem cells are in various stages of development.

Patients who have not benefited from conservative measures may benefit from invasive therapies, such as arthroscopy with joint debridement or lavage. The efficacy of lavage may result from the removal of debris and inflammatory mediators. Arthroplasty should be reserved for patients who continue to have persistent pain, loss of motion, and loss of function despite maximal medical management. The complication rate of this procedure is 2.5–3.5 times higher in the elderly than in younger patients. Thirty percent of older patients who are cognitively impaired experience a prolonged course of rehabilitation.

10. Which rheumatologic conditions can present with an acute monarthritis in the elderly?

When a joint becomes acutely inflamed and painful, it requires an immediate evaluation. Several arthritides can present with a single acutely swollen and painful joint:

Infectious arthritis	Neurogenic arthropathy (Charcot's joint)
Bacteria	Avascular necrosis
Mycobacteria	Tumor
Fungi	Systemic disease with monarticular flare
Spirochetes	(much less common)
Viruses	Rheumatoid arthritis
Crystal-induced arthritis	Systemic lupus erythematosus
Gout	Psoriatic arthritis
Pseudogout	AIDS
Hydroxyapatite disease	Inflammatory bowel disease
(Milwaukee shoulder)	Behçet's disease
Osteoarthritis	Reiter's syndrome
Foreign-body reaction	Reactive arthritis

11. What are the complications and mortality rate associated with septic arthritis?

Septic arthritis is the most life-threatening and destructive form of arthritis in all age groups. Joint destruction can occur in 1–2 days if the infection is unrecognized or inadequately treated. Approximately 25–40% of patients diagnosed with a septic arthritis are over age 60. Among the elderly, the mortality rate has been reported to be between 19 and 33%, as compared to 10% in the general adult population. Complications such as osteomyelitis, loss of joint motion and function, and osteoarthritis arise in the elderly. Three factors predicting poor outcome include old age, preexisting joint disease, and infected prosthetic joints.

12. Describe the clinical and diagnostic features of septic arthritis.

Physical findings include fever, joint swelling secondary to fluid distending the joint capsule, warmth, loss of motion, and severe pain. Constitutional symptoms may or may not be present. An investigation for an extraarticular site of infection should always be pursued.

Diagnosis is made by arthrocentesis of the involved joint. The presence of organisms on synovial fluid Gram stain or culture and evidence of an inflammatory synovial fluid help to confirm the diagnosis. Synovial fluid cell counts are often > 50,000 cells/mm^3 with > 80–90% neutrophils on the differential. Low white cell counts have also been reported, in the range of 6,000 cells/mm^3, but this is less frequent. Stains will be positive for organisms in approximately 75% of gram-positive infections and 50% of gram-negative infections. Other diagnostic tests include blood cultures, which may be positive in 25–78% of patients with nongonococcal bacterial arthritis but frequently negative in gonococcal arthritis. Appropriate imaging techniques, such as radiographs or MRI, should be obtained to evaluate for joint destruction and osteomyelitis. Antibiotic treatment should be started to cover organisms usually involved in septic arthritis. Treatment can be altered once culture results are available.

13. Which organisms are most commonly found in septic arthritis?

Gram-positive aerobes cause infection in approximately 85% of cases; *Staphylococcus aureus* accounts for 67%, *Streptococcus pneumoniae* for 3%, and non-group A, β-hemolytic streptococci for 15%. *Staphylococcus epidermidis* is frequently found in prosthetic joint infections. Gram-negative bacteria account for 18% of infections but also have been reported to occur in up to 30% of geriatric patients. Gram-negative and anaerobic infections are more commonly seen in parenteral drug users, immunocompromised hosts, and those with extremity wounds and GI cancers.

Although not considered common in the elderly, *Neisseria gonorrhoeae* can cause migratory arthritis, tendinitis, and acute monarthritis. This form of infectious arthritis is less destructive than that caused by nongonococcal organisms. *N. gonorrhoeae* needs to be considered in the elderly when appropriate clinical features are present. Tenosynovitis is the most frequent clinical presentation, although skin lesions in the form of pustules and macules also may be seen in two-thirds of the patients with disseminated gonococcal infection. In only 25% of patients with disseminated gonococcal infection will synovial fluid culture be positive.

Other agents, including fungi, viruses, spirochetes (Lyme disease), mycobacteria, and parasites, also have been reported to cause septic arthritis but usually have a more insidious course.

Microbiology of Septic Arthritis

ORGANISM	FREQUENCY
Gram-positive organisms	85%
Staphylococcus aureus	67%
Streptococcus pneumoniae	3%
Non-group A, b-hemolytic streptococci	15%
Gram-negative organisms	18%
Other agents	
Fungi	
Viruses	
Spirochetes	
Mycobacteria	
Parasites	

14. Discuss the pathogenesis of septic arthritis.

Septic arthritis most commonly occurs by hematogenous spread. Less frequent causes of infection include joint surgery, intraarticular injections, or penetrating trauma. The most common sites of infection involve the large joints, such as the knee and hip, but smaller joints also may be involved.

Risk factors predisposing the elderly patient to septic arthritis include:

Preexisting joint disease (rheumatoid arthritis and osteoarthritis)

Trauma

Intraarticular joint injection with glucocorticoids (infrequent; < 1/10,000 injections)

Concurrent extraarticular infection (skin, soft tissue, urinary tract, subacute bacterial endocarditis)

Illnesses or medications that impair host defenses:

Diabetes mellitus	AIDS
Chronic renal failure	Corticosteroid therapy
Cirrhosis	Cytotoxic agents

15. What are the common crystal-induced diseases in the elderly?

Crystal-induced arthritis often presents as monarticular arthritis. **Gout** is a metabolic disease characterized by recurrent attacks of arthritis affecting one or more joints of the extremity and is caused by deposition of monosodium urate crystals in the cartilage of synovial membrane, thereby provoking an inflammatory response. The prevalence of gout increases with age and approaches 4% among patients in the 50–74-year-old range. It frequently occurs in the first metatarsophalangeal (MTP) joint, ankle, metatarsals, or knee, although any joint may be involved. The involved joint is often extremely tender, hot, swollen, and red, resembling an acute infection.

Initial attacks are monarticular, but subsequent flares may be polyarticular and accompanied by fever. Tophaceous gout often occurs in elderly men, whereas diuretic-induced gout has been observed in elderly women. Diagnosis is made by demonstrating urate crystals in synovial fluid with a polarizing light microscope. Radiographs in early disease are usually normal, but in chronic disease they may demonstrate classic erosions with overhanging edges.

The prevalence of **calcium pyrophosphate deposition** (CPPD) disease, also called **pseudogout**, increases with age. Between the ages of 65 and 75 years, 10–15% of individuals have evidence of CPPD. This rate increases to 30–60% after age 85. Joints most commonly affected include the wrists and knees, but other joints also may be involved. The typical presentation is that of an acute self-limiting monarticular arthritis; however, asymptomatic disease with evidence of chondrocalcinosis on radiographs and a subacute chronic destructive arthropathy may develop. Radiographic changes often reveal the presence of chondrocalcinosis in the meniscus of the knee, the triangular ligament of the wrist, and occasionally the cartilage of the shoulder. Other findings resembling osteoarthritis include joint-space narrowing, bony sclerosis, subchondral cysts, and osteophyte formation. One should keep in mind that both gout and pseudogout also can present with a bursitis and tendinitis. Pseudogout has been associated with other conditions, including hypothyroidism, hyperparathyroidism, hemochromatosis, hypomagnesemia, and hypophosphatasia.

Apatite-induced arthritis, either secondary to hydroxyapatite (a component of bone) or other apatites, can cause an acute arthritis or periarthritis in joints affected by osteoarthritis. A rapidly destructive arthritis due to hydroxyapatite has been found in the elderly and is called **Milwaukee shoulder syndrome**, typically seen in women over age 70. Other joints, including the knee, also may be involved. The synovial fluid is often bloody with evidence of apatite crystals.

Common Crystal-Induced Arthritis

TYPE	CRYSTAL	PREVALENCE	PRESENTATIONS
Gout	Monosodium urate crystals	4% of 50–70 year olds	Most commonly affects first MTP joint, metatarsals, ankle, knee. Other joints may be affected. May be monarticular or polyarticular
CPPD	CPPD crystals	10–15% of 65–75-year-olds 30–60% after age 85	Commonly affects wrists, knees, but other joints may be affected. Usually monarticular but can be polyarticular
Apatite-induced arthritis	Hydroxyapatite or other apatite	Most common in 65–75-year-olds	Acute arthritis or periarthritis. Rapidly destructive arthritis called Milwaukee shoulder

16. How do you treat a crystal-induced arthritis?

Treatment of gout, pseudogout, and apatite disease is very similar. The first line of therapy is often an NSAID, which should be used cautiously in the elderly person, especially if other coexisting diseases are present. Prostaglandin analogs should be considered for gastric protection. Colchicine is used less often for the acute flare of crystal-induced arthritis but may be used for prophylaxis for gout and pseudogout. Systemic glucocorticoids also may be used in the acute attack, especially if polyarticular joint involvement is present or contraindications to NSAID use are present. Intraarticular corticosteroid injection is an alternative treatment if a single joint is involved. In chronic arthritis, treatment modalities are similar to those used for osteoarthritis. Allopurinol and probenecid are reserved for use in chronic gouty arthritis.

BIBLIOGRAPHY

1. AGS Panel on Persistent Pain in Older Persons: The management of persistent pain in older persons. Am Geriatr Soc 50:S205–S224, 2002.
2. Baker DG, Schumacher HR: Acute monoarthritis. N Engl J Med 329:1013–1020, 1993.
3. Brandt K, Smith CN, Simon CS: Intraarticular injections of hyaluronate in the treatment of patients with osteoarthritis of the knee: A randomized clinical trial. Arthritis Rheum 43:1192–1203, 2000.
4. Creamer P, Flores R, Hochberg M: Management of osteoarthritis in older adults. Clin Geriatr Med 14:435–454, 1998.
5. Hamerman D: Aging and the musculoskeletal system. Ann Rheum Dis 56:578–585, 1997.
6. Hughes SL, Dunlop D: The prevalence and impact of arthritis in older persons. Arthritis Care Res 8:257–267, 1995.
7. Lawrence RC, Helmick CG, Arnett FC, et al: Estimates of arthritis and selected musculoskeletal disorders in the United States. Arthritis Rheum 41:778–799, 1998.
8. McAdam PF, Ratella-Laawson F, Mardini IA, et al: Systemic biosynthesis of prostacyclin by cyclooxygenase (cox)-2: The human pharmacology of selective inhibitor of cox-2. Proc Natl Acad Sci USA 96:272–277, 1999.
9. Norman DC, Yoshikawa TT: Infections of the bone, joint, and bursa. Clin Geriatr Med 10:703–718, 1994.
10. Reginster JY, Derois R, Rorah LC, et al: Longterm effects of glucosamine sulphate on osteoarthritis progression: A randomized, placebo-controlled clinical trial. Lancet 357:251–256, 2001.
11. Schumacher HR: Osteoarthritis and crystal deposition disease. Curr Opin Rheumatol 10:244–245, 1998.
12. Apiegel B, Targowhite L, Dulai C, et al: The cost effectiveness of cyclooxygenase-2 selective inhibitors in the management of chronic arthritis. Ann Intern Med 138:795–805, 2003.
13. Towhead TE, Hochberg MC: A systematic review of randomized controlled trials of pharmacological therapy of the knee with an emphasis on trial methodology. Semin Arthritis Rheum 26:755–770, 1997.
14. Yelin E, Callahan LF: The economic cost and social and psychological impact of musculoskeletal conditions. Arthritis Rheum 38:1351–1362, 1995.

33. DIABETES MELLITUS

Tatyana Kemarskaya, MD, and Mary Ann Forciea, MD

1. What do the words "diabetes mellitus" mean?

Although the first description of diabetes goes back to the Egyptian papyrus of 1500 BC, the words "diabetes mellitus" are of Greek origin. "Diabetes" is derived from *diabainein*, meaning "a passer through" or "siphon" (*dia* = through and *bainein* = to go), and "mellitus" is derived from *meli*, which means "honey." Diabetes is a complex metabolic disease characterized by hyperglycemia caused by lack of insulin, resistance to insulin action, or both.

2. How common is diabetes mellitus (DM) in the elderly?

Recent surveys have indicated the prevalence of diagnosed diabetes at 13% of the population over 70 years. An almost equal percentage of patients with diabetes remains undiagnosed. Various ethnic and racial minorities as well as residents of long-term care facilities are at even greater risk of developing DM, with prevalence rates of 25% in some studies.

3. Is the pathophysiology of diabetes mellitus different in older persons?

There are two main types of DM. Type 1 diabetes mellitus (T1DM), known previously as insulin-dependent diabetes mellitus (IDDM), is characterized by defect in insulin production caused by autoimmune destruction of pancreatic beta cells. This type usually manifests itself in childhood and is rarely diagnosed in the elderly. Type 2 diabetes mellitus (T2DM) was previously known as non–insulin-dependent diabetes mellitus (NIDDM), although patients frequently used insulin. In the type 2 variant the initial defect is a decrease in the responsiveness of the somatic cells to insulin action. In the earliest stages of the disease, the beta cells of the pancreas respond to this "peripheral resistance" with increased production of insulin. Eventually, the production of insulin falls, leading to a combined deficiency in action and production of insulin. About 90% of patients with diabetes suffer from type 2 DM. This type of diabetes is by far most common among the elderly, and its prevalence in the community increases with aging.

4. Why is diabetes type 2 more common in older patients?

Age-associated factors that may contribute to increased peripheral resistance to the action of insulin are:

- Increased adiposity. Anthropomorphic studies have shown an increase in adiposity, especially in central (truncal) stores, in older people. Body composition of adipose tissue increases from 18% to 36% in males and 36% to 48% in females.
- Reduced physical activity. Common finding in older patients. Reductions in physical activity, even in the absence of changes in fat stores, are associated with decreased sensitivity of somatic cells to insulin.
- Genetic influences. The inheritance patterns of type 2 diabetes appear to be polygenic but are important both for the overall risk of obesity as well as for diabetes itself.

Elderly patients who are obese and sedentary, have family histories of DM, and belong to African-American, Latino, Native American or Pacific Island groups are at especially high risk of developing diabetes type 2.

5. What are the common signs and symptoms of new-onset diabetes in the elderly?

Manifestations of diabetes in the elderly can be both subtler and more dramatic than in younger adults. Human brain constantly requires glucose and is highly sensitive to the alteration of its quantity. Therefore, checking for hyper- or hypoglycemia is an important part of the initial assessment of the change in mental status in the elderly. With glucose acting as an osmotic diuretic, glucosuria is manifested by changes in urinary pattern, such as incontinence, frequency, and nocturia. Since these symptoms are common among the elderly, the clinician should consider an evaluation for possible diabetes, especially if there is a change in urinary patterns. Certain infections should also alert the clinician to new onset of DM in the elderly, such as frequent skin infections, especially fungal, recurrent urinary tract infections, and fungal vaginitis. The presence of a small quantity of insulin usually prevents the development of overt acidosis and ketone production. Diabetic ketoacidosis (DKA) is a very rare condition in the elderly. Instead they may develop hyperosmolar hyperglycemic non-ketotic coma (HHNK) characterized by a change in mental status, very high glucoses (may be in the 1000 range) and severe dehydration. Mortality from HHNK in the elderly is higher than that from DKA manifested in young people. Dehydration secondary to osmotic diuresis is far more common among the elderly than classical polydypsia due to an alteration in the thirst mechanism or inability to access water.

6. Which aspects of the physical examination of the older diabetic patient are especially important?

Certain areas of a physical exam should be performed at each visit.
- Special attention should be paid to the cardiovascular system. Blood pressure determination should include orthostatic measurements at onset and at least yearly, with the goal of 140/90 mmHg, as discussed below.
- High prevalence of local infections, poor healing, and high risk for falls warrant attention to the skin and foot examination at each visit. Examine skin for signs/symptoms of fungal skin infections, pressure ulcers, and signs of peripheral ischemia. Examine feet for pulses, ulcers, and sensation.
- Yearly examinations by a podiatrist and ophthalmologist, with fundoscopy, are recommended, with urgent visits for acute changes.

7. How is diabetes diagnosed in older patients?

The American Diabetes Association (ADA) defines the criteria for the diagnosis of diabetes. In the most recent ADA criteria, no age-specific adjustments are recommended. Measurement of glycosylated hemoglobin (often designated hemoglobin A1C) is not currently recommended as a diagnostic tool, but is widely used for monitoring the efficacy of treatment.

ADA Blood Glucose Criteria for the Diagnosis of Diabetes Mellitus (mg/dl)

	NORMAL	IMPAIRED GLUCOSE TOLERANCE	DIABETES MELLITUS
Fasting glucose after 8–12 hr fast (mg/dl)	< 110	> 110 but < 126	> 126 (two occasions)
Random glucose (mg/dl)	< 140		> 200 plus symptoms of diabetes

The diagnosis of diabetes mellitus is made after two consecutive readings of blood glucose > 126 mg/dl with a preceding fast of at least 8 hours. Patients must be free of active infection or acute illness during this measurement because illness is associated with transient deterioration in glucose tolerance. Criteria are published for the diagnosis of diabetes after oral glucose loading but are rarely used in routine practice in geriatric medicine.

8. What are the goals of treatment in the older patient with diabetes?

Older patients with T2DM are a heterogenous group, varying from robust, cognitively intact, functionally independent community-dwelling persons to frail, cognitively and functionally impaired nursing home residents. Therefore, consideration of life expectancy due to comorbid conditions, polypharmacy effects, and quality of life are crucial to defining the goals of treatment. Diabetes education needs to include risk/benefit discussions around several potential goals. The American Geriatrics Society (AGS) has recently published evidence-based guidelines for the treatment of the older person with diabetes (see references). These AGS criteria list possible goals in:

- Glycemic control
- Reductions in macro- and microvascular complications
- Recognition and treatment of common geriatric syndromes more prevalent in the diabetic population

9. What are reasonable goals for glucemic control in older patients?

The recent AGS guidelines suggest hemoglobin A1C goals of 7% or lower for older diabetics with good functional status. At least one large study of older patients found that a 1% reduction in hemoglobin A1C (HgbA1C) was associated with a 37% decline in microvascular complications, and a 21% reduction in macrovascular complications of diabetes. Despite these impressive results, risks associated with hypoglycemia and polypharmacy may alter benefits. For frail patients with a life expectancy of < 5 years, a goal of HgbA1C of 8% may be appropriate.

10. How can the macrovascular complications of diabetes be reduced?

Macrovascular complications of diabetes translate to increased risk for cardiovascular events, namely stroke and heart attack. Seventy percent of patients with DM die from a cardiovascular cause. Increased free fatty acids result in destabilization of the endothelium and acceleration of atherosclerotic disease. The latest AGS guidelines recommend more careful attention to cardiovascular risk reduction through:

- Aspirin use   • Blood pressure control
- Smoking cessation • Lipid management

Evidence-based guidelines suggest that older patients with DM should have target blood pressure (BP) goals of 140/80 mmHg. If patients can tolerate therapy, reduction to 130/80 mmHg may be even more beneficial in the older patient. Blood pressure should be lowered gradually (20 mmHg) per month unless severe hypertension is present. Many classes of antihypertensive medications are effective in lowering cardiovascular risks in these patients; angiotensin-converting enzyme inhibitors, cardioselective beta blockers, and angiotensin receptor blockers may offer added benefits for cardio- and nephroprotection.

Attention to the lipid profile has become increasingly important for the older diabetic patient. The goal of the low-density lipoprotein (LDL) portion of the total cholesterol is the same as for patients with known coronary disease and should be less than 100 mg/dl.

11. Microvascular impairment in diabetes: what does it cause?

In the U.S. diabetes is the leading cause of adult blindness, nontraumatic limb amputation, and end-stage renal disease (ESRD). Microvascular complications lead to neuropathy, nephropathy, and retinopathy. Another major complication of T2DM, peripheral vascular disease (PVD), is actually a combination of micro and macrovascular changes. Maintaining optimal glucose control has been proved to decrease the rate of microvascular complications.

Neuropathy. Nerve damage in diabetes mellitus may be due to either ischemic changes or exposure of the neurons to high glucose concentration. Neuropathy often presents as pain in the lower extremities. Besides pain, neuropathy increases the risk for injury due to lack of sensation in the feet. Another presentation of diabetic neuropathy is diabetic neurogenic atonic bladder, which is the most common cause of overflow incontinence in elderly women.

Peripheral vascular disease combined with neuropathy results in nonhealing ulcers, often leading to amputation. It is extremely important to teach the patient proper foot care and perform an exam of the feet every time the diabetic patient comes to the office. Referral to a podiatrist for at least a yearly exam is warranted for any elderly diabetic patient and is approved by Medicare.

Retinopathy. Diabetic patients are prone to diabetic retinopathy, macular degeneration, and cataract formation. Each elderly person with diabetes needs a yearly eye exam with fundoscopy. Early detection and laser photocoagulation therapy seem to be the best strategies to manage diabetic retinopathy.

Nephropathy. The average time of development of end-stage renal disease is 20 years from the onset of T2DM. Patients should be checked yearly for microalbuminuria (urinary albumin of 30–300 mg/24 hr). The current standard of care is to treat diabetic patients with an angiotensin-converting enzyme inhibitor or angiotensin receptor blocker (ARB), even in the absence of overt hypertension.

12. Which "geriatric" syndromes are important in older patients with diabetes?

Literature review showed that older patients with diabetes are at increased risk of depression, cognitive impairment, polypharmacy, urinary incontinence, injurious falls, and pain.

During the initial presentation period (first 3 months), annually, and with unexpected decline in functional status, the older patient with diabetes should be screened for:

• Depression using the geriatric depression scale (GDS)
• Cognitive function using Mini Mental Status Exam (MMSE) and other standardized tests
• Urinary incontinence
• Falls and injury

Medications should be reviewed at each visit to decrease polypharmacy. The use of assistive devices such as prefilled medication boxes or the involvement of caregivers helps to improve compliance in cognitively impaired patients.

13. Which lab tests should be performed and how frequently?

HbA1C: the most commonly used test for monitoring diabetes; should be checked every 6–12 months if the patient is stable.

Renal and lipid profiles: should be done yearly.

Urinalysis: checks for the presence of microalbuminuria should be performed at the time of diagnosis. If negative, they should be repeated annually except for nursing home residents or frail elderly with a life expectancy less than 5–7 years.

14. Does treatment of diabetes differ in older patients?

We continue to recommend dietary modification and increased activity for older patients with diabetes. A specialist in diabetes education best delivers dietary instruction in composition of diet and total number of calories. Even modest weight reduction can improve glucose tolerance (sensitivity to insulin) in many patients.

Exercise has benefits in cardiovascular fitness as well as in glucose control. Because of the incidence of coronary disease, older diabetics should undergo stress testing before beginning a serious exercise program. Exercise sessions should ideally last 30–40 minutes (including stretching) and should be performed 3–5 times weekly.

For many patients with type 2 diabetes, treatment with an oral agent instead of insulin injections can be managed. The major categories of medications available for older patients are discussed in question 15.

15. What should you know about antiglycemic medications use in the elderly?

CLASS OF MEDICATION	MECHANISM OF ACTION	CONTRA-INDICATIONS	SIDE EFFECTS	DECREASE IN HgbA1C	NAME	DOSE
Insulin secreta-gogues				1–2%		
Sulfonylureas (SU)	Increased insulin production	Caution with severe renal impairment	Weight gain of 2–5 kg Profound hypogly-cemia		Glyburide (Diabeta Micronase) Glipizide (Glucotrol) Glimeride (Amaryl)	0.625–10 mg daily or twice daily 2.5–10 mg daily or twice daily 0.5–8 mg

(Cont'd.)

CLASS OF MEDICATION	MECHANISM OF ACTION	CONTRA-INDICATIONS	SIDE EFFECTS	DECREASE IN HgbA1C	NAME	DOSE
Insulin secreta-gogues *(cont'd.)*						
Non-SU	Increased insulin production		As above, but less pronounced		Repaglinide (Prandin)	0.5–4 mg prior to meals day
					Nateglinide (Starlix)	60–180 mg before meals
Biguanides	Inhibits glucose release from the liver	Creatinine > 1.5 (males) > 1.4 (females) CHF, hepatic insufficiency	GI upset (diminishes with time) Lactic acidosis (rare)	1–2%	Metformin (Glucophage)	500–1000 mg 2 or 3 times/day Maximum: 2550 mg/ 24 hr
Alpha glucosidase inhibitors	Delays intestinal carbo-hydrate absorption	Careful with hepatic impairment	GI upset (flatulence, diarrhea)	0.5–1%	Acarbose (Precose)	25–100 mg before meals
					Miglitol (Glyset)	50–100 mg before meals
Thiazo-lidinedione	Insulin sensitizer	CHF class III–IV Liver impairment	Weight gain Edema	1–2%	Rosiglitiazone (Avandia)	2–4 mg/day or 2 times/ day or 8 mg max
					Pioglitazone (Acots)	15–45 mg/ day

CHF = congestive heart failure.

The first group, called **secretagogues**, consists of long-acting sulfonylureas (SU) and newer, shorter-acting non-SU drugs. Secretagogues bind to SU receptors of beta cells in the pancreas, causing insulin release at lower glucose concentrations. Their effect on improving peripheral resistance to insulin action is most likely secondary to a reduction in glucotoxicity. SUs (glyburide, glipizide, glimepride) have been used for over 2 decades and are relatively less costly. Dosage adjustment is required in mild renal failure. They should not be used in moderate or severe renal failure due to the risk of profound hypoglycemia. Hypoglycemia caused by SU secretagogues usually requires hospital admission, because it is a long-acting drug. Short acting non-SUs, such as repaglinide (Prandin) and nateglinide (Starlix), can be useful in diabetics who do not eat 3 regular meals a day. These drugs are given when the patient is actually eating. Since they are short-acting, they rarely cause significant hypoglycemia. All secretagogues cause weight gain.

Biguanide metformin (glucophage) has become widely used in older patients (when renal function permits) because of the low incidence of hypoglycemia. It works by inhibiting glucose release from the liver. The risk of lactic acidosis in severe illness or after IV contrast dyes requires caution. Metformin should be stopped during most hospital admissions and must be stopped 48 hr before imaging studies requiring contrast administration. It should not be used in males with creatinine > 1.5, females with creatinine > 1.4, or elderly patients with calculated creatinine clearance below 60%.

The **alpha glucosidase inhibitors** prevent disaccharide breakdown in the intestine and are associated with significant side effects of bloating and diarrhea in most patients. Their effect on glycemic lowering is less than with the other agents; they are seldom used in monotherapy.

The **thiazolidinediones** are insulin sensitizers. Decreased free fatty acids lead to an increase in insulin sensitivity in muscle and liver as well as improved glucose uptake in end-organs. They have been associated with both hepatic function loss and volume expansion. Caution should be exercised in patients with class II congestive heart failure (CHF); TZDs are contraindicated in class III and IV CHF due to their propensity to expand plasma volume. Liver function tests and weight should be closely monitored.

16. When is insulin used in older patients with diabetes?

Insulin is useful in acutely ill patients because of their changing requirements for glucose control. In office patients, insulin is used either when complications develop that preclude oral agents (renal failure, CHF, hepatic insufficiency) or when control cannot be achieved (presumably due to exhaustion of insulin production from the pancreas). The administration and varieties of insulin available are not significantly different in older and younger diabetics. Insulin glargine (Lantus) seems to be particularly beneficial in older adults. It can be given once a day, preferably at bedtime, lasts 24 hours, and has no significant peaks. Older patients may benefit from pre-filled and easy to use devices such as insulin pens and injectors.

17. How does management of the diabetic patient in long-term care differ from that of the patient in the office?

In guidelines developed by the American Medical Directors Association (AMDA), all new admissions to long-term care should be screened for the presence of DM. More attention should be directed to the macrovascular complications of diabetes since the life expectancy of most patients in this setting is < 5 years. For long-term care residents and terminally ill patients, quality-of-life issues are more important than intensive treatment of diabetes.

BIBLIOGRAPHY

1. Diabetes Control and Complications Trial (DCCT) Research Group: The effect of intensive treatment of diabetes on the development and progression of long-term complications in insulin-dependent diabetes mellitus. N Engl J Med 329:977–986, 1993.
2. Fritsche A, Schweige MH, Haring HU, for the 4001 Study Group: Glimepiride combined with morning insulin glargine, bedtime neutrin protamine Hagedorn insulin or bedtime insulin glargine in patients with type 2 diabetes: A randomized controlled trial. Ann Intern Med 138:952–959, 2003.
3. Gregg EW, Mangione CM, Cauley JA, et al: Diabetes and incidence of functional disability in older women. Diabetes Care 25:61–67, 2002.
4. Guidelines for Improving the Care of the Older Person with Diabetes Mellitus. California Healthcare Foundation American Geriatrics Society Panel on Improving Care for Elders with Diabetes. J Am Geriatr Soc 51:S265–S280, 2003.
5. Harris MI: Diabetes in America: Epidemiology and scope of the problem. Diabetes Care 21(Suppl 3):c11–c14, 1998.
6. Heart Outcome Prevention Evaluation Study Investigators: Effects of ramipril on cardiovascular and microvascular outcomes in people with diabetes mellitus: Results of the HOPE Study and MICRO-HOPE substudy. Lancet 335:253–259, 2000.
7. Highlight from 62nd Scientific Session of the American Diabetes Association. Resident Staff Physician March(Suppl), 2003.
8. Hogikyan RV, Halter JB: Aging and diabetes. In Ellenberg & Rifkin's Diabetes Mellitus, 6th ed. New York, McGraw-Hill, 2003, pp 565–580.
9. Insucchi SE: Oral antihyperglycemic therapy for type 2 diabetes. JAMA 287:360–372, 2002.
10. Managing diabetes in the long-term care setting: Clinical practice guidelines. Orlando, AMDA, 2003.
11. Nathan DM: Initial management of glycemia. N Engl J Med 347:1342–1349, 2002.
12. Poletsky L (ed): Principles of Diabetes Mellitus. New York, Kluwer Academic Publishers, 2002.
13. UK Prospective Diabetes Study (UKPDS) Group: Intensive blood-glucose control with sulfonylureas or insulin compared with conventional treatment and risk of complications in patients with type 2 diabetes (UKPDS33). Lancet 352:837–853, 1998.
14. United Kingdom Prospective Diabetes Study (UKPDS) Group: Tight blood pressure control and risk of macrovascular and microvascular complications: UKPDS 39. BMJ 317:703–713, 1998.

34. URINARY INCONTINENCE

Mary Ann Forciea, MD, and Grace Cordts, MD

1. What is urinary incontinence?

Urinary incontinence (UI) is the involuntary loss of urine in a quantity or frequency sufficient to cause a social or hygienic problem.

2. How big a problem is urinary incontinence in older patients?

In the National Survey of Self-Care and Aging, 41% of Medicare recipients over the age of 65 years who were living in their communities listed UI as a problem. In other studies, approximately 50% of patients with UI have never reported the problem to their physician. The reasons given range from simple embarrassment and ignorance of treatment options to the assumption that UI is a normal part of growing older. In nursing facilities, the national average prevalence of UI is approximately 40%; in some facilities the prevalence may be as high as 80%.

Urinary incontinence can lead to many other problems in older patients:
- Skin breakdown and pressure ulcers
- Falls (especially in nocturnal trips to the bathroom)
- Social isolation (distance to an available toilet)
- Depression

The development of UI can be the major factor in the decision to pursue placement in a nursing facility for a chronically ill older patient.

3. What are the causes of UI in older patients?

UI can be acute (and usually reversible) or chronic and persistent. Acute incontinence has a sudden onset and is often associated with a medical illness; persistent incontinence occurs over time. Acute factors may worsen persistent UI.

The causes of **acute incontinence** can be remembered with the help of the mnemonic **DRIP:**

Delirium. Patients are temporarily unaware of the urge to void or cannot communicate the need to use the bathroom

Restricted mobility. Any condition, such as trauma or stroke, that restricts mobility may cause incontinence. This type of incontinence is sometimes called functional incontinence, since it is the impairment in functional ability that causes incontinence rather than a problem with the anatomy of voiding.

Infection, Inflammation, or Impaction. Acute cystitis is the most common cause of acute UI in the elderly. Fecal impaction is a common cause in residents of nursing facilities

Pharmaceuticals. Diuretic use is the most common drug in this category. Others include alpha-adrenergic agonists and blockers, narcotics, anticholinergics, and psychotropic agents.

Chronic UI is usually divided into four types:

Stress incontinence: leakage of urine with any increase in intra-abdominal pressure: coughing, sneezing, or bending over. The amount of urine lost can vary from inconsequential to substantial. In women, the most common cause of stress incontinence is relaxation of the pelvic floor muscles. In men, stress incontinence can develop after prostate surgery or radiation due to damage to sphincters. Stress incontinence is the most common type of UI in patients under the age of 75.

Urge incontinence (detrusor instability): loss of urine after an uncontrollable desire to void. Patients often complain that they do not have enough time to get to the toilet after the urge to void or that they have "small bladders." In addition to increased irritability of the detrusor muscle, urge incontinence can develop in patients with neurologic disorders such as dementia, stroke, and Parkinson's disease. Urge incontinence is the most common type of UI in patients over the age of 75.

Overflow incontinence: leakage of urine from a distended bladder. The bladder enlargement may be caused by outlet obstruction, such as that seen with prostatic enlargement in men, or by an atonic, neurogenic bladder, as seen in spinal cord injury or autonomic neuropathy of the nerves controlling bladder function. Medications such as narcotics and anticholinergics can also produce an atonic bladder.

Functional incontinence: loss of urine due to the inability of the patient to move to the toilet, undress, and coordinate movements required for normal toileting. Common causes are dementia, musculoskeletal problems, and stroke.

Often UI in older patients can be multifactorial; identification of the individual components and appropriate treatment can improve continence in most patients.

4. What anatomic structures control voiding?

The nervous system plays a major role in the control of voiding. Cerebral function is required to govern appropriate times and places of voiding. Spinal cord function of both autonomic and somatic nerve function is necessary. Activity of the sympathetic nerves enhances continence; parasympathetic activity promotes voiding. Somatic nerves and skeletal muscle control the pelvic floor muscles as well as the external sphincters.

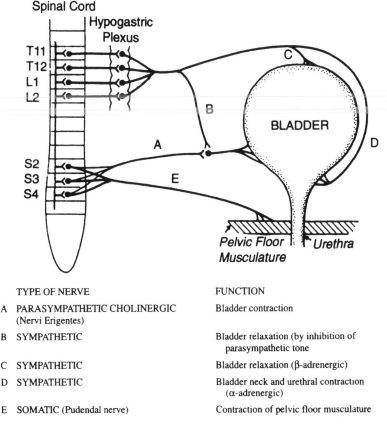

TYPE OF NERVE	FUNCTION
A PARASYMPATHETIC CHOLINERGIC (Nervi Erigentes)	Bladder contraction
B SYMPATHETIC	Bladder relaxation (by inhibition of parasympathetic tone
C SYMPATHETIC	Bladder relaxation (β-adrenergic)
D SYMPATHETIC	Bladder neck and urethral contraction (α-adrenergic)
E SOMATIC (Pudendal nerve)	Contraction of pelvic floor musculature

Parasympathetic, sympathetic, and somatic innervation of the bladder. (From Ouslander JG: Geriatric urinary incontinence. Dis Mon 38:67–149, 1992, with permission.)

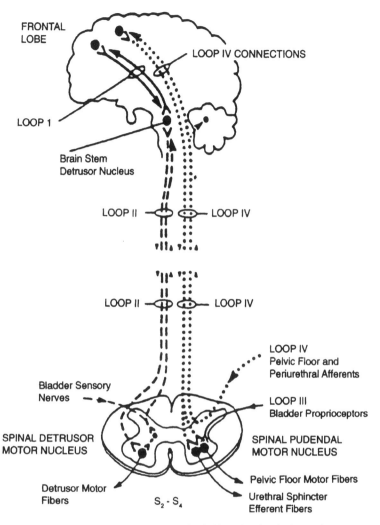

FRONTAL
LOBE

LOOP IV CONNECTIONS

LOOP 1

Brain Stem
Detrusor Nucleus

LOOP II — LOOP IV

LOOP II — LOOP IV

LOOP IV
Pelvic Floor and
Periurethral Afferents

Bladder Sensory
Nerves —

LOOP III
Bladder Proprioceptors

SPINAL DETRUSOR
MOTOR NUCLEUS

SPINAL PUDENDAL
MOTOR NUCLEUS

Pelvic Floor Motor Fibers

Detrusor Motor
Fibers

$S_2 - S_4$

Urethral Sphincter
Efferent Fibers

Central nervous system connections to the bladder and periurethral musculature.

5. What normal changes in the urinary tract are associated with aging?

Aging involves decreases in estrogen, bladder capacity, and urethral pressure. Prostate size increases with aging. The changes may predispose to incontinence, but do not cause incontinence. *Incontinence is not a normal part of aging.*

6. What is the best way to ask older patients about urinary incontinence?

Although older patients may be reticent to initiate conversations about incontinence, they can be appreciative of questioning that opens the topic. Useful questions can include the following, especially if preceded by the statement, "Many patients in this practice have trouble controlling their urine flow":

- Do you ever lose urine when you cough, laugh, or sneeze?
- How often do you have difficulty holding your urine until you can get to the toilet?
- How often do you lose control of your urine completely?

7. What special items in the history of a patient with UI are important?

In addition to the initial questions noted above, questions about the onset of the incontinence (gradual or sudden), duration, timing, frequency, and quantity of urine lost are useful. Is dysuria or hematuria present? How does the patient currently manage fluid intake? What is the current pattern of bowel regularity? In addition, medication history, especially as related to the timing of the onset of the incontinence, is especially important in the elderly. Questions about current medical illness can lead to clues about the etiology of the incontinence (for example, new congestive heart failure can lead to nocturia). Finally, questions about the environment of the home or nursing facility, such as distance to the toilet, can lead to therapeutic interventions that improve continence (e.g., bedside commodes, urinals, grab bars near toilet). Questions about use and type of protective padding can be useful indicators of quantity of urine lost.

Voiding diaries are logs (usually kept for 1–2 days) of timing of toilet visits with indicators of wet/dry status at each visit to the toilet. These diaries can be useful in some patients for the diagnosis of UI and can also be used to monitor therapy.

8. What special components of the physical examination are important in the older patient with UI?

To identify causes that may have precipitated incontinence and to help establish pathophysiology, a general physical exam is indicated in the initial examination of the patient with UI. Special attention should be paid to the following areas:

Key Aspects of the Physical Exam

Abdominal exam	Identify bladder fullness, tenderness, masses, surgery
Rectal exam	Identify stool impaction, sphincter tone, perineal sensation, bulbocavernous reflex, prostate nodules, rectal masses
Genital exam	Identify anatomic abnormalities, skin condition
Pelvic exam	Identify muscle atrophy, genital atrophy, masses, pelvic organ prolapse, muscle tone
Neurologic exam	Identify treatable disorders, spinal cord compression, stroke Evaluate cognitive status
Functional status	Identify ability to use bathroom, dress and undress, ambulate

9. What is the initial step in the evaluation of UI in the older patient?

The urinalysis remains the initial test for all patients with UI to indicate the presence of hematuria, glycosuria, proteinuria, and pyuria. Testing strips also include markers of infection such as the presence of leukocyte esterase. Urinalysis samples that indicate the possibility of infection should be sent for culture.

10. Do special considerations apply to the urinalysis of an older patient?

The best sample for urinalysis is clean-catch, midstream urine. Patients are instructed in perineal cleansing and asked to initiate urination, then insert the receptacle into the urine stream for collection. Many older patients have difficulty with optimal collection and may need family members or office staff to assist them.

In some frail patients who are unable to participate in midstream urine collection, obtaining a diagnostic urine sample via Foley catheterization may be the only practical alternative. Care for sterile technique should always be taken. Some older women are catheterized more comfortably in the left lateral lithotomy position than in the standard lithotomy position.

In patients with chronic, indwelling Foley catheters, urine samples obtained from the Foley or drainage bag are rarely useful because of chronic colonization of the drainage system. If an acute infection is suspected, the chronically indwelling catheter should be removed, a new catheter inserted, and the initial urine obtained through the catheter sent for analysis and culture.

11. What additional tests can be done by the primary care provider?

Bladder filling and emptying can be assessed with bladder ultrasonic scanning. In most hospital units, nursing facilities, and geriatric medicine outpatient practices, simple bladder ultrasound equipment is available. Ultrasound is also useful in the noninvasive estimation of postvoid residual filling and bladder capacity. Direct visualization of leaking with cough in the standing and lithotomy positions can also be done.

12. When is referral indicated?

Most older patients with UI can be helped by their primary care providers without extensive testing. Patients should be referred to specialists for the following situations:

- Hematuria without infection
- UI with recurrent symptomatic urinary infections
- PVR > 200 ml
- Prostate nodule
- Uncertain diagnosis after initial evaluation
- Failure to respond to adequate therapeutic trial
- Symptomatic pelvic prolapse
- Recent history of pelvic surgery or radiation therapy

13. What therapies are available for UI in the older patient?

Behavioral, pharmacologic, and surgical therapies are available for the treatment of UI.

14. Describe the behavioral therapies useful for older patients with UI.

Behavioral techniques present little risk to the patient and have produced improvements in continence equal to pharmaceuticals in some studies. Patient or caregiver education and reinforcement are critical to the success of behavioral strategies. Specific techniques, which can be offered in most primary care sites, include pelvic muscle exercise, bladder retraining, and prompted voiding. High-tech measures, which are usually available through specialty referral, include biofeedback, electrical stimulation, and vaginal cone retention. An adjunct to any of these behavioral techniques is improvement in the physical environment, such as improved toilet access, clothing that makes disrobing easier, and accessible call systems.

Pelvic muscle (Kegel) exercises involve repetitive contractions of pelvic floor muscles. Patients are instructed in the identification of target muscles through maneuvers such as Valsalva or urine flow interruption. Patients are then instructed to contract and release the target muscles in 10-second cycles (10-second contraction, 10-second release). Ten repetitions constitute a set. Patients with UI should perform at least 5 sets/day. Maintenance therapy is 3 sets/day. Pelvic muscle exercises have been repeatedly demonstrated to improve continence in women. If done by men prior to prostrate resection, postsurgical continence rates can be improved.

Bladder retraining involves progressive increases in the intervals between mandatory voiding with distraction or relaxation techniques. It requires that the patient resist or inhibit the sensation to void. It has been shown to be helpful in urge and stress incontinence.

Prompted voiding attempts to teach patients to recognize their continence status and request toileting. It has been used successfully in patients with cognitive impairment in nursing facilities.

15. Which medications are helpful in the treatment of UI in the elderly?

Several drugs have been developed that, especially when used in conjunction with behavioral techniques, can aid continence. Initial doses should always be low, and careful monitoring of side effects is necessary.

Stress incontinence can be improved with topical (vaginal) estrogen in many women.

Urge incontinence is treated with drugs with anticholinergic and smooth muscle-relaxant properties. Oxybutinin, the classic drug in this category, is now available in a long-acting preparation. Common side effects are dry mouth and mild confusion. Tolterodine, a newer agent, is also available in a sustained-release preparation. Calcium channel blockers have also been used for urge incontinence.

Overflow incontinence is treated with drugs that relax the sphincter or stimulate bladder contractions. Examples include alpha-adrenergic blockers such as terazosin. In men with prostatic enlargement, alpha agonists, which cause reduction in the prostatic capsule, can be used.

In many older patients who have combination etiologies of incontinence, more than one agent may be required.

16. When is surgical intervention appropriate?

Older patients must be evaluated with special care for surgical corrections. The etiologies of UI in these patients may be mixed, and the surgical risks are greater. Patients with anatomic etiologies of UI such as bladder prolapse or prostatic hypertrophy may ultimately require surgical correction to restore continence. Improvements in artificial sphincters continue and might ultimately benefit selected older patients. Injections of collagen at the urethral-pelvic junction can provide short-term improvements in selected patients with stress incontinence.

The placement of an appropriate pessary in a frail older woman with bladder or uterine prolapse may improve continence adequately to improve function and care.

17. Which treatment methods do patients prefer?

A large community survey of older people indicated that 44% of women and 15% of men preferred using disposable pads to manage UI: 37% limited fluids for the management of UI. In a study of nursing facility residents given the choices of catheters, medications, and prompted voiding, patients chose medication and diapers, families chose catheters and diapers, and nursing staff chose prompted voiding.

18. When is an indwelling Foley catheter an appropriate choice?

Indwelling catheters can be uncomfortable, can interfere with social functioning, and are associated with increased risk of infection. The use of an indwelling catheter is appropriate when:

- Urinary retention is resistant to other therapy
- Wounds are present in the perineum
- The patient is terminally ill or unconscious
- The patient expresses a preference for catheter treatment.

Indwelling catheters should not be routinely irrigated. Sustained antibiotic coverage in patients with indwelling catheters does not reduce the incidence of infection and is associated with antibiotic resistance.

BIBLIOGRAPHY

1. Johnson TM, Ouslander JG, Uman GC, Schnelle J: Urinary incontinence preferences in long-term care. J Am Geriatr Soc 49:710–718, 2001.
2. Newman D: Managing and Treating Urinary Incontinence. Health Professions Press, Baltimore, 2002.
3. Nicholle LE: Management of urinary tract infection in the elderly. Home Health Care Consult 8:10–20, 2001.
4. Ouslander JG, Schnelle SF: Incontinence in the nursing home. Ann Intern Med 122:438–449, 1995.
5. Ouslander JG, Schnelle JF, Al-Samarrai N: Prompted voiding for nighttime incontinence in nursing homes: Is it effective? J Am Geriatr Soc 49:706–709, 2001.
6. Resnick NM, Yalla SV: Management of urinary incontinence in the elderly. N Engl J Med 313:800–805, 1985.

35. PROSTATE DISEASE

George W. Drach, MD

BASIC CONCEPTS

1. Where is the prostate?

The prostate gland surrounds the male urethra as it exits below the urinary bladder. Its normal size is about 20 grams, and it has three zones: central, peripheral, and transition. The peripheral zone, which lies posteriorly and inferiorly, is the site of most prostate cancers. The central zone is posterior and superior. The transition zone surrounds the urethra centrally, mostly superior and anterior. Benign prostatic hyperplasia occurs in the transition zone.

2. What is hyperplasia of the prostate?

Prostate tissue grows in response to stimulation by the hormone testosterone and its derivative dihydrotestosterone (DHT), which is created through action of the enzyme 5-alpha-reductase on testosterone. DHT stimulates growth factors—for example, epidermal growth factor (EGF). The stromal (muscular and fibrous) and glandular tissues of the prostate respond by growing. Because it contains muscle, the stroma also responds to nervous stimuli, especially $alpha_1$ adrenoceptors. Prostate cell death (apoptosis) normally happens regularly in early years so that the growth/death balance is maintained. After approximately age 40, this process no longer achieves balance with cell death and results in overall transitional zone growth or what is called benign prostatic hyperplasia (BPH).[1]

3. What causes prostate cancer?

There is no clear answer. Genetics seem to play a part, because prostate cancer may be strongly present in some families. Most cases, however, are sporadic and without family history. One theory implicates the failure of apoptosis as an inciting factor for cancer.

4. Is there a way to avoid prostate problems through diet or other health maneuvers?

Some experts suggest that a diet low in cholesterol and fat, similar to the heart diet, decreases the risk of prostate cancer and BPH. In addition, intake of substances such as lycopenes (found in tomatoes, certain juices), selenium, or vitamin E may decrease risk of prostate cancer. Others feel that diets emphasizing vegetables contribute to lower risk of BPH.

5. How do we evaluate patients for bladder outlet trouble or difficulty with voiding?

At present, initial evaluation comes from a review of the patient's symptoms, referred to as lower urinary tract symptoms (LUTS). LUTS have two major categories: obstructive and irritative symptoms.

OBSTRUCTIVE SYMPTOMS	IRRITATIVE SYMPTOMS
Hesitancy	Frequency
Decreased or thin urinary stream	Urgency
Prolonged urination with intermittency	Nocturia
Incomplete bladder emptying	Urge incontinence

These symptoms may exist with other urinary diseases, such as infection, carcinoma, bladder stones, urethral stricture, or neurogenic bladder. Thus, one cannot assume that all such symptoms in older men are caused by BPH.

A useful means of estimating severity of LUTS is to use the validated Prostate Symptom Score sheet developed by the American Urological Association (AUA).

Prostate Symptom Score Sheet

	NEVER	LESS THAN 1 TIME IN 5	LESS THAN HALF THE TIME	ABOUT HALF THE TIME	MORE THAN HALF THE TIME	ALMOST ALWAYS
1. Over the past month or so, how often have you had a sensation of not emptying your bladder completely after you finished urinating?	0	1	2	3	4	5
2. Over the past month or so, how often have you had to urinate again less than two hours after you finished urinating?	0	1	2	3	4	5
3. Over the past month or so, how often have you found you stopped and started again several times when you urinated?	0	1	2	3	4	5
4. Over the past month or so, how often have you found it difficult to postpone urination?	0	1	2	3	4	5
5. Over the past month or so, how often have you had a weak urinary stream?	0	1	2	3	4	5
6. Over the past month or so, how often have you had to push or strain to begin urination?	0	1	2	3	4	5
7. Over the past month, how many times did you usually get up to urinate from the time you went to bed at night until the time you got up in the morning?	0 never	1 time	2 times	3 times	4 times	5 times or more

In addition to the symptoms above, most questionnaires add an overall "bother" score that helps physicians decide when to consider medical or interventional therapy. If the bother value is significant (3–5 out of 5), one usually initiates some type of therapy.

Physical examination of the abdomen, especially for palpable bladder or kidney enlargement, and a focused lower-body neurologic examination follow the symptom analysis. Thereafter the prostate is evaluated by digital rectal examination (DRE) to estimate prostate size and to rule out nodularity. Large glands (over 50 cm^3), however, may be greatly underestimated by this DRE technique. Perhaps the best technique to estimate true prostate size is transrectal ultrasound imaging, but this approach is seldom necessary initially.

6. Of what importance is the physical examination for prostate enlargement?

As noted above, it serves as an estimate of prostatic size, which may correlate with risk for acute urinary retention. In addition, any finding of nodularity, asymmetry, or induration should lead to urologic consultation in appropriate older patients whose quality of life could be affected by discovery of significant cancers.

7. Are additional tests necessary after symptom analysis and examination?

Laboratory evaluation should always include at least urinary dipstick testing, with microscopic examination of the sediment and urinary culture for any finding of red blood cells, white blood cells, or positive nitrites (bacteria). The AUA recommends a baseline serum creatinine if one has not been performed recently. Determination of prostate-specific antigen (PSA) (see below) may help predict likelihood of retention and level of need to initiate medical therapy. If the PSA value is over 1.6 ng/ml and the prostate larger than 40 cm^3, the patient may well benefit from administration of 5-alpha-reductase inhibitors (see below).

Imaging for determination of postvoid residual urine should be done if there is any concern about the degree of retention. It is now done reliably by transabdominal ultrasound with little discomfort to the patient. Renal evaluation by ultrasound must be performed also for any patient with bladder obstructive disease and elevated serum creatinine. Complex pressure/flow studies of the bladder, or urodynamics studies, need be done only for imprecise findings or when one considers intervention. Urologic consultation should be arranged at this time.

8. How can the primary care physician or geriatrician initiate treatment of LUTS associated with BPH?

Once the provider has made the decision to initiate treatment, the first step is to decide which medical therapy might be best for the patient. Usual urologic practice predicts first-level treatment with alpha-adrenergic drugs. At present, three major drugs are used to decrease periprostatic alpha-adrenergic muscle tone: doxazosin, terazosin, and tamulosin.

The first two are available in generic form, the last as a patented drug. However, it is advisable to start doxazosin and terazosin slowly at 1–2 mg at bedtime and to titrate upward because of hypotensive and orthostatic side effects or development of fatigue. Patients should report noticeable improvement in urination within 72 hours and should have a decrease in symptom scores when reassessed about every 2–3 weeks until stable. Amounts can be increased if necessary to 4–5 mg or more, up to a maximum of 8–10 mg.

Tamulosin does not usually involve orthostatic problems and can be given at its full 0.4-mg starting dose 30 minutes after the same daily meal (drug information pamphlet). Some patients require 0.8 mg for full effect.

As noted above, patients with larger prostate glands may benefit from the addition of finasteride or dutasteride to the alpha blocker. Doses for finasteride are 5 mg and for dutasteride 0.5 mg daily.

9. When should referral for possible procedure or surgical intervention be considered?

Certain problems predict poor results from medical therapy of BPH and LUTS and should lead to urologic consultation. Examples include persistent severe symptoms (AUA symptoms score over 20, with a high "bother" score of 4 or 5), recurrent gross hematuria, uncontrollable urinary infections, high residual urine volumes that do not improve with therapy, urinary retention, progression of renal failure, bladder calculi, or discovery of prostate cancer.

10. What types of intervention are now available?

Treatment choices vary greatly. In the past, transurethral resection of the prostate (TURP) dominated. This procedure used cystoscopic instruments and radiofrequency ("hot") wire loops to remove obstructing prostate tissue. Over the past 2 decades, many other methods of removing, vaporizing, or eliminating prostatic tissue have appeared and can be chosen by the urologist.

11. What about the use of phytotherapy (plant and other natural agents)?

Popular literature extols use of many natural agents such as saw palmetto and pygium to relieve LUTS related to BPH. No substantial studies show clear benefits of any of these agents. It is not, therefore, possible to recommend their use until such definitive studies are reported.

12. What complications may result from untreated progressive BPH with obstruction?

Prolonged bladder outflow obstruction can lead to stone formation, chronic infections, development of bladder diverticula, chronic retention of urine, and (rarely) deterioration of renal function. Perhaps the most distressing result is urinary retention or inability to void. Factors that increase the risk of acute retention include significantly enlarged prostate, high "benign" PSA level (above), postvoid residual urine of > 200 ml, maximum urinary flow rate below 10 ml/sec, prior episode of retention, and severe LUTS.

PROSTATITIS

13. What are the forms of prostatitis?

Classically, prostatitis was placed into one of four forms: acute, chronic bacterial, nonbacterial, and prostatodynia. These categories were proposed years ago and served to allow organization for purposes of treatment and for study.[2] Recently, the National Institute of Health, through a consensus process, proposed revised categorization that improved upon the prior classification.[3]

NIDDK Classification of Prostatitis

I. Acute bacterial prostatitis	Acute severe illness with fever, chills, urinary tract infection
II. Chronic bacterial prostatitis	Subclinical illness with bacteria proven in prostate
III. Chronic abacterial prostatitis	Chronic pelvic pain syndrome (CPPS)
IIIA. Inflammatory CPPS	White blood cells in semen, expressed prostatic secretions, voided bladder-3
IIIB. Noninflammatory CPPS	No white blood cells
IV. Asymptomatic inflammatory prostatitis	Discovered during other studies

14. How do we diagnose the various forms of prostatitis?

Once again, studies have shown that use of a symptom index questionnaire can be helpful in diagnosis of prostatitis. The Chronic Prostatitis Symptom Index (CPSI) has been validated in primary care and urologic offices.[2,3] Unfortunately, LUTS and prostatitis symptoms can be similar; thus, some degree of clinical suspicion must be applied.

As noted above, acute prostatitis presents as severe illness, with significant dysuria, difficult voiding, fever, chills, pyuria, and urinary infection. For chronic bacterial prostatitis, in the past, diagnostic algorithms recommended evaluation of the afebrile patient with mild urinary symptoms and included collection of two initial urinary specimens: the first 5–10 ml passed, followed by the usual midstream urine. These were labeled VB-1 and VB-2, referring to voided bladder 1 (urethral specimen) and voided bladder 2 (midstream specimen). Both were examined microscopically and by culture.[4]

Prostatic examination and massage were then performed while an open-mouthed cup was held under the tip of the penis. If the massage resulted in passage of some few drops of prostatic fluid, this expressed prostatic excretion (EPS) was sent for microscopic examination and culture. If no fluid came forth, a third specimen (VB-3) of urine was collected soon after the massage. This was called the post-prostatic massage urine and again was submitted for microscopic analysis and culture.

One can see that a possible four specimens resulted from the evaluation. Stamey and colleagues published elaborate results of such studies and proposed that bacterial prostatitis existed when the VB-1 and VB-2 had few white blood cells and few bacteria and the prostatic fluid and/or VB-3 had significant numbers (at least 10-fold greater than the VB-1 and VB-2). This approach still appears in many texts and reports.[4] However, the NIH prostatitis study group, which initiated the above symptoms questionnaire, remains unable to validate the above method of diagnosis.[5]

15. Summarize the diagnostic recommendations.

Presently, the best summary of diagnostic recommendations includes the following steps:
• Confirm that symptoms are consistent with one of the prostatitis syndromes (standardized symptom questionnaire).

- Examine lower abdomen, genitalia, perineum and rectum, and lower-body neurologic status.
- Exclude nasty mimics of prostatitis:
  - Inguinal hernia
  - Perirectal abscess
  - Interstitial cystitis/bladder carcinoma
  - Detrusor/sphincter dyssynergia
  - Distal ureteral stone
  - Müllerian duct (utricle) cyst stone
  - Prostatic/ejaculatory duct stone(s)

16. How do we treat bacterial prostatitis?

We must remember that treatment of bacterial prostatitis assumes that we have recovered bacteria from some prostatic specimen and that we have sensitivity studies available. Many drugs do *not* penetrate the prostate/blood barrier. Those mentioned below do so and form the basis of most therapy.

ANTIBIOTIC	USE
Tetracyclines	100 mg doxycycline 2 times/day for 21 days; if not improved, repeat × 1; especially useful for suspected chlamydial infection
Trimethoprim/ sulfamethoxazole	One double-strength tablet 2 times/day for 21 days, repeated as above if needed; inexpensive, useful for gram-negative bacteria
Macrolides	Erythromycin, 250 mg 4 times/day for 21 days, with repeat course if needed; especially used for the unusual gram-positive infection, such as streptococci
Fluoroquinalones	Ciprofloxacin, 500 mg 2 times/day for 21 days, with repeat course as necessary; perhaps best for gram-negative infection

17. Summarize the treatment approaches to NIH types III A&B.

- Antimicrobials may be tried
- Alpha blockers
- Prostatic massage
- Anti-inflammatories
- Pain control measures, pain clinic referral
- Biofeedback
- Alpha-reductase inhibitors

BIBLIOGRAPHY

1. Kirby RS, McConnell JD: Benign Prostatic Hyperplasia, 4th ed. Oxford, Health Press, 2002.
2. Drach GW, Fair WR, Meares EM Jr, Stamey TA: Classification of benign diseases associated with prostatic pain: Prostatitis or prostatodynia. J Urol 120:266, 1978.
3. Litwin MS, McNaughton-Collins M, Fowler J Jr, et al: The National Institutes of Health Chronic Prostatitis Symptom Index: Development and validation of a new outcome measure. J Urol 162:369–375, 1999.
4. Meares EM Jr, Stamey TA: The diagnosis and management of bacterial prostatitis. Br J Urol 44:175–179, 1972.
5. Turner JA, Ciol MA, Von Korff M, Berger R: Validity and responsiveness of the National Institutes of Health Chronic Prostatitis Symptom Index. J Urol 169:580–583, 2003.

36. PROSTATE CANCER

George W. Drach, MD

1. How do we detect prostate cancer?

Most patients with prostate cancer undergo prostate needle biopsy indicated after elevation of prostate-specific antigen (PSA) on a screening blood test. A few others have biopsy because of nodularity of the prostate on digital rectal examination (DRE). Rarely, routine bone films for some other reason show osteoblastic metastases that are characteristic of prostate cancer. No matter which process points to prostate cancer, the ultimate diagnosis in the U.S. requires biopsy of the prostate, most often by means of transrectal needle biopsy controlled by transrectal ultrasound.

2. How does one determine if a prostate nodule exists?

DRE experience ultimately leads the physician to recognize abnormalities of density of the prostate: nodularity, induration, or asymmetry. Also available are models of the prostate that demonstrate the tactile sensations for normal, benign hyperplastic and nodular prostates. If there is any question about prostatic abnormality, urologic consultation should be requested.

3. What if there is only asymmetry or induration of the prostate without a discreet nodule?

Asymmetry is least likely to indicate prostate cancer, and induration may occur with other diseases such as prostatitis. Both problems require urologic consultation.

4. What are the guidelines for PSA screening of geriatric patients?

PSA is a glycoprotein protease that liquifies the semen clot after ejaculation; it is secreted by prostate epithelial cells. Most laboratories accept the range of 0–2 ng/ml as clearly normal and 2–4 ng/ml as probably normal. Values above 4 ng/ml are considered abnormal, but there is a gray zone of about 4–10 ng/ml in which many patients have no prostate cancer but show significant benign prostatic hypertrophy (BPH) or prostatitis.

PSA exists in bound and free forms in the serum. Some experts advise measurement of free and total PSA as one means of predicting risk of prostate cancer. Larger percentages of free PSA (especially above 25%) predict a higher likelihood of benign hyperplasia. Guidelines for screening PSA differ among major national organizations in the United States. Often, the decision to perform a screening PSA results from an informed discussion between physician and patient. In general, men over the age of 65 should have yearly or every other yearly PSA screens if they have good general health and a life expectancy of 10 years. In addition, they must accept the concept that the result of the screening PSA may lead to prostate biopsy and may affect decisions about how any cancer that is discovered might be treated.

5. How is prostate cancer classified pathologically?

Most transrectal biopsies recover 6–12 needle slivers. Specific areas of the prostate are biopsied separately. If the pathologist identifies prostate cancer, he or she estimates the best and worst areas seen in terms of cellular dedifferentiation, with grade 1 being best and grade 5 being worst. The two numbers are then added to give a Gleason score. The pathologist also estimates the volume of disease. One positive biopsy with only 5% of the core involved is clearly low-volume disease, whereas biopsies with 10 or 12 cores showing prostate cancer depict high-volume disease. As one can see, the possible Gleason scores range from 2 (well-differentiated) to 10 (undifferentiated). In general, patients with Gleason scores of 4 or less, with PSA values below 8–10, have less than a 10% chance of dying from prostate cancer within 15 years, and many such patients are followed by watchful waiting. Patients with Gleason scores of 5–7 have a 30–60% risk of death in 15 years and may be candidates for surgery and/or radiation. Therefore, such options may be discussed. Patients with Gleason scores at 8 or above tend to have more significant disease and are not considered good candidates for surgery. They may choose radiation therapy, often with the addition of hormonal therapy.

6. How does one present treatment options to patients with prostate cancer?

Decisions about treatment options are individualized for each patient. Major contributory factors include PSA level, Gleason score, volume of disease, patient age, and comorbid diseases. The major categories of treatment options include:

- Watchful waiting for patients with low PSA, low Gleason score, and low disease volume.
- Definitive therapy by surgical removal or radiation (either external beam or brachytherapy [seeds]). At present, there is great controversy about whether surgery or radiation has greater cure rates or lower complication rates. Both are viable alternatives and should be offered to the patient.
- Patients with existing metastatic disease at the time of diagnosis usually do best with hormonal (testosterone suppression) therapy of some type.

7. What are the hormonal treatment options for prostate cancer?

Charles Huggins of the University of Chicago remains the father of the concept of hormonal therapy for prostate cancer. He performed bilateral orchiectomy (castration) on many patients and demonstrated significant relief of symptoms and prolongation of life. Since this procedure is surgical and maiming, treatment by suppression of testosterone through administration of oral estrogens became more common until the late 1980s. However, it became clear that such treatment led to significant cardiac and thromboembolic side effects in about 6–8% of patients. Then came luteinizing hormone-releasing hormone (LHRH) agonists such as luprolide, which cause increased luteinizing hormone excretion by the pituitary gland, overdriving and exhausting the production of testosterone by the Leydig cells of the testis. Subsequent depletion of testosterone results in levels that mimic castration and lead to suppression of prostate cancer. It is the most common form of hormone therapy today, and the side effects are annoying but not dangerous. Luprolide, however, does not suppress production of all male hormone analogs: about 15% of total male hormones continue to be secreted by the adrenal glands. Several agents to suppress adrenal male hormones now exist. One example is biclutamide. Not all patients require total male hormone ablation (administration of luprolide and biclutamide simultaneously), but this technique can benefit selected patients. Some experts advise total suppression in *all* patients when hormonal therapy is selected. However, castration and/or use of low dose estrogens remain, in many ways, viable and inexpensive alternatives to expensive drug therapy.

8. Does patient age affect the treatment options?

Clearly it does. If life expectancy is limited and the degree of prostate cancer is low, watchful waiting seems best. If the patient is 85 years of age and in good health and has a PSA of 30, a Gleason score of 9, and high-volume tumor but no clinical manifestations of disease, he still has a high risk of death from cancer within 5 years. Since he has at least that many years of life expectancy, nonsurgical therapy should be considered. In addition, some patients cannot tolerate the idea that they are living with a cancer and demand treatment despite counseling to the contrary.

BIBLIOGRAPHY

1. Albertsen PC, Hanley JA, Gleason DF, Barry MJ: Competing risk analysis of men aged 55 to 74 years at diagnosis managed conservatively for clinically localized prostate cancer. JAMA 280:1008–1010, 1998.
2. Canto EL, Slawin KM: Early management of prostate cancer: How to respond to an elevated PSA. Annu Rev Med 53:355–368, 2002.
3. Jani AB, Hellman S: Early prostate cancer: Clinical decision making. Lancet 361:1045–1053, 2003.

37. SEXUAL FUNCTIONING

Fran E. Kaiser, MD

1. How does the sexual response cycle change with aging?

Changes in Human Sexual Response with Aging

PHASE	MALE	FEMALE
Excitement	Reduced scrotal vasocongestion Decreased testicular elevation Delayed penile erection	Reduced breast and genital vasocongestion Diminished vaginal secretions Delayed arousal
Plateau	Prolonged Diminshed pre-ejaculatory secretions	Reduced elevation of uterus and labia majora
Orgasm	Short duration Reduction in prostatic and urethral contraction	Short duration Fewer and weaker uterine and vaginal contractions
Resolution	Rapid detumescence and testicular descent Prolonged refractory period	Rapid reversal to prearousal stage

As defined by Masters and Johnson, the stages of sexual response change with aging, although these changes do not preclude sexual activity. In 1992, the National Institutes of Health (NIH) defined erectile dysfunction as "the inability of the male to attain and maintain erection of the penis sufficient to permit satisfactory intercourse." Erectile dysfunction has replaced the term *impotence.*

2. Are loss of sexual function and erectile dysfunction normal consequences of the aging process?

No. While some older adults experience a decrease in sexual activity with age, many individuals remain sexually active. Erectile dysfunction, though common with age (occurring in 52% of all men aged 40–70 and > 95% of diabetic men > 70), indicates underlying organic disease. An estimated 30 million men in the United States have erectile dysfunction.

3. Is the most common cause of erectile dysfunction psychogenic?

No. Prior to the 1980s, it was thought that 90% of erectile dysfunction was due to psychogenic causes. Although underlying organic etiologies are more common than psychogenic problems, one cannot discount a psychological overlay to a chronic problem. Depression, performance anxiety (fear of failure), and "widower's syndrome" (a widower's entering a new relationship may evoke guilt about the deceased partner, as bereavement may not be completed) may occur.

We now know that the most common cause of erectile dysfunction is vascular. Over 50% of men have vascular dysfunction, which can relate to poor arterial inflow, excessive venous outflow, or a combination of these factors. Neurologic, hormonal, and medication effects can also play a role. Neurologic problems such as stroke, multiple sclerosis, spinal cord lesions/traumas, and peripheral and autonomic neuropathy may cause erectile dysfunction. Diabetes, hypo- and hyperthyroidism, hyperprolactinemia, and Cushing's syndrome are associated with erectile dysfunction. No one knows the frequency of these conditions—it depends on the setting. An endocrinologist will see more hormonal problems than an internist, and a psychiatrist may see more depression than another specialist. More information about the physiology of erection is now known. Altered nitric oxide, vasoactive intestinal peptide, and neuropeptide Y are implicated in erectile function.

Etiology of Impotence

Vascular	Psychologic	Medications *(cont'd.)*
Arteriosclerotic	Depression	Antidepressants
Venous leakage	"Madonna" syndrome	H_2 blockers
Arteriovenous malformations	Performance anxiety	**Systemic defects**
Local trauma	Widower's syndrome	Renal failure
Nervous system	Stress	Chronic obstructive pulmonary
Central	**Endocrine**	disease
Stroke	Diabetes mellitus	Cirrhosis
Multiple sclerosis	Hypogonadism	Leprosy
Temporal lobe epilepsy	Hyperprolactinemia	Myotonia dystrophica
Spinal cord	Hypothyroidism	**Nutritional disorders**
Trauma	Hyperthyroidism	Obesity
Tumor	Cushing's syndrome	Protein-calorie malnutrition
Peripheral	**Medications**	Zinc deficiency
Autonomic neuropathy	Antihypertensive agents	**Peyronie's disease**
Sensory neuropathy	Anticholinergics	**Prostatectomy**

4. What is the role of medication in causing erectile dysfunction?

Ten percent of commonly prescribed medications result in erectile dysfunction. In nearly 25% of men with erectile dysfunction, medications play a role. *All* antihypertensives, regardless of class, have been associated with impotence. The most common medications to cause potency problems are thiazide diuretics. These drugs drop penile pressures and lower testosterone and bioavailable testosterone levels.

5. How does hypogonadism cause erectile dysfunction?

Hypogonadism can be defined as a low testosterone level (generally < 300 ng/dl) and a low bioavailable testosterone level. Bioavailable testosterone is the fraction of testosterone not bound to sex hormone-binding globulin (SHBG) and is the "testosterone equivalent" of the relationship of the free thyroxine index to total thyroxine. That is, since testosterone is bound to SHBG, a measure of the total testosterone alone is not especially helpful in defining gonadal status. Low testosterone and low bioavailable testosterone levels are linked to low libido (sex drive) but not, per se, to erectile dysfunction. Young men who have been castrated may get erections. However, improvement in libido with testosterone treatment may be enough to overcome lack of sexual interest and erectile problems in some individuals.

6. What tests are helpful in diagnosing and determining the cause of erectile dysfunction?

All patients should be screened for sexual problems. A nonjudgmental question such as "Do you have any difficulty with your ability to have sex?" may be a good opener.

A careful sexual, medical, and medication history and a depression assessment using the Beck Depression Inventory or the Yesavage Geriatric Depression Scale are all beneficial. Penile tissue should be examined for fibrous plaques or bands that would occur with Peyronie's disease (plaques or bands causing penile bending). Small or soft testicles, gynecomastia, and increased hip girth suggest hypogonadism. Decreased penile sensitivity or abnormal cremasteric or bulbocavernosus reflexes suggest neuropathy. Penile Doppler testing can be helpful to diagnose abnormal vascular status, especially when an exercise component is added. This test measures pressure in the penis and compares it to pressure in the arm. A ratio < 0.65 (penis to brachial pressure) is diagnostic of vascular problems.

Testosterone, bioavailable testosterone, and luteinizing hormone should be measured. Thyroid function tests should be obtained. Nocturnal penile tumescence testing (sleep study of erectile function) is not especially helpful in those over age 50, as it is often impaired in older subjects despite an ability to get and maintain erections adequate for intercourse.

7. How can you treat erectile dysfunction?

When an etiology such as hypogonadism with decreased libido or depression is found, management is clear. In most cases, however, the etiology is multifactorial, and various alternatives are available. Noninvasive choices include sildenafil and vacuum tumescent devices. **Sildenafil** (Viagra), an oral type V phosphodiesterase inhibitor, results in penile vasodilation when stimulation occurs. It is contraindicated in patients taking nitrates and also may impair color vision. Care and caution should be used in patients with known or suspected cardiac disease, even if they do not take nitrates. **Vacuum tumescent devices** (the creation of negative pressure using a pump attached to a plastic tube placed over the penis) create an erection. A band or ring is then placed at the base of the penis, the vacuum is released, and the tube is removed. The erection lasts 15–30 minutes. **Penile injection therapy** (prostaglandin E1, alprostadil [Caverject]) is used when the man wishes to get an erection. **Surgery** or the implantation of bendable or inflatable rods into the penis is another method of treatment. Each method has benefits as well as problems, and often individual lifestyle and preference dictate therapeutic choice. Oral agent use remains the preferred choice.

8. What is the effect of estrogen loss in women?

Estrogen deficiency is associated with a reduction in vaginal blood flow, decreased vaginal lubrication, and increased vaginal fragility with thinning of vaginal mucosa. These changes can result in dyspareunia (painful intercourse). To treat estrogen deficiency locally, Estrace cream (or its equivalent) is inserted into the vagina 2–4 gm once daily for 2 weeks and then as maintenance 1 gm 1–3 times a week. Estrogen and progesterone have minimal effects on libido, and levels do not predict desire, sexual function, or sexual response. Estrogen has a positive and beneficial effect on vaginal lubrication and tissue strength (stronger and less friable) and from that aspect can improve sexual function. Testosterone does seem to play a major role in libido in women.

9. Is hysterectomy associated with an alteration in sexual function?

Hysterectomy is the most commonly performed surgery in women, with one-third of women over age 60 having had this procedure. However, it tends not to be associated with a decline in sexual function. For women who feel that sex is primarily a procreative function, the loss of the uterus may impact on the psychological importance and influence sexual response. For women in whom uterine contractions play an important role in orgasm, hysterectomy may impair orgasmic sensation but generally does not result in anorgasmia.

10. Does medication use affect sexual function in women?

This is relatively unknown, because few studies of medication effect explore sexual function in women. However, data suggest that antidepressants and antihypertensive agents are at least implicated in sexual dysfunction in women.

11. What reasons do older women give for changes in their sexual activity?

- Lack of a partner
- Partner erectile dysfunction
- Personal health problems
- Vaginal dryness

Masturbation is a common form of sexual expression, especially when one does not have a partner or the partner's health or abilities are impaired. Many older individuals find this an acceptable and enjoyable experience.

12. What about sexuality in a long-term care setting?

There is no age at which sexual activity and expression ends. It is important to recognize that a nursing home is still home. Staff need to provide opportunities for privacy for mutually desired sexual activities or for masturbation. The only true problem is coercive or aggressive behavior.

BIBLIOGRAPHY

1. Bretschneider JG, McCoy NL: Sexual interest and behavior in healthy 80- to 102-year-olds. Arch Sex Behav 17:109–129, 1988.
2. Diokno AC, Brown MB, Herzog AR: Sexual function in the elderly. Arch Intern Med 150:197–200, 1990.
3. Feldman HA, Goldstein I, Hatzchristou G, et al: Impotence and its medical and psychosocial correlates: Results of the Massachusetts Male Aging Study. J Urol 151:54–61, 1994.
4. Goldstein I, Lue TF, Padma Nathan H, et al: Oral sildenafil in the treatment of erectile dysfunction. N Engl J Med 338:1397–1404, 1998.
5. Kaiser FE, Viosca SP, Morley JE, et al: Impotence and aging: Clinical and hormonal factors. J Am Geriatr Soc 36:511–519, 1988.
6. Kaplan HS, Owett T: The female androgen deficiency syndrome. J Sex Marital Ther 19:13–24, 1993.
7. Krane RJ, Goldstein I, de Tejada IS: Impotence. N Engl J Med 321:1648–1659, 1989.
8. Morley JE, Kaiser FE: Impotence: The internist's approach to diagnosis and treatment. Adv Intern Med 38:151–168, 1993.
9. Rendell MS, Rajfer J, Wicker PA, et al: Sildenafil for treatment of erectile dysfunction in men with diabetes. JAMA 281:421–426, 1999.
10. Roughan PA, Kaiser FE, Morley JE: Sexuality and the older woman. Clin Geriatr Med 1:87–106, 1993.

38. ALCOHOL

David Oslin, MD

1. Is alcohol use safe in late life?

Generally, most people over age 65 do not have problems associated with alcohol consumption. No evidence suggests that the responsible use of alcohol in moderate amounts is deleterious to one's physical health. In fact, it may reduce cardiovascular mortality and overall mortality in all age groups. Less is known about any associations between moderate alcohol intake and the risk for mental illnesses, such as cognitive impairment or affective disorders. In patients with chronic illnesses such as diabetes, hypertension, or major depression, even moderate alcohol use should be avoided. Small amounts of alcohol can interfere with pharmacologic treatment or exacerbate illness.

2. Define heavy and moderate alcohol use.

Moderate alcohol use in older persons is an average of 1 drink/day. The typical pattern of drinking for most people is to consume 2 or 3 drinks once or twice per week, on the weekend, or when dining out. Others may have 1 glass of wine or a nightcap every evening. Although this amount of drinking is typically nonproblematic, patients should be educated about and monitored for the development of any problems indicative of alcohol abuse. **Heavy** alcohol use is > 1 drink/day.

3. What is alcohol abuse or dependence, and how prevalent is it in late life?

Alcohol abuse is defined by DSM-IV as a maladaptive pattern of drinking that leads to significant impairment in a person's life, including health, legal, or occupational problems or disruption in social or family functioning. **Alcohol dependence** represents a greater severity of impairment as manifested by three or more of the following:

- Tolerance
- Withdrawal symptoms
- Drinking more than intended
- Persistent desire or attempts to cut down
- A great deal of time spent in acquiring or recovering from alcohol
- Important social, occupational, or recreational activities ignored
- Continued use despite adverse problems related to alcohol

Epidemiologic studies have shown that "heavy" drinking is present in 3–9% of people over 65, with the current prevalence of alcohol abuse or dependence in the elderly being between 2–4%. There is about a 5:1 male-to-female ratio for alcohol abuse or dependence.

Alcohol use disorders are much more prevalent in clinics and hospitals. The prevalence of alcohol abuse and dependence among older primary care patients ranges from 4–13% with a lifetime prevalence of 33%. The prevalence for a current diagnosis of alcohol abuse or dependence among older inpatients on medical or surgical units ranges from 5–43%.

4. Did older patients with alcohol problems always begin drinking when they were younger?

No. Patients with an alcohol use disorder can be divided into two categories: those who have had problems most of their lives (early-onset group) and those who started having problems after age 50 (late-onset group). About one-third of older persons who are alcohol-dependent have the onset of their disease in late life. The incidence of alcohol abuse and dependence in late life has been estimated at 0.63 cases/100 person-years. The late-onset group may start problem drinking in relation to life stressors, such as affective disorders, retirement, loss of a spouse, or financial problems, but these are not the entire cause.

5. What are some risk factors that cause a person to start drinking in late life or relapse?

Change in social situation	Demographic factors
Death of spouse	Caucasian
Retirement	Male
Death of friends	Higher income
Increased leisure time	Higher education
Change in financial status	

A family history of alcohol dependence is less common in late-onset alcoholism than early-onset.

6. How can late-onset alcohol use disorders be prevented?

Prevention of excessive alcohol use is enhanced by a good **physician-patient relationship**. Routinely asking a patient about alcohol use, about significant stressors or losses, and about major changes in a patient's life such as retirement or loss of independence are keys to recognizing the onset of many problems, including problems with alcohol use. Recognition of these risk factors is paramount in preventing the escalating use of alcohol. This type of clinical relationship is becoming difficult as less time is spent with patients and as patients transfer care between many physicians.

The **community** can also play a role in preventing alcoholism. Programs at senior centers, churches, or community colleges can provide educational activities as well as social support networks for all elders. Health care providers should routinely inquire about a patient's leisure time management and hobbies and help to support community involvement. An intact social group of non–alcohol-abusing peers is an important aspect to preventing late-onset problem drinking.

7. Do changes in alcohol metabolism and degree of intoxication occur with aging?

The older person is more likely to have a higher blood alcohol level and suffer more acute intoxicating effects, such as trouble with balance, changes in fine motor skills, and cognitive dysfunction. This effect may be more pronounced in older women than in older men but has not been thoroughly studied. This effect represents a change in the volume of distribution of alcohol and not changes in hepatic metabolism. Also, changes in body mass and fat distribution occur with aging that will cause an increase in the blood alcohol level for a given amount of alcohol. Age-associated changes in the blood-brain barrier may make an older person more vulnerable to the intoxicating effects of alcohol. The increased intoxicating effect seen with older people is consistent with findings that the quantity of consumption but not the frequency decreases as people age. The older individual may reduce the amount consumed because less alcohol is necessary to produce a similar effect as when the person was 20 years younger.

8. What is the best way to identify patients with alcohol problems?

The **clinical interview** is the best tool for identifying persons with alcohol-related problems. Alcohol abuse and dependence have been shown to be underdiagnosed among the elderly in hospitals and primary care clinics. Several easily administered screening instruments have both good sensitivity and specificity. The **SGMast** is recommended as quick and sensitive. The patient is first asked if he currently drinks any alcohol. If the patient answers "yes," he is asked the following 10 questions:

	YES	NO
1. When talking with others, do you ever underestimate how much you actually drink?	(1)	(0)
2. After a few drinks, have you sometimes not eaten or been able to skip a meal because you didn't feel hungry?	(1)	(0)
3. Does having a few drinks help decrease your shakiness or tremors?	(1)	(0)
4. Does alcohol sometimes make it hard for you to remember parts of the day or night?	(1)	(0)

(Cont'd.)

	YES	NO
5. Do you usually take a drink to relax or calm your nerves?	(1)	(0)
6. Do you drink to take your mind off your problems?	(1)	(0)
7. Have you ever increased your drinking after experiencing a loss in your life?	(1)	(0)
8. Has a doctor or nurse ever said they were worried or concerned about your drinking?	(1)	(0)
9. Have you ever made rules to manage your drinking?	(1)	(0)
10. When you feel lonely, does having a drink help?	(1)	(0)

TOTAL SMAST-G SCORE (0–10) _____

Reprinted with permission of the University of Michigan Alcohol Research Center. © The Regents of the University of Michigan, 1991

If the person answers yes to three of these questions, a detailed alcohol use history should be taken, with careful attention to how alcohol use has affected the patient's life. The use of clinic brochures and educating clinic staff about alcohol use problems are also effective ways of recognizing early problems. Prevention is the key to treating late-onset alcoholism.

9. List the medical problems associated with alcohol use.

Alcohol-related medical problems can be one of the best ways of identifying patients with alcohol use disorders, which have been associated with toxic effects on almost every organ system.

Hepatic dysfunction
Gastrointestinal disorders (varices, gastritis, pancreatitis, esophagitis)
Central and peripheral nervous system dysfunction
Anemia (macrocytic)
Myopathy
Cardiomyopathy
Aspiration pneumonia
Malnutrition (specifically thiamine deficiency)
Cancer (hepatic, GI, head and neck)

10. What is the best treatment for acute alcohol withdrawal?

Acute alcohol withdrawal, alcohol withdrawal seizures, and alcohol withdrawal delirium are preventable disorders. Careful history-taking to identify patients at risk is the key to prevention. In the event that alcohol is not available to a patient, such as after admission to the hospital or when required to stop drinking for tests, proper detoxification can prevent significant morbidity to the patient. Onset of acute confusion or other mental status changes after several days in the hospital also should alert the clinician to the possibility of alcohol withdrawal. The standard treatment for detoxification or for treating withdrawal symptoms is the use of **benzodiazepines** such as oxazepam. The dose of benzodiazepine should be titrated for each individual. The clinician should avoid overmedicating the patient and can use autonomic signs, such as heart rate and blood pressure, to guide the treatment.

11. Discuss the best treatment plan for a patient with an alcohol use disorder.

After you recognize that a patient has an alcohol problem, most patients are best treated in a structured **outpatient addiction program**. Also recognize that for some patients, the stigma associated with being in an addiction program makes them refuse to participate in a program. There also is evidence that the late-onset alcoholic is much less likely to seek treatment, although such individuals do respond to treatment. Some of these patients can be managed as outpatients in a primary care clinic using brief interventions. Brief interventions are workbook-based treatment sessions focused on reducing alcohol consumption. If a patient does not achieve abstinence or remission of the abuse or dependence, then convincing the patient of the merits of a treatment program becomes a key element in overall care. Although being firm about recommending treatment is important, it also is important for the physician to maintain a relationship with the patient so that he or she can continue to work with the patient on treating the illness.

Although alcohol use disorders are chronic illnesses and patients are prone to remissions and exacerbations, the long-term outcome for patients can be good. With close attention to drinking, family support, and management of leisure time, patients can change drinking habits. The literature suggests that older patients are as likely as younger patients to respond to treatment. The benefits of abstinence are not only improved quality of life and improved relationships, but also that many of the toxic physical effects of alcohol are reversible.

12. Which types of medications should be avoided in patients with alcohol use problems?

Many medications interact with alcohol causing an increase in side effects or toxic effects. Medications that are hepatically metabolized or are active in the CNS should be used with caution in patients who are actively drinking. In patients with an alcohol use disorder that is in remission, it is important to realize that medications such as benzodiazepines and opiates are also addicting and have the potential for abuse or causing a relapse. However, these medications may be used to treat an illness that warrants their use, such as acute pain or anxiety disorders, or for the short-term relief of insomnia. The key to using these medications is the careful monitoring of both the medications and alcohol use.

Medications with potential drug–alcohol interactions include:

H$_2$ blockers	β-blockers	Antihypertensives
Aspirin	NSAIDs	Nitroglycerin
Warfarin	Acetaminophen	Certain antibiotics
Benzodiazepines	Oral hypoglycemics	

13. Should naltrexone or disulfiram (Antabuse) be prescribed?

Medications that reduce a person's craving for alcohol or cause adverse effects after drinking have been demonstrated effective only in the context of an addiction program. They should not be used as the sole method of treatment.

14. How can the clinician respect patient confidentiality while involving the family in treatment?

The family may be one of the best allies in identifying and treating patients with addiction problems. Patients have the right to refuse any discussions with family, and consent from the patient should be obtained before discussing issues about substance use with family members. Care providers should educate patients, however, about eliciting the assistance of family members. As with any chronic condition, emotional support from family members and close friends is an important predictor of treatment response. Patients and physicians also should realize that family members are usually aware of a patient's alcohol use, and refusal to allow family members to help is often a way for a patient to obstruct treatment consciously or unconsciously.

BIBLIOGRAPHY

1. Anton RF: Pharmacologic approaches to the management of alcoholism. J Clin Psychiatry 62:11–17, 2001.
2. Barry KL, Oslin DW, Blow FC: Prevention and Management of Alcohol Problems in Older Adults. New York, Springer Publishing, 2001.
3. Frances A: Diagnostic and Statistical Manual of Mental Disorders, 4th ed. Washington, DC, American Psychiatric Press, 1994.
4. LaCroix AZ, Guralnik JM, Berkman LF, et al: Maintaining mobility in late life. Am J Epidemiol 137: 858–869, 1993.

5. Lakhani N: Alcohol use amongst community-dwelling elderly people: A review of the literature. J Adv Nurs 25:1227–1232, 1997.
6. Liberto J, Oslin D, Ruskin P: Alcoholism in older persons: A review of the literature. Hosp Commun Psychiatry 43:975–984, 1992.
7. Nelson HD, Nevitt MC, Scott JC, et al: Smoking, alcohol, and neuromuscular and physical function of older women. JAMA 272:1825–1831, 1994.
8. O'Loughlin JL, Robitaille Y, Boivin J-F, Suissa S: Incidence of and risk factors for falls and injurious falls among the community-dwelling elderly. Am J Epidemiol 137:342–354, 1993.
9. Reid MC, Anderson PA: Geriatric substance disorders. Med Clin North Am 81:999–1016, 1997.

39. THE OLDER DRIVER

Sheila Pasupathy and Risa Lavizzo-Mourey, MD, MBA

1. Is driving an important issue among older adults?

The ability to drive defines independence and provides a sense of self-esteem for many older adults. Suggesting that it is unsafe to drive is a major threat to their sense of control in everyday life. On a pragmatic level, driving represents the sole means of transportation for many seniors. Studies in 1994 show that 88% of older Americans rely on a private automobile for most of their transportation needs. The trend to "gray in place" represents the desire of older adults to remain in rural or suburban communities where mass transit is not easily accessible.

Driving cessation often leads to decreased quality of life because people lose the ability to participate freely in social opportunities, visit family, go to the grocery store, or engage in essential activities independently. The resulting increase in loneliness and isolation may adversely affect health and well-being. Hardest hit are couples in cohorts over the age of 80. Women of this generation often never learned to drive and depend completely on their husbands for mobility. Unfortunately, many older people do not have a strong network of support or access to appropriate social/community supports to maintain independent living. Thus, research in this area generally focuses on two objectives: (1) to identify and rehabilitate people with impairments to prolong driving independence and (2) to identify and create viable driving alternatives for people who need to compensate for mobility loss.

2. What are the costs of poor driver safety among the elderly?

Studies by the National Highway Traffic Administration show that the number of traffic fatalities is on the rise for older cohorts.

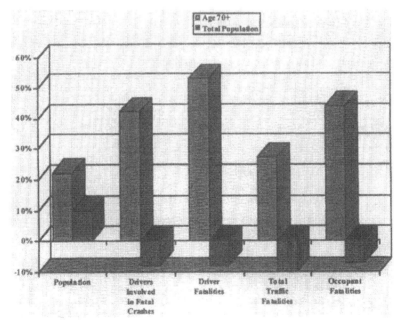

Percent Change, 1987–1997. Source: National Highway Traffic Safety Administration.

Although older adults drive substantially less than younger drivers, they incur a disproportionate number of fatalities per mile driven due to increasing fragility. These statistics illustrate
the seriousness of driving risk for the elderly—a trend that must be reversed in the face of a burgeoning senior population.

Traffic Deaths per 100,000 Population

Motor vehicle traffic fatality rates by age group, 1990–2000 (National Center for Statistics & Analysis).

3. The ability to drive depends on which functions?

Driving is a highly integrative task that depends on psychomotor, cognitive, and sensoriperceptual
functions. Specifically, vehicle operation requires the interaction of sustained visual attention, adequate speed of mental processing, timely and accurate responses, and adequate sensory motor control.

4. Does normal aging have an impact on driving skills?

Normal aging results in a number of basic functional changes that affect driving skills.
Fortunately, evidence indicates that older drivers exhibit good judgment by adjusting their driving practices to accommodate declining function.

FUNCTION	AGE-RELATED CHANGES	DRIVING-RELATED IMPAIRMENTS
Psychomotor	Decreased number and size of muscle fibers Decreased responsiveness to electrical stimulation Decreased myosin adenosine triphosphatase activity Degradation of joints and tendons	Reductions in musculoskeletal function result in: • Slowing • Deteriorated strength • Reduced dexterity and coordination • Increased reaction time
Sensoriperceptual	Decreased visual acuity Drop in peripheral field vision Decreased retinal illuminance Increased light scattering Reduced amplitude of accommo-dation—presbyopia Loss of retinal photoreceptors Loss of retinal ganglion cells as well as other age-related cortical changes	Changes in optical and visual function result in: • Decreased night visual acuity • Decreased resistance to glare • Decreased contrast sensitivity • Increased dark-adaptation time interval

5. What medical conditions affect driving ability?

Studies show that certain medical conditions, prevalent in older adults, increase crash risk:

Seizure disorders. People afflicted with epileptic seizures may experience loss of motor function and/or total loss of consciousness. Every U.S. state has varying restrictions against driving for people with epilepsy.

Stroke. Presenting symptoms of stroke include motor, sensory, and cognitive deficits—all essential for safe driving. Recommendations from the American Medical Association suggest that changes of higher cerebral functions in association with cerebrovascular accidents should be an indication to stop driving.

Diabetes. Hyperglycemia may result in symptoms of fatigue and sluggishness. In addition, chronic complications of diabetes such as macroangiopathy, microangiopathy, and diabetic retinopathy may have a detrimental impact on driving.

Cardiovascular disease. Many conditions classified under cardiovascular disease impair driving ability. For instance, sick sinus syndrome causes lethargy, weakness, light-headedness, dizziness, and episodes of near-syncope or actual loss of consciousness.

Arthritis. Arthritis may generate pain causing unconscious hesitancy and total restriction of motion, which can greatly affect braking, turning, and gripping the wheel.

Dementia. Dementia, depending on severity, affects cognitive functions necessary for competent driving. Loss of cognitive function affects judgment, memory, and attention.

Parkinson's disease. Parkinson's disease is characterized by resting tremor, pill rolling of the fingers, forward flexion of the trunk, and muscle rigidity and weakness. These motor impairments affect overall vehicle control.

Foot abnormalities. Foot abnormalities such as toenail irregularities, calluses, bunions, and toe deformities such as hammer toes increase crash risk because they may affect the ability to maneuver between the accelerator and brake.

Bursitis. Bursitis, especially of the shoulder or elbow, may cause severe pain and limitation of mobility.

6. How do eye problems affect driving ability?

According to the Framingham Eye Study, the four leading causes of vision impairment among older adults are age-related macular degeneration, cataract, glaucoma, and diabetic retinopathy. Driving involves the simultaneous use of central and peripheral vision. Thus, the effects of these conditions critically affect crash risk.

CONDITION	EFFECT ON VISION
Age-related macular degeneration	Distortion and/or loss of central vision
Cataract	Loss of vision acuity, contrast sensitivity Increased sensitivity to glare, nearsightedness
Glaucoma	Gradual loss of peripheral vision Eventual damage to central vision
Diabetic retinopathy	Gradual development of severe blurred vision–macular edema Potential loss of vision via retinal detachment

7. Which medications can affect the ability to drive safely?

Any medication has the potential to affect driving ability profoundly. The following groups of medications are especially risky:

MEDICATION	POTENTIAL EFFECT ON DRIVING ABILITY
Benzodiazepines	Impaired vision, attention, information processing, memory, motor coordination, ability to perform combined skills task, and driving under controlled conditions

(Cont'd.)

MEDICATION	POTENTIAL EFFECT ON DRIVING ABILITY
Antidepressants	Impaired attention, memory, motor coordination, and open road driving
Opioid analgesics	Impaired vision, attention, and motor coordination Sedation
Antihistamines	Sedation Impaired coordination, simulated driving, and open road driving
Hypoglycemics*	Impaired cognition, memory, vision, information processing, and motor control

* A threat only if hypoglycemia is induced.

8. What is the physician's role in evaluating driver safety?

Physicians have a duty to protect their patients' lives. Thus, when a patient's health impairs the ability to drive, physicians have a duty to recommend limitations or cessation if driving poses a threat to the patient. The good news is that many elders self-regulate—they limit their driving based on their own limitations. Unfortunately, some are not fully aware of their limitations and continue to drive under unsafe conditions. To distinguish safe drivers from unsafe drivers, physicians should include an assessment of driving skills in the normal evaluation of the geriatric patient. Evaluating driving competency is a particular challenge for physicians faced with resolving the conflict between an elderly patient's quality of life and public safety. Unnecessary limitations on driving ability may have a detrimental effect on the patient's well-being, whereas failure to recommend driving cessation when it is appropriate may lead to a crash that harms the patient and/or others. Therefore, a physician must take care in assessing and making judgments about driving performance and must be prepared to discuss recommendations with patients and their families.

9. How is driving safety evaluated?

Criteria for determining who is at risk for crashes have not been validated, but questions related to driving can serve as triggers for further evaluation. A targeted listing may assess the following:
- Impact of driving on quality of life
- Driving frequency and distances
- Driving patterns (e.g., freeway vs. local roads, day vs. night driving)
- Changes in driving patterns in the past year
- Use of medications known to impair driving
- Alcohol use
- Presence of driving-impairing medical conditions
- Condition of driving-related functions
- Number of accidents
- Use of seatbelts

Based on the history, physicians must be prepared to question and examine further patients whose responses indicate potential risk. This next level of assessment should attempt to elucidate problem areas and uncover additional medical conditions through basic examinations. Examples of tests that may be used include:
- Mini-Mental State Exam for dementia
- Neurologic exam and gait and balance test for Parkinson's disease
- Snellen eye chart for vision
- Whisper test for hearing
- Cervical spine, hip, and knee mobility test for arthritis
- "Get-up-and-go" test to test musculoskeletal response

If the presence of a driving-impairing condition is confirmed, the physician must perform another level of assessment to determine severity of illness. At this point, the physician may need to gather more information about the nature of the uncovered condition, or he/she may refer the patient to other professionals who can better determine whether the condition poses a threat to driving ability. Referral to an occupational therapist for a formal driving screening is recommended.

Driving screenings at best simulate driving with video and at the least probe specific cognitive and motor skills required during driving for comparison with age-appropriate norms. Poor performance on a driving screen may be enough to convince an unsafe driver to stop. Many states have legislation requiring physicians to report disabled patients to the registry of motor vehicles, even if they are unable to drive only temporarily. If reported by a physician, a patient must participate in a more complete medical evaluation.

10. Which medical conditions are physicians obligated to report to the Department of Transportation?

Almost all states have established regulations regarding drivers with impairments. The Department of Transportation states that physician reporting is a highly effective mechanism for identifying medically impaired drivers. Over 40,000 reports are submitted each year, of which 72% signify impairments that are significant enough to merit temporary or permanent recall of driving privilege. Policies vary from state to state and may be obtained through the Bureau of Driver Licensing. Pennsylvania's reporting requirements include the following:

- A person with visual acuity of less than 20/100 combined vision with best correction may not be qualified to drive. Other vision policies restrict driving to daylight hours and certain areas.
- A person with a seizure disorder shall not be qualified to drive unless the person has been free from seizure for at least 6 months from the date of the last seizure, with or without medication. Waivers of the freedom-from-seizure requirement may be made on recommendation by a physician under specific conditions.
- A person with any of the following conditions shall not be qualified to drive:
    1. Unstable or brittle diabetes or hypoglycemia, unless the patient has been free from any related syncopal attack for at least 6 months.
    2. Cerebral vascular insufficiency or cardiovascular disease, which, for the preceding 6 months, has resulted in either (1) syncopal attacks or loss of consciousness or (2) vertigo, paralysis, or loss of qualifying visual fields.
    3. Periodic episodes of loss of consciousness that are of unknown etiology or not otherwise categorized, unless the person has been free from such episodes for the year immediately preceding.
- Providers may make recommendations to restrict driving if the patient has a condition that, in the opinion of the provider, is likely to impair the ability to drive safely.

11. What options are available to rehabilitate drivers at risk for crashes?

Many older adults who are forced to limit or stop driving based on functional impairments are often not aware of retraining options that allow them to get behind the wheel safely once more. Several options are available:

1. Occupational therapists have developed comprehensive programs that not only assess a patient's capacity to drive but also analyze deficits that may improve through training. For example, an occupational therapist may design an exercise program to increase physical strength, endurance, and mobility if a physical condition hampers driving. Such programs are comprehensive and give patients a chance to become mobile again.

2. Specialized adaptive equipment may be used to compensate for functional limitations. Many older adults without cognitive deficits respond well to such implements. For example, people who do not have adequate strength in their legs may benefit from hand controls that facilitate use of gas and brake pedals. Other commonly prescribed equipment compensates for reduced range of motion, reaction time, dexterity, and peripheral vision.

3. Several organizations offer driver training programs that cover a variety of issues, including new safety rules and common traffic problems associated with age. Such programs are usually 4–8 hour courses and are sponsored by associations such as the National Safety Council, the American Automobile Association, and the American Association of Retired Persons. New pilot projects have been launched by companies such as General Motors. These courses have limitations

in improving driving ability because they do not address the debilitating effects of medical conditions in conjunction with normal aging and generally do not impart skills training to overcome functional impairments.

BIBLIOGRAPHY

1. Johansson K, Lundberg C: The 1994 International Consensus Conference on Dementia and Driving: A brief report. Alzheimer Dis Assoc Disord 11:62–69, 1997.
2. Messinger-Rapport B: How to assess and counsel the older driver. Cleve Clin J Med 69:184–192, 2002.
3. Morgan R, King D: The older driver—a review. Postgrad Med J 71:525–528, 1995.
4. Owsley C, Ball K, McGwin G, et al: Visual processing impairment and risk of motor vehicle crash among older adults. JAMA 279:1083–1088, 1998.
5. Owsley C, Stalvey B, Wells J, Sloan M: Older drivers and cataract: Driving habits and crash risk. J Gerontol 54:M203–M211, 1999.
6. Retchin S (ed): Medical Considerations in the older driver. Clinics in Geriatric Medicine, vol. 9. Philadelphia, W.B. Saunders, 1993.
7. Wallace R: Cognitive change, medical illness and crash risk among older drivers: An epidemiological consideration. Alzheimer Dis Assoc Disord 11:31–37, 1997.

40. COMPLEMENTARY AND ALTERNATIVE MEDICINE

Elizabeth R. Mackenzie, PhD

1. What is complementary and alternative medicine?

The National Center for Complementary and Alternative Medicine (NCCAM) at the National Institutes of Health (NIH) defines complementary and alternative medicine (CAM) as "those treatments and health care practices not taught widely in medical schools, not generally used in hospitals, and not usually reimbursed by medical insurance companies." This definition covers a wide array of modalities, from chiropractic manipulation, therapeutic massage, and reflexology to homeopathy, herbal medicines, Traditional Chinese Medicine (including herbs, acupuncture, tai chi, qigong), Ayurvedic medicine, yoga, meditation, spiritual healing, and shamanism. These examples are only a small fraction of the kinds of unconventional healing practices available in the U.S. However, most have some underlying assumptions or perspectives in common. CAM purports to be holistic; that is, it treats the whole person, including physical, mental, emotional, and spiritual dimensions.

Biomedicine has been the dominant form of health care in the U.S. since the mid-nineteenth century. It relies largely on sophisticated surgical techniques, vaccines, antitoxins, and other pharmaceutical preparations. Biomedicine rose to dominance in large part because of its many impressive successes (e.g., vaccines to reduce childhood diseases, antibiotics to treat infection). Despite growing interest in biopsychosocial approaches to health among providers and health researchers, conventional medicine typically has compartmentalized the practice and study of medicine into separate specialties and subspecialties. Although allowing greater intellectual precision, this compartmentalization has resulted in a somewhat fragmented approach to understanding health and disease. Generally speaking, "holism" is one way to differentiate CAM from conventional biomedicine. A corollary is that CAM seeks to heal the person rather than to cure the disease.

CAM systems focus on prevention and health promotion (or wellness) rather than on treating symptoms after they have arisen. Because conventional health care has a growing interest in health promotion and because consumer demand for access to holistic forms of medicine has increased, certain facets of CAM are gradually finding their way into the mainstream, often making it difficult to distinguish among systems that are alternative, complementary, integrated, integrative, or conventional. For example, the use of vitamin E for Alzheimer's disease began as a CAM intervention but has been largely adopted by mainstream medicine. Acupuncture used to be viewed askance by the medical community and is now practiced in many large hospitals nationwide. Many health systems are adding CAM clinics or holistic programming. This pattern of inclusion of CAM modalities into conventional medicine, shown to be effective, is part of the process of creating "integrated medicine," a health care system that uses the perspectives and techniques of both biomedicine and CAM.

Ambiguities surrounding the categorization of particular modalities and systems probably will become even more pronounced as managed care organizations and insurers begin to cover CAM modalities and as medical schools offer courses in CAM or integrated medicine, according to their own definitions of the category.

An often overlooked characteristic of CAM modalities is that many originated in the healing traditions of specific cultural or ethnic groups, typically from non-Western societies. In fact, these healing traditions (or ethnomedicine) have engendered a vast array of CAM systems. Traditional Chinese medicine or traditional Oriental medicine, the Indian Ayurvedic tradition, and herbal and shamanic healing from tribes across North and South America, Africa, Australia, and Eurasia have contributed much to our knowledge of nonbiomedical healing systems. Only a few modalities have their roots in Western Europe (e.g., chiropractic manipulation, homeopathy, naturopathic medicine, European folk medicine, and certain religious healing traditions). Various modalities developed in the past few decades do not have explicitly ethnomedical roots, such as numerous body work techniques designed to help people achieve enhanced structural balance (e.g., Rolfing, Alexander, and Feldenkrais techniques, cranial-sacral therapy), treatments that require special technology (e.g., biofeedback, transcutaneous electrical nerve stimulation), and the use of various nutritional supplements (e.g., glucosamine sulfate to treat arthritis). Nonetheless, there is a significant overlap between CAM and ethnomedicine.

2. Do older adults use CAM?

Over one-third of older adults (aged 50+) in the U.S. use CAM. In a survey of 101 primary care physicians treating persons diagnosed with probable Alzheimer's disease, Coleman et al. found that over one-half administered at least one CAM therapy. Among the most popular CAM therapies for Alzheimer's disease are vitamins, health foods, herbal medicine (especially ginkgo biloba), music therapy, and home remedies. Patients with osteoarthritis also appear to be frequent users of CAM modalities; both acupuncture and glucosamine sulfate are popular CAM treatments for arthritis. Because so many of the chronic conditions most likely to be treated with CAM modalities are prevalent in older adults, and because the highest reported use nationally is in the 35–49-year-old group, CAM use among older adults can be expected to increase over the next several years.

3. How can the physician discuss CAM use with patients?

Despite the de facto integration of CAM into the health care landscape, a 1990 survey found that approximately 70% of persons who use CAM modalities do not discuss the topic with their physicians. Given the high probability that CAM use will affect conventional treatment plans and health outcomes, clinicians should include questions about CAM use. Eisenberg recommends the following approach: "Patients with [chief complaint] frequently use other kinds of therapy for relief. For example, some patients use chiropractic, massage, herbs, vitamins, etc. Have you used or thought about using any of these or other therapies for your [chief complaint] or for any other reason?" It is extremely important that the question be asked in a nonjudgmental and nonthreatening manner. Patients who sense that their medical provider disapproves of, ridicules, or disparages attempts to explore the potential benefits of CAM usually conceal their interest. Concealment may have seriously adverse consequences for the physician–patient relationship, possibly leading to lower quality of care. Clinicians should keep in mind that it is possible to acknowledge patients' beliefs about CAM without sharing them. Creating a psychological environment that supports forthright, respectful dialogue is the first step toward better understanding of CAM by both patients and providers.

4. To integrate or not to integrate?

Given the current trends in use of CAM, most clinicians probably will have to face the question of how comfortable they are with discussing and perhaps integrating aspects of CAM into their practice. There are three salient dimensions to this question: (1) Does it work? (2) Can it harm? (3) By whom should it be delivered?

5. Are CAM modalities efficacious?

Perhaps the most important piece of information about CAM from the point of view of the practicing clinician is, "Does it work?" The past decade or so has seen numerous U.S. studies of the efficacy of CAM modalities for particular conditions, many funded by the NIH. Although many studies have been inconclusive and some modalities have been shown to have dubious therapeutic value, investigations into a wide array of therapies indicate some promise. CAM modalities previously suggested to be efficacious for conditions common within the population of older adults are summarized in the following tables.

CONDITION	CAM TREATMENT	STUDY
Cognitive decline	Ginkgo biloba (herb)	Kanowski et al: Proof of efficacy of the ginkgo biloba special extract Egb 761 in outpatients suffering from primary degenerative dementia of the Alzheimer type and multi-infarct dementia. Pharmacopsychiatry 4:149–158, 1995.
Frailty, poor balance, falls	Tai chi	Wolf et al: Reducing frailty and falls in older persons. J Am Geriatr Soc 44:489–497, 1996.
Depression	Exercise	Moore, Blumenthal: Exercise training as an alternative treatment for depression among older adults. Alt Ther Health Med 4:48–56, 1998.
Osteoarthritis	Acupuncture	Bareta: Evidence presented to consensus panel on acupuncture's efficacy. Alt Ther Health Med 4: 22–30, 102, 1998.
Coronary artery stenosis	Support groups/ lifestyle changes	Ornish et al: Can lifestyle changes reverse coronary heart disease? The Lifestyle Heart Trial. Lancet 336:129–133, 1999.
Fibromyalgia	Acupuncture	Berman et al: Is acupuncture effective in the treatment of fibromyalgia? J Fam Pract 48:213-238, 1999.

CAM Modalities Recently under Investigation via NIH-NCCAM Grants

CONDITION	TREATMENT	STUDY
Sleep disorders (Parkinson's disease)	Melatonin	University of California at San Francisco (Dowling)
Agitation	Music and massage	University of Massachusetts (Remington)
Knee osteoarthritis	Acupuncture	University of Maryland (Berman)
Depression	Hypericum (St. John's wort)	Duke University (Davidson)
Alcoholism	Acupuncture	Minneapolis Medical Research Foundation (Bullock)
Depression	Acupuncture	University of Arizona (Allen)

For a complete list of current research, see <www.nccam.nih.gov/research/extramural/index.htm>.

6. Can CAM modalities harm the patient?

For providers interested in integrating some CAM modalities into their practice, it is important to be aware of contraindications, herb-drug interactions, and other potential harmful effects of CAM use. Of greatest concern, especially in terms of toxicity, is herbal medicine or phytomedicine. Although herbal preparations often have fewer side effects than synthetically produced drugs and many are so benign that they can be used in large quantities under most circumstances (e.g., chamomile, red clover), some have the potential to harm when used improperly. For example, licorice root is known to raise blood pressure and should not be used by hypertensive patients. St. John's wort must be stopped 1 week before anesthesia/surgery. Echinacea, an herb used as an immune system booster, is contraindicated for persons with autoimmune disorders. Ginkgo biloba inhibits platelet-activating factor and therefore can interact adversely with antithrombotic drugs. Many herbs can induce menstruation (e.g., pennyroyal, feverfew), and pregnant women are well advised to use herbal teas, tinctures, and extracts with caution. Essential oils used in aromatherapy, although plant-derived and therefore a type of phytomedicine, are the extremely concentrated volatile oils of a plant (the "essence" of the plant) and should rarely if ever be taken internally.

Patients also may stop taking their prescribed medication, replacing it with a CAM treatment without their physician's knowledge. Although the hypertensive patient whose blood pressure becomes significantly lowered as a result of biofeedback or meditation may actually no longer require antihypertensive medication, it is best for this transition to occur gradually and under a physician's supervision.

7. By whom should CAM be delivered?

Because CAM covers such a broad array of modalities, philosophies, and cultural traditions, it is not always clear how to judge a practitioner's competence. Some modalities have rigorous licensing and training requirements (e.g., traditional Chinese medicine, massage, naturopathy), and licensed practitioners can be assumed to have reached a certain level of competence. National and state level associations usually publish lists of licensed and certified practitioners. However, some modalities have no such oversight, and many of the most skilled practitioners may be self-taught or educated under an informal apprenticeship (e.g., herbal medicine and various forms of ethnomedicine, such as curanderismo, santeria, Native American healing). Knowing whom to trust is often best determined by the practitioner's local reputation among patients and health professionals alike. Another method for choosing a CAM practitioner is to seek out physicians or nurses who have undergone training in a specific modality. Numerous physicians now practice as acupuncturists, homeopaths, herbalists, or other CAM specialists.

8. What reliable resources are available for accurate information about CAM?

1. The NIH's National Center for Complementary and Alternative Medicine (NCCAM) offers information about use of CAM, including current and past research into efficacy and definitions. Their clearinghouse for information can be reached at 1-888-644-6226: their Web address is http://nccam.nih.gov. The National Cancer Institute also has an Office of Cancer Complementary and Alternative Medicine at www3.cancer.gov/occam/.

2. The American Holistic Health Association (AHHA) serves as a national association for CAM practitioners and a clearinghouse for information about CAM for the public. Web site: http://ahha.org; telephone: 714-779-6152.

3. Fleming T (ed): PDR for Herbal Medicines. Montvale, NJ, Medical Economics Company, updated each year.

4. Blumenthal M (ed): The Complete German Commission E Monographs: Therapeutic Guide to Herbal Medicines. Newton, MA, Integrative Medicine Publishers/American Botanical Council, 1998.

5. Dossey L (ed): Alternative Therapies in Health and Medicine. Aliso Viejo, CA, Innovision Communications. Telephone: 1-800-899-1712.

6. Gordon J: Manifesto for a New Medicine: Your Guide to Healing Partnerships and the Wise Use of Alternative Medicine. Reading, MA, Perseus Books, 1996.

7. Eisenberg D: Advising patients who seek alternative medical therapies. Ann Intern Med 127:61–69, 1999 [includes an appendix listing information resources].

8. NIH, Office of Alternative Medicine: Alternative Medicine: Expanding Medical Horizons [Workshop on Alternative Medicine's Report to the NIH, Chantilly, VA]. Washington, DC, U.S. Government Printing Office, 1992.

BIBLIOGRAPHY

1. Astin JA: Why patients use alternative medicine: Results of a national study. JAMA 279:1548–1553, 1998.
2. Coleman LM, Fowler LI, Williams ME: The use of unproven therapies by people with Alzheimer's disease. J Am Geriatr Soc 43:829–830, 1995.
3. Eisenberg DM: Advising patients who seek alternative medical therapies. Ann Intern Med 127:61–69, 1997.
4. Eisenberg DM, Davis RB, Ettner SL, et al: Trends in alternative medicine use in the United States, 1990–1997: Results of a follow-up national survey. JAMA 280:1569–1575, 1998.
5. O'Connor BB: Implications for the health professions. In Healing Traditions: Alternative Medicine and the Health Professions. Philadelphia, University of Pennsylvania Press, 1995, pp 161–195.

IV. Hospital Care of the Geriatric Patient

41. PERIOPERATIVE MANAGEMENT IN THE ELDERLY

Joan Weinryb, MD, CMD, and Jerry Johnson, MD

1. What impact does chronologic age have on surgical outcome?

With the increasing life expectancy of our society, older people are more likely to undergo surgical procedures. Although studies show higher rates of mortality and morbidity for elderly persons, this finding appears to be based, at least in part, on the increasing incidence of comorbidities in old people. Comorbid conditions make the likelihood of poor outcome 4 times higher. Understanding of the risks is confounded by the fact that many studies of postoperative outcome in the elderly combine patients undergoing emergency and elective procedures. Others combine low-risk patients with those who have coexisting underlying diseases. The presence of other illnesses, especially cardiac and pulmonary diseases, is predictive of perioperative morbidity and mortality. Also predictive is the urgency of the procedure, with fewer complications for elective surgery. Emergency surgery is 20 times riskier than an elective procedure. Age is a predictor of longer length of hospitalization and of cardiac and noncardiac complications; however, with the improvements in anesthetic and perioperative management, rates of complication do not preclude surgery in elderly persons.

2. How does the type of surgery affect the perioperative outcome?

Anatomic location confers risk. The least risky procedures are cataract surgeries, hernia repairs, and transurethral prostatectomy, with mortality rates of less than 1%. Cardiac and vascular procedures, such as repair of abdominal aortic aneurysms, are more risky, with mortality rates from 3–10%. Certain procedures, such as carotid endarterectomy, are less risky if undertaken in a hospital that does a high volume of the procedure. Emergency surgery increases the risk of any procedure.

3. What are the major causes of perioperative morbidity and mortality in the elderly?

Failure of the cardiac, pulmonary, or renal system is most likely to lead to perioperative morbidity and mortality. Multiple chronic conditions increase surgical risk. Age-related changes also contribute. For example, diabetes mellitus is associated with increased risk of accelerated atherosclerosis, leading to cardiac complications and peripheral vascular problems. Elevated serum glucose levels are associated with postoperative bleeding and impaired wound healing. Respiratory muscle weakening is part of normal aging and may lead to diminished pulmonary reserve, atelectasis, and pneumonia postoperatively. Decreasing renal function, due to age and disease, affects ability to survive diagnostic procedures using radiographic contrast materials and response to medications.

4. Why is preoperative assessment important in elderly people?

As the population ages, it is increasingly likely that a person will require a surgical procedure to treat disease or accident. Surgical rates are 55% higher in persons over 65. Forty percent of older general hospital admissions are to surgical services. Older patients account for 75% of postoperative deaths. Surgical mortality of patients over 65 undergoing cardiac revascularization is about 5%, compared with 1% in younger patients. Intra-abdominal surgical mortality rates of 3–5% are about twice that in younger people. Since surgical complications are more common in persons over the age of 65 and seem to be related to underlying illnesses, risk assessment is increasingly important in enabling appropriate treatment planning.

5. How can the general medicine or geriatric consultant contribute to the preoperative assessment?

Although often termed "clearing" the patient for surgery, no patient or physician can be assured of zero risk. Preoperative assessment involves evaluating the patient to determine what underlying conditions contribute to the risk of poor outcome, whether these factors are correctable, or whether appropriate perioperative planning can diminish the risk implicit in the condition.

6. Which medical problems should be considered in evaluating the older preoperative candidate?

Patients should be evaluated for acute medical problems known to contribute to surgical morbidity and mortality. Acute myocardial infarction, pulmonary embolus, and decompensated diabetes mellitus are examples of conditions known to contribute to poor outcome and are good reasons to postpone elective procedures. Chronic conditions should also be considered in evaluating the elderly person. Dementia is known to be a risk factor for the development of perioperative delirium. Delirium can lead to dehydration, malnutrition, inability to cooperate with therapy, increased rates of infection, and other complications, leading to prolonged hospitalization, increased mortality, and increased likelihood of discharge to a nursing home. Depression can also lead to dehydration, malnutrition, deconditioning, inability to cooperate with care, and poor outcome. Poor nutrition is associated with poor surgical outcome. A 10% loss of body weight is associated with impaired immunity, 20% with decreased healing and infection, 30% with weakness that precludes sitting, pneumonia and a 50% mortality rate, and 40% with a nearly 100% mortality rate. Some studies indicate improved outcome for patients with normal preoperative nutritional status receiving supplemental nutrition perioperatively. Little evidence supports postponing procedures to provide nutritional support for all but the most severely affected. Parkinson's disease can contribute significantly to perioperative complications, with increased risk of aspiration, obstipation due to constipation, delirium, hypotension, and myocardial infarction as well as deconditioning and falls, all prolonging recovery. Prostate enlargement is associated with urinary retention and increased rates of infection.

7. Does decreased mobility or exercise tolerance affect postoperative outcome?

Decreased exercise tolerance is a nonspecific indicator of increased surgical risk. It is associated with cardiac disease and with mortality in general. Patients who are not active enough to leave their homes at least twice a week by their own efforts have been shown to have more frequent complications of all kinds than more active persons. The inability to exercise sufficiently to attain a heart rate of 100 beats/min predicts cardiac ischemic events.

8. What information should be obtained by the medical history?

The frequency of multiple comorbidities in the elderly necessitates a comprehensive history and physical examination. The **cardiac history** should attempt to identify the past evidence of coronary artery disease or congestive heart failure. A myocardial infarction in the previous 6 months, active congestive heart failure, arrhythmia, and unstable angina confer substantial risk of postoperative cardiac complications. Chronic hypertension does not confer increased risk of postoperative complications except as a marker for cardiac disease. However, very elevated blood pressure, evidence of recent fluctuations in blood pressure, or new-onset hypertension may predict instability during the procedure.

It is estimated that a fourth of deaths that occur within 6 days of surgery are related to pulmonary complications. The **pulmonary history** should attempt to identify the presence of chronic obstructive pulmonary disease (COPD) or asthma, a history of smoking, and long-term steroid use. Other risk factors for postoperative pneumonia include altered sensorium, cerebrovascular accident (CVA), alcohol use, and the type of procedure planned. Abdominal aortic repair and upper abdominal and intrathoracic procedures confer the greatest risk.

Previous **thromboembolic events** including deep venous thrombosis (DVT) involving either upper or lower extremities or pulmonary emboli are significant risk factors for postoperative thromboembolic events. These complications are seen most frequently in orthopedic surgery of the knee and hip and pelvic or intra-abdominal surgery for malignant conditions.

Hypertension, diabetes, and other atherosclerotic risk factors may indicate need for concern about the patient's **renal function**. Even though the records may indicate a normal serum creatinine, the elderly person with reduced muscle mass may still have renal insufficiency and require modification of usual medication doses.

A **functional history** determines status and ability to recover mobility and self-care postoperatively. A **nutritional history** may disclose underlying feeding problems, including dysphagia, GI diseases, and involuntary weight loss. Interestingly, underestimation of actual weight loss is associated with poor outcome, whereas overestimation is not.

9. What information can be obtained from the physical examination?

A general impression of the level of **frailty and deconditioning** can be deduced from observing the patient moving around the exam room. The **cardiopulmonary exam** can detect the presence of active heart failure or a cardiac murmur, particularly aortic stenosis, the most common valvular disease in the elderly. The presence of an S_3 heart sound, increased jugulovenous pulse, bradycardia, tachycardia, and irregularities suggesting ectopic beats may alert the clinician to potential risk factors. Examination of the lower extremities may reveal peripheral pulse abnormalities or evidence of edema indicating underlying cardiac or circulatory problems.

Decreased breath sounds may suggest COPD. Rales or bronchospasm may suggest **pulmonary disease** or heart failure. Assessment of the **skin** helps determine if peripheral vascular disease, delayed wound healing, or the development of pressure sores is likely to be a problem. **Musculoskeletal abnormalities** from arthritic changes, Parkinson's disease, or stroke may be associated with mobility problems, functional disability, and other factors that can impede recovery.

The **neuropsychiatric exam** is aimed at determining whether there is acute or chronic cognitive impairment, depression, evidence of Parkinson's disease, or focal weakness that would indicate underlying cerebrovascular disease. A **BMI** of 22 or less is an indication of compromised nutritional status and may lead to further laboratory evaluation.

10. What preoperative indexes are useful in predicting postoperative complications?

Anesthesiologists have long used **Dripp's Physical Status Scale** to classify patients in five groups from class I, healthy persons, to class V, patients who are moribund and not expected to survive 24 hours with or without the operation. This scale is more useful in predicting the outcomes of patients at the ends of the spectrum than as a predictor in classes II, III, and IV. Furthermore, it gives no insight into correctable factors.

The **Goldman Cardiac Risk Index** (CRI), a predictor of postoperative cardiac outcomes in noncardiac surgery, is the best known predictive tool. Nine independent factors that assess the level of hemodynamic stress imposed on the vital organ systems and the risk of adverse cardiac outcomes are assigned points:

VARIABLE	ASSIGNED POINTS
Third heart sound	11
Elevated jugular vein pressure	11
Myocardial infarction in past 6 mo	10
EKG shows more than 5 PVCs per min	7
EKG-PACs or any rhythm other than sinus	7

(Cont'd.)

VARIABLE	ASSIGNED POINTS
Age greater than 70	5
Emergency procedure	4
Intrathoracic, intra-abdominal, or aortic surgery	3
Poor general status—metabolic or bedridden	3

PVC = premature ventricular contracture, PAC = premature atrial contraction.

These nine factors are used to classify patients into 4 categories of risk:

CLASS	POINT TOTAL	NO OR MINOR COMPLICATION (%)	LIFE-THREATENING COMPLICATION (%)	CARDIAC DEATH (%)
Class I	0–5	99	0.7	0.2
Class II	6–12	93	5	2
Class III	13–25	86	11	2
Class IV	> 26	22	22	56

Generally, with individuals over age 70 who undergo an intra-abdominal, intrathoracic, or aortic procedure and who have any of the first five factors above will total 13 points, placing them in one of the two highest risk categories by this scale. Detsky modified the CRI, adding points for unstable angina, pulmonary edema, and class II or III status by the Canadian Cardiovascular Society Scale for angina. Eagle derived a third, simpler cardiac index (discussed below in question 12) in persons undergoing vascular surgery. Note that high scores on the CRI or Detsky indexes are greater than 12 or 15 points, and a high score on the Eagle index is greater than 3 criteria. Multiple studies have indicated that low-risk categories in these clinical indexes tend to underestimate the risk of cardiac complications in patients undergoing peripheral vascular procedures.

11. Which routine preoperative tests should be obtained?

The purpose of preoperative testing is to discover diseases or problems unrecognized by the history and physical examination or to confirm the diagnosis suspected by the history and examination. Routine tests that should be obtained in all elderly patients include the following:
- Fasting glucose (screens for diabetes)
- Complete blood count (may indicate the presence of an infection or anemia)
- Electrolytes (may indicate the risk of arrhythmias)
- Blood urea nitrogen and creatinine (useful in calculating the creatine clearance to delineate renal function)
- Chest x-ray (screens for occult pulmonary disease)
- EKG (detects ischemia or arrhythmias)

12. When are noninvasive cardiac tests indicated?

Because of the concern about postoperative ischemic events, **thallium testing**, most often with dipyridamole, has become almost a routine procedure before all surgery in the elderly in some medical centers (15–90%). Such an approach is not indicated, since patients at low risk require no intervention and those at high risk are already designated as candidates for revascularization.

Imaging studies are most useful for those at intermediate risk, defined by Eagle as two or more of the following: Q waves on the resting EKG, history of ventricular ectopy requiring treatment, diabetes, and known angina. The guideline from the American College of Cardiology/American Heart Association (ACC/AHA) combines the type of procedure (e.g., vascular procedures carry high risk), exercise capacity, prior evidence of coronary disease, and other clinical indicators such as diabetes into an algorithm that determines whether screening tests are indicated. The American College of Physicians has created a similar, less complex guideline. What is clear is that preoperative cardiac imaging to lower the risk of surgery should be obtained only in patients for whom a prophylactic cardiac surgical intervention would be indicated, regardless of the preoperative context.

An **echocardiogram** may be useful in persons in whom a systolic murmur is suspicious for aortic stenosis. Measures of left ventricular ejection fraction are useful in quantifying risks in persons undergoing cardiac procedures. In noncardiac procedures, these studies are not indicated preoperatively for asymptomatic patients. Holter monitoring and exercise testing are not consistently useful in asymptomatic individuals.

13. When is invasive monitoring required?

Right-heart catheterization is indicated in patients undergoing major vascular procedures or in those with active heart failure, significant aortic stenosis, unstable angina, or recent MI. Under other circumstances right-heart catheterization adds marginal information to that which can be obtained by a careful and thorough history and physical examination and testing as described above. An increasing body of evidence indicates that under many conditions right-heart catheterization is associated with more complications than the information gained would warrant.

14. When are pulmonary function tests indicated?

Age alone is not an absolute indication for pulmonary function testing. All procedures do not confer an increased risk of pulmonary complications. Patients undergoing lung resection always undergo pulmonary function testing to determine if the remaining lung will be adequate. Procedures that involve incisions of the upper abdomen or thorax impair respiratory function. Patients preparing for such procedures should probably undergo pulmonary function testing, especially if they have cough, COPD, cigarette smoking, dyspnea, or other known pulmonary disease. Orthopedic procedures and procedures of the lower abdomen confer minimal risk of pulmonary compromise; thus pulmonary function tests are not indicated in asymptomatic individuals.

Body size and age affect pulmonary function tests. There is a paucity of data on what constitutes normal pulmonary function tests in individuals over age 75. Appropriate ranges as predictors of respiratory complication are uncertain in the elderly. Most studies of pulmonary risks have enrolled individuals with known lung disease, particularly COPD. These data may not apply to the elderly in general. Nevertheless, as predictors of significant respiratory complications, the data suggest:

- $PCO_2 > 45$ mmHg
- $FEV_1 < 2$ liters (particularly less than 1 liter)
- Maximal ventilatory volume < 50% predicted

15. Summarize useful preoperative recommendations.

General: Cessation of smoking before surgery is helpful but should be undertaken at least 2 weeks before surgery. Training before surgery in coughing and deep breathing may be undertaken. If COPD is present, aggressive use of bronchodilators can be implemented both pre- and postoperatively. Any pulmonary infections should be treated before the operation.

Thromboembolism: Prophylaxis of thromboembolic events is connected to the risk inherent in the procedure and the individual risk of the patient. In many cases, low-molecular-weight (LMW) heparin, low-dose unfractionated heparin, and warfarin are effective in lowering the risk of thromboembolus. LMW heparin has the advantage of requiring no monitoring, and has a lower incidence of thrombocytopenia than unfractionated heparin, but it is more expensive. In general, when started preoperatively, once-daily LMW heparin is effective, but when started postoperatively, twice-daily dosing has been shown to be superior. Warfarin has the disadvantage of requiring extensive monitoring. Hirudin, a polypeptide derived from leeches that directly inactivates thrombin, is an expensive alternative that may cause fewer bleeding complications than LMW heparin. Minidose warfarin (1 mg) daily and aspirin are considered ineffective compared with alternatives. Pneumatic compression stockings, while more effective than placebo, are less effective than other options but carry no risk of bleeding.

For **high-risk general surgery patients** and for most nonorthopedic surgery, low-dose un-fractionated and LMW heparin are comparable. For patients undergoing surgery for intra-abdom-inal or pelvic malignancy, low-dose heparin begun on the day of surgery is indicated. LMW heparin with or without intermittent pneumatic compression is also effective.

Among **high-risk orthopedic surgery patients**, recommendations vary with the type of procedure. For persons undergoing hip replacement, LMW heparin and warfarin produce compa-rable reductions in thromboemboli. Both are more effective than low-dose unfractionated hep-arin. The dose of LMW heparin varies with the compound used. Results are comparable among the agents tested if used twice daily starting postoperatively (12–24 hr) or once a day starting pre-operatively (8–12 hr). Warfarin should be initiated the evening before surgery at 10 mg and ad-justed subsequently to maintain the international normalized ratio (INR) in the 2.0–3.0 range. Hirudin is an expensive alternative but may cause fewer bleeding complications than LMW hep-arin. It is useful for patients with heparin-induced thrombocytopenia. Patients undergoing repair of a **hip fracture** also require anticoagulation, but which agent is optimal is unclear. In a meta-analysis, low-dose unfractionated heparin was comparable to LMW heparin. Low-dose warfarin (prothrombin time 1.5 times control) confers a reduction in DVT comparable to heparin. In pa-tients undergoing **total knee replacement**, LMW heparin is superior to warfarin, and should begin 12 hours postoperatively to prevent bleeding complications. Minidose warfarin (1 mg) and aspirin are much less effective than the other alternatives for any of these types of orthopedic surgery. Pneumatic compression stockings should be used in patients undergoing **neurosurgery** and patients with contraindications to anticoagulation.

Cardiac medications: In patients at risk of postoperative ischemic, antianginal medica-tions should be maximized. Antihypertensive therapy, particularly with a beta blocker or alpha$_2$ blocker (e.g., clonidine), should be continued up to and including the day of surgery. Heart fail-ure and clinically significant arrhythmias (most commonly atrial fibrillation) should be con-trolled before surgery. Individuals with coronary artery disease or at risk of coronary artery disease should be treated with a beta blocker to lower the heart rate to 55–60 beats per minute before and up to 7 days after surgery. Antihypertensives should be continued at the preopera-tive dose.

Coronary artery revascularization: Prophylactic coronary artery bypass surgery for the sole purpose of preventing a perioperative event is unwarranted. No randomized clinical trials have tested the hypothesis that prophylactic coronary artery bypass grafting or angioplasty in the preoperative period prevents complications, and the morbidity and mortality of the prophylactic coronary procedure must be considered in comparing the risks of revascularization to the risks of no revascularization. In general, the physician should perform a revascularization procedure only if it would be performed in the absence of the surgical procedure.

16. How should pain be prevented and controlled during the perioperative period?

Pain is one of the major components of a wide range of neural, endocrine, metabolic, im-munologic, and inflammatory changes that constitute the stress response to surgery. Recent evi-dence has shown that surgical trauma induces processes of nervous system sensitization that contribute to and enhance postoperative pain and lead to chronic pain if inadequately treated. Proactive, preoperative analgesic strategies may avoid this problem, as well as the precipitous postoperative rise in catecholamines and corticosteroids that elevates the risk of a cardiac is-chemic event. Pain after operation is the most important factor responsible for regional impair-ment of ventilation, leading to pulmonary complications. Abdominal pain activates a spinal reflex arc with sympathetic hyperactivity that inhibits intestinal propulsive activity. Elderly patients are more sensitive to the effects of analgesia and sedatives. Once pain is fully developed, higher anal-gesic doses are required to control it, increasing the likelihood of adverse events.

The optimal form of pain treatment is one that is applied pre-, intra-, and postoperatively to preempt the establishment of pain hypersensitivity. Systemic opioid analgesia given on demand postoperatively is often poorly effective and should not be used as the mainstay of treatment. Practitioners have several options to manage pain effectively beginning preoperatively. NSAIDs can be initiated preoperatively. Morphine, 5–10 mg preoperatively, can be given intravenously. Tramadol, which can be given orally, intramuscularly, or intravenously, may offer an advantage over standard opioids. Lastly, many types of intraoperative regional blocks, administered by trained personnel, are effective.

Once pain has developed, many techniques have been used with varying degrees of success. Preoperative analgesics should be continued on a routine schedule. Patient-controlled analgesia allows patients to self-administer small boluses of an opioid, but patients must be mentally and physically capable of managing the process. Intraoperative regional blocks can be continued postoperatively.

BIBLIOGRAPHY

1. Ahsan A, Khuri S: Development and validation of a multifactorial risk index for predicting postoperative pneumonia after major noncardiac surgery. Ann Intern Med 135:847–857, 2001.
2. American College of Cardiology and American Heart Association: Guidelines for perioperative cardio-vascular evaluation for non-cardiac surgery. J Am Coll Cardiol 27:3, 1996.
3. Bailes B: Perioperative care of the surgical patient. AORN 72:185–207, 2000.
4. Dalen J, Hirsh J: Fourth American College of Chest Physicians Consensus Conference on Antithrombotic therapy. Chest 108(4 Suppl):225–522S, 1995.
5. Eagle KA, Coley M, et al: Combining clinical and thallium data optimizes preoperative assessment of cardiac risk before major vascular surgery. Ann Intern Med 110:859–886, 1989.
6. Johnson J: Surgical principles in the aged. In Gallo J, Busby-Whitehead J, Rabins P, et al (eds): Reichel's Care of the Elderly: Clinical Aspects of Aging. Philadelphia, Lippincott Williams & Wilkins, 1999, pp 536–542.
7. Mangano D, Goldman L: Preoperative assessment of patients with known or suspected coronary disease. N Engl J Med 333:1750–1757, 1995.
8. Mangano D, Layung E, Wallace A, Tateo I: Effect of atenolol on mortality and cardiovascular morbidity after non-cardiac surgery. N Engl J Med 335:1713–1720, 1996.
9. Morrison RS: The medical consultant's role in caring for patients with hip fracture. Ann Intern Med 128:1010–1020, 1998.
10. Polanczyk C, Marcantonio E: Impact of age on perioperative complications and length of stay in patients undergoing noncardiac surgery. Ann Intern Med 134:637–643, 2001.
11. Richardson J, Bresland K: The management of postsurgical pain in the elderly population. Drugs Aging 13:17–31, 1998.
12. Weitz J: Low-molecular weight heparins. N Engl J Med 337:688–697, 1997.
13. Zibrak JD, O'Donnell CK, Morton K: Indications for pulmonary function testing. Ann Intern Med 112:763, 1990.

42. STROKE

Steven E. Arnold, MD, and Joan Weinryb, MD, CMD

1. What is a stroke?

Stroke is an injury to the brain caused by occlusion or rupture of a cerebral artery. It is the third most common cause of death, after coronary artery disease (CAD) and cancer, in the United States; it is also the leading cause of adult disability. The challenges of stroke prevention and care are particularly compelling for geriatricians, given the burgeoning elderly population and the fact that the most significant risk factor for stroke is age.

2. What are the major categories of stroke? Why are they important to recognize?

The stroke syndrome is characterized by rapid onset and a pattern of focal neurologic signs and symptoms that reflect injury in a specific vascular territory. The two broad categories of stroke are (1) ischemic stroke, which results from thrombosis or embolism, and (2) hemorrhagic stroke, which is due to primary intracerebral hemorrhage or subarachnoid hemorrhage. Thrombotic strokes are the most common and account for approximately 65% of all strokes, whereas embolic strokes account for 20–25%. Intracerebral hemorrhage accounts for 5% and subarachnoid hemorrhage for 5%.

Diagnosing the type and location of stroke is critical for appropriate management and prevention of recurrence. The mortality rate of hemorrhagic stroke is 3–5 times greater than the mortality rate of ischemic stroke and requires different therapies. Although information about the early course may be difficult to obtain, mode of onset can yield clues about whether the lesion is thrombotic, embolic, or hemorrhagic in origin. The symptom profiles for stroke vary according to type of stroke and vascular territory.

3. How does onset differ for different types of strokes?
Thrombotic strokes
- Variable onset of neurologic symptoms
- Frequently preceded by transient ischemic attacks (TIAs) heralding permanent deficits with temporary symptoms
- Neurologic deficits are often rapid in onset but may be fluctuating, stepwise, or stuttering ("stroke in evolution")

Embolic strokes
- Sudden onset
- Maximum neurologic deficit present from the beginning

Intracerebral hemorrhage
- Sudden onset
- Often occurs in setting of elevated blood pressure and during activity

Subarachnoid hemorrhage
- Sudden onset
- Tends to occur during activity and may be associated with elevated blood pressure
- Accompanied by a crashing headache (which is a rare or minor symptom in other stroke types)
- Often proceeds to coma, from which the patient may emerge in a confusional state

4. What are the major clinical syndromes of stroke ?
Middle cerebral artery
- Contralateral hemiplegia
- Contralateral hemisensory loss
- Contralateral homonymous hemianopia

- Ipsilateral gaze preference
- Aphasia (dominant hemisphere)
- Affective disturbance (especially nondominant hemisphere)
- Neglect (failure to respond to stimuli presented to the side opposite a brain lesion; especially nondominant hemisphere)

Anterior cerebral artery
- Contralateral leg/foot paralysis
- Gait disturbance
- Abulia (loss or impairment of volition)
- Ideomotor apraxia (inability to perform purposeful movements)
- Perseveration (inappropriate repetition of word, phrase, or behavior)
- Urinary incontinence

Posterior cerebral artery
- Contralateral homonymous hemianopia
- Dyslexia
- Memory impairment
- Contralateral hemiparesis (mild)
- Contralateral hemisensory loss
- Variable brainstem signs (e.g., ipsilateral third-nerve palsy, contralateral involuntary movements, hemiplegia, ataxia)

Internal carotid artery
- Transient monocular blindness
- "Watershed" signs: homonymous hemianopia, aphasia (dominant hemisphere), neglect (nondominant hemisphere, variable sensorimotor deficit
- Signs of middle, anterior, and posterior cerebral artery infarction (as above)

Vertebral artery
- Ipsilateral cerebellar ataxia
- Ipsilateral face dysesthesia
- Contralateral trunk and limb dysesthesia
- Vertigo
- Nystagmus
- Ipsilateral vocal cord paralysis
- Dysphagia
- Nausea and vomiting
- Ipsilateral Horner syndrome

Basilar artery
- Wide spectrum of clinical symptoms
- Contralateral hemiplegia or quadriplegia
- Contralateral sensory loss
- Horizontal gaze palsies
- Ipsilateral facial paralysis
- Internuclear ophthalmoplegia (inability to adduct contralateral eye with voluntary eye movement)
- Nystagmus
- Nausea, vomiting
- Deafness, tinnitus
- Coma
- "Locked-in" syndrome (intact consciousness but total paralysis except for eyelid and vertical eye movements)

Lacunar syndromes
- Pure motor hemiparesis
- Pure sensory stroke
- Dysarthria/clumsy hand syndrome
- Hemichorea/hemiballismus
- Homolateral ataxia and crural paresis

5. What causes stroke?

Primary thrombotic occlusion typically occurs in a blood vessel already partially occluded by atherosclerosis. The earliest lesion is a "fatty streak" that evolves into a fibrous plaque. The rate of progression from atheromatous stenosis to virtual occlusion is highly variable but may be as short as weeks. The source of most **cerebral embolisms** is the heart. Less commonly, embolic material may be released from ulcerated atherosclerotic plaques in the aortic arch and origin of the great vessels. The sites of embolic occlusion within the brain are more variable than in atherothrombotic disease, although there is some predilection for right hemisphere lesions, based on tendencies of blood flow. **Lacunar infarcts** are a particular type of ischemic stroke involving the deep perforator arterial and arteriolar branches of the major cerebral blood vessels. Pathologically, they are due to lipohyalinosis or microatheroma.

Intracerebral hemorrhage is usually due to either rupture of the small penetrating arteries of the brain in the setting of hypertension or to amyloid angiopathy. Rupture of a congenital saccular aneurysm, which typically occurs at sites of arterial bifurcation or branching, is the most common cause of subarachnoid hemorrhage. Most aneurysms are asymptomatic until they rupture. Arteriovenous malformation or tumors may also cause subarachnoid hemorrhage.

Thrombotic stroke

1. Atherosclerotic plaque (may be due to stenotic ischemia or "local" ulcerated plaque embolization)
   - Common carotid bifurcation
   - Proximal vertebral artery
   - Internal carotid siphon
   - Middle cerebral artery stem
2. Unusual causes
   - Antiphospholipid antibodies
   - Clotting inhibitory factor deficiencies
   - Arteritides
   - Cerebral vein thrombosis
   - Polycythemia vera

Embolic stroke

1. Cardiac source
   - Mural thrombus (atrial fibrillation, myocardial infarction)
   - Valvular disease
   - Patent foramen ovale
   - Bacterial endocarditis
   - Libman-Sacks endocarditis
   - Atrial myxoma
2. Atherosclerotic plaques in aortic arch or origin of great vessels

Lacunar stroke: strongly associated with the following:

1. Age
2. Diabetes mellitus
3. Hypertension

Intracerebral hemorrhage

1. Rupture of small penetrating vessels in setting of hypertension
   - Putamen
   - Thalamus
   - Pons
   - Cerebellum
2. Amyloid angiopathy (tends to be lobar)
3. Hemorrhagic conversion of an ischemic infarct

Subarachnoid hemorrhage

1. Cerebral aneurysm
   - Anterior communicating artery
   - Internal carotid artery at origin of posterior communicating artery
   - Middle cerebral artery bifurcation
2. Arteriovenous malformation
3. Tumor

6. What other conditions can mimic TIAs or stroke?

A number of other neurologic processes that cause transient as well as permanent deficits may be confused with TIA or stroke. It has been estimated that 10–15% of initial diagnoses of stroke are incorrect. Seizures (especially simple and complex partial seizures), confusional states, and cardiogenic syncope are the disorders most often misdiagnosed as stroke. Other conditions that can simulate stroke or TIA include migraine and migraine equivalents, subdural hematoma, brain tumor, hypoglycemia, demyelinating disease, brain abscess, encephalitis, and panic attack. Because management of these various conditions differs greatly, correct diagnosis is crucial.

7. What are the major modifiable risk factors for stroke?

Much of the steady decline in stroke mortality in the past 50 years may be attributed to the identification and treatment of risk factors, particularly hypertension. This decline has been most prominent in the elderly, but it appears to be slowing or may even reversing in recent years. Stroke remains the third leading cause of death. The risk factors of age, male gender, African-American heritage, and heredity are not modifiable. Other medical and lifestyle factors may be modified. A greater emphasis on education and management of the modifiable risk factors will decrease the high incidence of stroke.

Major Risk Factors for Stroke

MODIFIABLE MEDICAL FACTORS	RELATIVE RISK	LIFESTYLE FACTORS	RELATIVE RISK
Systolic and diastolic hypertension	3- to 4-fold	Cigarette smoking	1.5- to 2.9-fold
Cardiac disease		Excessive alcohol	4-fold
Atrial fibrillation	5- to 17-fold	Physical inactivity	Not certain
Coronary artery disease	2- to 4-fold		
Congestive heart failure	2- to 4-fold		
Left ventricular hypertrophy	2- to 4-fold		
Diabetes mellitus	2- to 4-fold		
Hyperlipidemia	Not certain		
Hypercoagulable state	Not certain		
Elevated homocysteine	Not certain		

Other potential risk factors for stroke include atrial septal aneurysm, patent foramen ovale, aortic arch atheroma, antiphospholipid antibodies, and chronic inflammation. These factors may be especially important in younger populations with cryptogenic stroke. Their significance in the geriatric population is undetermined.

8. What are the options for primary stroke prevention?

Stroke prevention strategies target the modifiable risk factors noted above. In general, although the risk factors for stroke are not exactly the same as those for CAD, the main cause of death in patients with cerebrovascular disease is cardiac disease. Therefore, the same recommendations are made for stroke as for CAD. Hypertension, diabetes mellitus, hyperlipidemia, tobacco abuse, alcoholism, and obesity should be managed with a combination of dietary and lifestyle changes and medication . Statins appear to be useful in stroke prevention, both by lowering cholesterol and by other, less understood mechanisms

Control of hypertension, including isolated hypertension, with thiazides, beta blockers, angiotensin-converting enzymes inhibitors, and dihydropyridine calcium channel blockers reduces stroke risk, even in people over 80.

Smoking cessation reduces risk with disappearances of elevated risk within 5 years. Anticoagulation in patients with atrial fibrillation can reduce risk. Aspirin does not appear to be useful for primary prevention.

9. When should anticoagulation be considered for primary stroke prevention in patients with cardiac disease?

For primary prevention of stroke in patients with a well-established cardiac source for embolic stroke (chronic atrial fibrillation, dilated cardiomyopathy, valvular heart disease, prosthetic valves), anticoagulation with warfarin is clearly effective and generally has an acceptable risk of bleeding complications. People over the age of 75 share in this decreased risk, although they experience a significantly higher risk of major hemorrhage . The decision to anticoagulate is an individual one that must be based on the risk of stroke and the risk of complications in a particular patient. Antiplatelet therapy with aspirin (325 mg.) has fewer bleeding complications and has been shown to reduce the risk of stroke in patients with atrial fibrillation, albeit with significantly less efficacy (about half) than warfarin. Initial results from recent trials combining low dose warfarin and aspirin have not been encouraging.

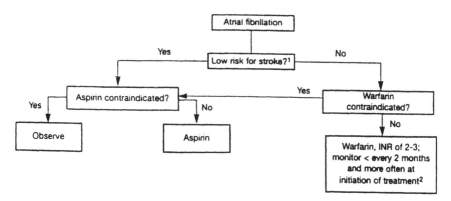

[1] Low stroke risk: age < 60 years with none of the following: previous transient ischemic attack/stroke, hypertension, diabetes mellitus, congestive heart failure, echocardiogram with left atrial enlargement or global left ventricular dysfunction.

[2] INR: International Normalized Ratio is a measure of prothrombin time that adjusts for differences in thromboplastin reagents used by different laboratories. INRs between 2 and 3 are currently considered optimal for atrial fibrillation patients.

Atrial fibrillation.

10. Describe the initial management of patients with acute stroke.

For all patients with acute stroke, rapid clinical evaluation and initiation of treatment are critical, especially now that thrombolytic therapy for hyperacute stroke is widely available. Patients should be offered treatment with tissue-type plasminogen activator if onset of stroke is less than 3 hours before presentation. Beyond the history and physical examination, the initial emergency department evaluation should include an EKG, chest x-ray, complete blood count, platelet count, prothrombin and partial thromboplastin times, chemistry profile, erythrocyte sedimentation rate, syphilis serology, and arterial blood gases. It is imperative to distinguish hemorrhage from infarction as soon as possible because further acute management decisions depend on this distinction. A noncontrast CT scan of the head should be performed and interpreted urgently because it easily differentiates hemorrhage from infarction in almost all cases.

The utility of magnetic resonance imaging (MRI) in the early management of stroke has been controversial. Conventional MRI methods (T1-, T2-, and proton density-weighted images) can detect ischemic lesions much sooner after stroke and with much greater anatomic resolution than CT, but the advantages of MRI over CT have not been demonstrated by clinical outcome studies. However, new MRI methods have been developed, including diffusion-weighted imaging and perfusion imaging, which can detect within minutes the territory undergoing infarction and the ischemic territory still at risk for infarction. These techniques offer the promise of identifying which patients are best able to benefit from acute thrombolytic therapy. The choice of test may depend on its availability as an emergency service.

In patients with ischemic infarction, high blood pressure (BP) should not be lowered rapidly. Asystolic BP < 220 mmHg or mean arterial pressure (MAP) < 130 mmHg is acceptable unless there are other intervening variables, such as heart failure or aortic dissection. For patients with hemorrhage, elevated BP should be lowered and maintained in the normal range. Other general management strategies should include treatment of hypoglycemia or hyperglycemia (> 170 mg/dl), monitoring of cardiac status, oxygen for hypoxemia, avoidance of dehydration, treatment of fever, and monitoring for cerebral edema and seizures. Specialized stroke units can save lives and improve outcome and should be used if available.

11. Discuss the guidelines for thrombolytic treatment of hyperacute stroke.

The National Institute of Neurologic Disorders and Stroke has found that tissue-type plasminogen activator treatment is effective for minimizing damage from acute ischemic stroke and preserving functional status in a select group of patients, if initiated within 3 hours of initial symptom onset. Much depends on the expediency of stroke recognition and triage by the patient, family, emergency medical transport services, and hospital emergency services.

Tissue-type plasminogen activator treatment should be offered if the following conditions are met:

1. The diagnosis is acute ischemic stroke.
2. A definite time of initial symptom onset is known and treatment can be initiated within 3 hours.
3. The patient has significant acute focal neurologic deficit.
4. A neurologist has been consulted and concurs with treatment and will participate in ongoing inpatient management.
5. A CT scan of the head has been obtained and interpreted by an experienced physician.

Tissue-type plasminogen activator treatment should not be offered under the following conditions:

1. The time of onset is unclear (including patients who wake from sleep with symptoms).
2. Sustained blood pressure is greater than 185/110 mmHg at the time that treatment is to be administered.
3. CT scan shows any hemorrhage.
4. Neurologic deficits show significant spontaneous improvement before initiation of treatment (includes TIAs).
5. Only minor neurologic deficit is present.
6. Other contraindications pose a risk for hemorrhage.

After treatment, emergent ancillary care in a skilled care facility (intensive care unit or acute stroke care unit) that permits close observation, frequent neurologic assessments, and cardiovascular monitoring must be available.

12. Does a TIA or minor stroke require immediate diagnosis and management?

TIAs and minor strokes should be evaluated and treated according to the same principles as stroke. TIAs are warning signs of stroke, and aggressive management may prevent permanent disability or death. The rate of a completed stroke after TIA may be as high as 57% within 2 years. Most occur within the first year. The risk of stroke in the first few days after a TIA is unclear, although it is considered to be highest during this period. Therefore, all patients with a recent TIA (within 10 days) should be evaluated urgently.

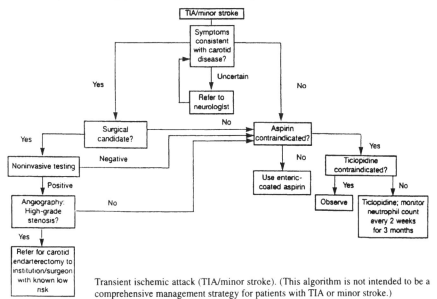

Transient ischemic attack (TIA/minor stroke). (This algorithm is not intended to be a comprehensive management strategy for patients with TIA or minor stroke.)

13. What diagnostic tests are useful in the evaluation of new stroke or TIA?

No algorithm for diagnosis of stroke is uniformly accepted. Which tests to perform is a decision based on the clinical factors of age, clinical presentation, risk factors, other health considerations, and intent to treat. At a minimum, evaluation should include the above admission tests, head CT, and noninvasive carotid artery evaluation to identify atherosclerotic carotid artery disease. Duplex scanning is the most revealing noninvasive method, combining ultrasound real-time imaging with a Doppler probe. It is quite accurate in detecting significant disease up to the carotid bifurcation. Ultrasound techniques are of little utility for vertebrobasilar disease. Additional diagnostic tests and procedures for selected patients include transthoracic echocardiography (and transesophageal echocardiography when a cardioembolic source is highly suspect); transcranial Doppler, MRI, and MR angiography to assess suspected intracranial arterial stenoses; cerebral angiography to identify cerebrovascular disease with the greatest sensitivity; and tests for coagulopathies (e.g., proteins C and S, antiphospholipid antibodies, antithrombin III deficiencies, and Leiden factor V, especially in younger patients without another obvious cause). For cases of suspected subarachnoid hemorrhage, lumbar puncture is indicated if clinical suspicion is high and CT is nondiagnostic. Early angiography is also indicated in subarachnoid hemorrhage, especially in more robust, less impaired patients for whom early aneurysm repair would be the treatment of choice. Positron emission tomography and single photon emission CT, although not widely available, may be useful in assessing TIAs in which there is no anatomic lesion and in early stroke prior to tissue infarction.

14. What is the role of anticoagulation in acute stroke?

Although randomized controlled trials have shown that heparin and low-molecular-weight heparin have no benefit in acute ischemic stroke not due to cardiac emboli, anticoagulation is clearly effective in preventing recurrent cardioembolic stroke. Patients with cardioembolic stroke due to atrial fibrillation, recent myocardial infarction, valvular disease, or patent foramen ovale should be anticoagulated if they have no contraindications. Heparin should be administered on admission for at least 48 hours before being replaced by warfarin if no systemic contraindications are present, no hemorrhage is seen on imaging studies, the infarct is not large (hemorrhagic conversion is a higher risk in larger than in smaller strokes), and no evidence of bacterial endocarditis is seen. For patients with atrial fibrillation who are not candidates for long-term anticoagulation, low-dose heparin may be considered. Aspirin alone also reduces the risk of further embolization in atrial fibrillation, although not nearly as effectively as warfarin. The role of anticoagulation is more controversial for atherothrombotic ischemic stroke. In patients with atherothrombotic stroke in evolution, many physicians feel compelled to anticoagulate, but the value of this approach has not been demonstrated. Anticoagulation is of no benefit in completed stroke.

15. What is the role of neuroprotective agents in acute stroke?

Various neuroprotective agents are under study for their potential role in interrupting the cascade of molecular events that lead to neuron death after ischemic injury. Examples include calcium channel antagonists, glutamate antagonists, sodium channel antagonists, glycine antagonists, opioid antagonists, and antioxidants/free radical scavengers. Although this strategy is appealing, to date there is little convincing clinical evidence that any neuroprotective drug is effective in either reducing size of infarction or improving outcome.

16. What are the major complications of acute stroke ?

The most common and significant medical complications after stroke include deep vein thrombosis and pulmonary embolism, aspiration pneumonia, urinary tract infections, and pressure sores. Cardiac arrhythmias are also common. EKG monitoring is indicated in the first few days. Three major neurologic complications, common in large strokes, are cerebral edema, seizures, and hemorrhagic transformation of ischemic infarcts. Cerebral edema is especially threatening in cerebellar infarctions because it can cause brainstem herniation. Hyperventilation, osmotic therapy, or even surgery may be needed for cerebral edema. Corticosteroids have not been shown to be effective in cerebral infarction or hemorrhage with or without edema. Seizures should be treated with anticonvulsants. If anticoagulation is considered for stroke in evolution or other circumstances, a repeat CT scan should be performed before initiation of heparin to rule out hemorrhagic conversion.

17. When should carotid endarterectomy be recommended?

Major controlled studies have clearly demonstrated that carotid endarterectomy (CEA) reduces the risk of subsequent stroke in patients who have had TIAs or minor stroke and who have arteriographically confirmed stenotic lesions > 70%. It appears to be of no benefit in patients with less than 50% stenosis. Patients in this group should be more vigorously evaluated for cardioembolic and other causes of stroke. If no other cause emerges, they should be treated medically with risk factor reduction and antiplatelet therapy. For patients with moderate degrees of stenosis (50–69%), CEA may yield a moderate reduction in risk for subsequent stroke, but treatment for this group must strongly consider surgical skill and recognized surgical risk factors. If ulcerated plaque is present in the setting of moderate stenosis, the risk of stroke increases and patients benefit from CEA. Surgical decisions in this setting should be made on an individual basis.

Recommendations for Carotid Endarterectomy

GRADE (%) OF STENOSIS	RECOMMENDATION	RISK REDUCTION
< 50%	No. Search for cardioembolic or other sources	
50–69%	Individualized decision Yes, if ulcerated plaque is present	27%
> 70%	Yes	48%
Asymptomatic, > 60%, low surgical risk	Yes	

Risks of CEA include stroke and death as well as local complications such as hematoma, infection, or false aneurysm formation. Although successful CEA confers a relative risk reduction in the incidence of stroke over the ensuing 5 years, perioperative and arteriography-related risk for mortality and stroke must be taken into account. There should be an approximately 3% aggregate risk of stroke or death in the perioperative period with an experienced team, including the risk of stroke associated with arteriography.

The results of CEA for the elderly are controversial. Some studies indicate an increased risk of complications with advanced age, whereas a recent study of CEA in octogenarians found the procedure to be as safe and effective as for the general population. Patients with prohibitive surgical risk should be treated with antiplatelet agents and risk factor reduction. It appears that female sex, age > 75 yr (?), systolic BP > 180 mmHg, history of peripheral venous disease, contralateral occlusion, and intracranial stenosis of the ipsilateral internal carotid increase the risk of poor outcome with CEA

18. What medical therapy can prevent recurrent stroke in patients with established atherothrombotic cerebrovascular disease?

Numerous controlled clinical trials have demonstrated the efficacy of antiplatelet agents for the secondary prevention of stroke in patients who have had TIAs or previous stroke. Aspirin has been the most extensively studied, and its use is associated with a 23% decrease in the risk of subsequent stroke or myocardial infarction. Controversy continues over the optimal dose, with recommendations ranging from 30 mg to 1300 mg. A recent survey found that most neurologists recommend 325 mg per day in deference to gastrointestinal symptoms; however, recent studies have suggested that higher doses may be better for secondary stroke prevention.

Ticlopidine and clopidogrel are two other platelet antiaggregants with efficacy in secondary stroke prevention. They work by inhibiting adenosine diphosphate (ADP) linkage of fibrinogen to platelets and have a greater global inhibitory effect than aspirin. Ticlopidine has been reported to be modestly more effective than aspirin in preventing strokes. Adverse reactions, including diarrhea, rash, GI upset, and neutropenia, have limited its widespread use. Monitoring for neutropenia , which occurs in 2.4% of patients and is fully reversible on discontinuation of the medication, requires checking every 2 weeks for the first 3 months. Clopidogrel is at least as effective as aspirin with a somewhat better safety and side-effect profile.

The role of warfarin for carotid atherothrombotic stroke prevention is unclear It is more expensive than aspirin and more difficult to use, requiring monitoring by frequent blood tests. A multicenter center (Warfarin Aspirin Recurrent Stroke Study) found no superiority of warfarin over aspirin in prevention of recurrent ischemic stroke. It is possible that subgroups with aortic arch atheroma and cardioembolic causes and others would have increased benefit. Dipyridamole and sulfinpyrazone have no efficacy in secondary stroke prevention, either when used alone or in combination with aspirin.

19. How should asymptomatic carotid artery disease be managed?

Bruits heard during physical examination, vascular studies done for other reasons, or screening tests for unusual symptoms may identify carotid stenosis in asymptomatic patients. Asymptomatic carotid stenosis is an indicator of more extensive atherosclerosis and is associated with an increased risk of stroke. The Asymptomatic Carotid Atherosclerosis Study (ACAS) reported that for asymptomatic people with high-grade stenoses, Carotid endarterectomy in combination with aspirin and risk factor reduction reduces the relative risk for stroke compared with medical therapy alone. The relative risk reduction is not as great as for patients who have had TIAs or minor strokes. Consequently, consideration of other factors, such as age, other medical illnesses, and surgical and arteriographic complication risks, become even more important in reaching a surgical decision. Whether or not surgery is recommended, risk factor modification and antiplatelet therapy should be initiated.

20. Who should be referred for rehabilitation after stroke?

Sensory, motor, cognitive, and language deficits are the presenting symptoms of stroke and may be permanent . Mortality from stroke has declined with advances in technology and treatment. As a consequence, a greater proportion of patients survive with substantial neurologic impairment. The goal of rehabilitation is not cure but rather adaptation to functional handicap—to maximize function in the service of enhancing quality of life. A host of factors should be considered in determining the appropriateness of referral for rehabilitation. Consultation with a physiatrist, physical therapist, occupational therapist, and/or speech therapist is recommended to delineate the appropriate rehabilitation needs of the patient. Patients with mild deficits may not need specialized rehabilitative services. Patients who are stuporous, completely immobile, severely cognitively impaired, or severely ill medically will derive little benefit. Type and severity of neurologic deficit, presence and degree of cognitive impairment, physical endurance, patient and family goals, available social support, and psychological make-up contribute to the success of rehabilitative efforts and need to be carefully assessed. Age is not a factor; patients of all ages have shown substantial benefit in outcome from rehabilitation.

21. How common are depression and other psychiatric complications after stroke? How should they be managed?

Mood disturbances are common after stroke due to both organic and psychological factors. Depression can play a critical role in the success of a patient's recovery, rehabilitation, and adjustment to disability after stroke and should be assessed and treated aggressively. Depending on the diagnostic criteria used, prevalence estimates for depression after stroke range from 23% to 63%. Because of the frequent impairments in communication and cognition and because of the common bias that "anyone would be depressed after a stroke," clinical depression is underdiagnosed and undertreated. Yet its importance is underscored by studies indicating that depression in the post-acute phase has an impact on physical recovery and subsequent function in the chronic phase. Treatment with antidepressant medication is as effective in post-stroke depression as in other depressive disorders and should be used. The selective serotonin reuptake inhibitors (SSRIs), such as sertraline, paroxetine, and fluoxetine, are especially well tolerated and effective. Methylphenidate (Ritalin) has also been shown to be helpful.

Other neuropsychiatric complications of stroke include delirium with agitation, paranoid reactions (especially in association with Wernicke's aphasia) poor impulse control, and pseudobulbar affect (emotional incontinence). These complications can be highly distressing to patients, family, and caregivers alike and are often amenable to psychiatric management.

BIBLIOGRAPHY

1. Adams HP, Brott TG, Crowell RM, et al: Guidelines for the management of patients with acute ischemic stroke. A statement for health care professionals from a special writing group of the Stroke Council, American Heart Association. Stroke 25:1901–1914, 1994.
2. Anderson DC: Primary and secondary stroke prevention in atrial fibrillation. Semin Neurol 18:451–459, 1998.
3. Barnett HJ, Taylor DW, Eliasziw M, et al: Benefit of carotid endarectomy in patients with symptomatic moderate or severe stenosis. North American Symptomatic Carotid Endarterectomy Trial Collaborators. N Engl J Med 339:1415–1425, 1998.
4. Barnett HJM (ed.): Stroke: Pathophysiology, Diagnosis, and Management. New York, Churchill Livingstone, 1998.
5. Barnett HJM, Eliasziw M: Aspirin benefit remains elusive in primary stroke prevention [editorial]. Arch Neurol 57:306–308, 2000.
6. Biller J, Feinberg WM, Castaldo JE, et al: Guidelines for carotid endarterectomy: A statement for healthcare professionals from a special writing group of the Stroke Council, American Heart Association. Stroke 29:554–562, 1998.
7. Dyken ML: Antiplatelet agents and stroke prevention. Semin Neurol 18:441–450, 1998.
8. Gorelick PB, Sacco RL, Smith DB, et al: Prevention of a first stroke: A review of guidelines and a multidisciplinary consensus statement from the National Stroke Association. JAMA 281:1112–1120, 1998.
9. Hart RG, Halperin JL, McBride R, et al: Aspirin for the primary prevention of stroke and other major vascular events: Meta-analysis and hypotheses Arch Neurol 57:326–332, 2000.
10. Meschia JF: Thrombolytic treatment of acute ischemic stroke. Mayo Clinic Proc 77:542–551, 2002.
11. National Institute of Neurological Disorders and Stroke rt-PA Stroke Study Group: Tissue plasminogen activator for acute ischemic stroke. N Engl J Med 333:1581–1587, 1995.
12. Robinson RG: Treatment issues in poststroke depression. Depress Anxiety 8(Suppl 1):85–90, 1998.
13. Strauss S: New evidence for stroke prevention. JAMA 288:1388, 2002.

43. HIP FRACTURES

John Bruza, MD

1. Who is at risk for hip fracture?

Over 90% of hip fractures result from falls with the majority occurring in people over 70 years old. Nevertheless, only a small minority of falls (around 5%) result in a fracture of the hip. (See Chapter 12 to understand who is at risk for falling and why.) Other independent risks for hip fracture include osteoporosis, female sex (which persists across all ethnic subgroups but especially white and Asian women), chronic corticosteroid use, urban residence, residing in a nursing home, and dementia.

2. Discuss the morbidity and mortality associated with hip fractures.

Functional dependence and death are important consequences of hip fracture. Over 250,000 hip fractures occur annually in the United States. This number is projected to double by year 2040 as the elderly population expands. Mortality among the elderly 1 year after hip fracture ranges from 14% to 36%. Mortality data from the Medicare population are probably most reliable and demonstrate rates of 7% at 1 month, 13% at 3 months, and 24% at 12 months after fracture.

Approximately 35–50% of patients with a fractured hip do not regain their previous level of ambulating, and up to 20% may become nonambulatory. Rates of returning home after hip fracture vary widely from 40% to 90% and probably reflect regional differences in availability of home care services, skilled nursing facilities, and the value placed on returning home. At 6-month survival after hip fracture: 60% of patients regain walking ability, about 50% recover prefracture activities of daily living (ADL), and about 25% recover prefracture instrumental activities of daily living (IADLs). Since the advent of the prospective payment system, which has shortened the in-hospital length of stay, the rate of institutionalization at 1 year after hip fracture has increased significantly.

Factors associated with death after hip fracture
- Advanced age
- Male sex
- Poorly controlled medical illness (especially cardiac, pulmonary, and cerebrovascular disease)
- Psychiatric illness
- Poor preoperative stabilization
- Postoperative complications

Factors to predict recovery of walking after hip fracture
- Male sex
- Younger age
- Absence of dementia
- Use of assistive device before injury (brings previously learned skills to therapy)

Factors associated with nursing home placement after hip fracture
- Age over 80
- Delirium or dementia
- Need for assistance with ADLs prior to fracture
- Lack of family involvement
- Inadequate physical therapy postoperatively

3. How do you evaluate a patient with a painful hip and a reported normal hip x-ray?

Think of a hip fracture until proven otherwise. Patients with painful hip and difficulty standing or walking despite normal anteroposterior pelvis and lateral hip radiographs should be suspected of occult fracture. Other diagnoses to consider include acetabular fracture, pubic ramus fracture, isolated trochanteric fracture, and trochanteric bursitis or contusion. Try repeating the anteroposterior view with the leg internally rotated 15–20°. If still normal, consider magnetic resonance imaging of the hip. Bone scanning is also a possibility but is more costly and may require the fracture to be 2 or 3 days old to appear on scan.

4. Discuss important perioperative considerations peculiar for patients with hip fracture.

The medical consultant plays an important role in clearance for hip surgery. As patients are often brought to medical attention many hours or days after the injury, identifying the time of injury helps to guide the evaluation for dehydration, rhabdomyolosis, and delirium. Medical stabilization of fluid and electrolyte imbalances, cardiovascular stabilization (especially congestive heart failure), identifying delirium and comorbid infections (pneumonia, urinary tract infections [UTIs]), and assessing nutritional status should be completed before surgery.

The timing of surgery for an early repair within 24–48 hours after admission is associated with a reduction in 1-year mortality rates and lower incidences of pressure sores, delirium, and fatal pulmonary embolism. Hence prompt identification and treatment of medical problems may prevent surgical delay and the attendant risks of immobilization (deep venous thrombosis [DVT], atelectasis, pneumonia, UTIs, deconditioning, and skin breakdown). However, some patients may have medical conditions such as unstable angina that clearly benefit from delay for further stabilization and subsequent surgery in a timely manner.

Thorough evaluation of preinjury functioning in ADLs and IADLs helps in deciding the type of surgical repair and the plan for rehabilitation. As the treatment goal of all hip fractures is the return to prior level of functioning, establishing that prior level guides all treatment decisions. For example, a nonambulatory nursing home resident with advanced dementia and minimal discomfort following hip fracture may have no significant change in level of functioning and may best be treated with nonoperative management.

Successful return to premorbid functioning depends on good fracture reduction, maintaining range of motion in the hips, preventing weakness and muscle atrophy, adequate pain control, supporting nutritional requirements, and preventing complications.

5. What are the considerations for a particular type (location) of hip fracture?

Femoral neck fractures account for 30% of hip fractures and can be treated by internal fixation with multiple screws or prosthetic replacement. Femoral neck fractures are intracapsular and risk disruption of the blood supply to this region. Some controversy exists over the best surgical procedure for this type of fracture with consideration of bone quality, patient age and prior level of functioning, displacement, comminution, and risk of delayed ambulation. Incomplete to minimally displaced fractures may be treated with internal fixation. Displaced fractures pose a greater risk (up to 40%) of avascular necrosis and nonunion and generally require prosthetic total hip replacement in the elderly population. Prosthetic replacement allows weight bearing usually on the following morning and thus a more rapid return to full function.

Intertrochanteric fractures are most common, accounting for up to two-thirds of hip fractures in the elderly. Standing falls deliver their impact most commonly on this region. Bleeding into the soft tissue is common and sometimes severe, requiring close following of blood counts and monitoring for hypotension. Its treatment is less controversial and consists of internal fixation with a sliding nail or screw mechanism. Ambulation begins soon after surgery but is often more gradual with higher demands for pain management, and returning to full unassisted ambulation may take a few months.

6. Is antibiotic prophylaxis necessary?

Prophylactic antibiotics reduce postoperative deep wound infections by 44%. First- and second-generation cephalosporins are most commonly used and should be dosed 0–2 hours before surgery and continued for 24 hours. Most studies have not shown any added benefit for longer routine courses of antibiotics. A commonly used regimen in a patient with normal renal function is 1 gm of cefazolin every 8 hours, started just before surgery for a total of 3 doses.

7. Which type of thromboembolic prophylaxis should be used?

Much controversy and wide variability in practice exist over which type of thromboembolic prophylaxis is most indicated. Most DVTs occur in the first week after hip fracture, but an increased risk can remain for over 6 weeks. Without prophylaxis, the prevalence of DVT is about 50%. Reviews of the literature suggest that low-molecular-weight heparin (LMWH) may reduce the incidence of thrombosis more than other regimens. A new synthetic factor Xa inhibitor, fondaparinux, has been approved with similar efficacy to LMWH but has limited use at present. Both LMWH and low-dose warfarin are considered first-line treatments. Risks accompany each strategy and have to be individualized for some frail, high-risk elderly patients. Compression stockings have negligible risk and can add benefit to all strategies. The regimens should be started immediately on admission.

DVT Prophylaxis for Hip Fractures

Low-molecular-weight heparin	Lowest reduction of thrombosis risk but also higher bleeding risk. Expensive.
Unfractionated heparin	Inexpensive and proven effective in numerous studies.
Factor Xa inhibitor	Limited experience. Studies suggest as effective or better than LMWH with similar bleeding risk. Most expensive regimen. No antidote available for reversal.
Low-dose warfarin	Effective but more likely than others to be over- or underdosed and requires regular monitoring. Goal for international normalized ratio (INR) is 1.5 times control.
Aspirin	Not as effective as above four. May be suitable alternative for patients at high bleeding risk that makes others contraindicated.
Pneumatic compression stockings	Of added benefit to all above regimens and should be used routinely.

8. Discuss important postoperative considerations.

The most important issue after surgery is early mobilization. The first day after surgery the patient should be moving from bed to chair and standing or walking during the first or second day. Some difficult surgical fixations may warrant an exception to limiting weight bearing but should be avoided as much as possible due to higher rates of complication associated with immobilization and delay in rehabilitation participation. Common complications of hip fractures include:

- Delirium
- DVT
- Pain
- Functional decline
- Catheter-associated UTI
- Urine retention and incontinence
- Unsuccessful fracture union, instability and dislocation
- Pneumonia or atelectasis
- Malnutrition
- Surgical infection (wound, joint or bone)

Indwelling urinary catheters are best removed within 24 hours after surgery to reduce the common problems of urinary infections, retention, and incontinence and to assist in early mobilization. Periodic straight catheterization for bladder-scanned volumes greater than 200 ml of urine may be necessary on removal but is preferable to continued use of indwelling catheters.

9. What causes delirium after hip fracture?

Delirium is a common complication of hip fractures, occurring in up to 50% of cases (see Chapter 8). Advanced age, dementia, alcohol use, and prior functional status are the most important risk factors for delirium. Few prospective studies have examined the causes of delirium specifically in patients with hip fracture. Looking at combined medical and surgical patients, common causes include fluid and electrolyte imbalances, adverse drug reactions (especially among opioids, sedative-hypnotics, and anticholinergics), infection, metabolic disorders, and decreased brain perfusion. One retrospective study of delirium specific to hip fracture found a greater likelihood to develop delirium after admission and especially after surgery, more multifactorial causes, more spontaneous resolution, and lower rate of delirium on discharge. Goals of treatment include early recognition, identification of cause, prompt treatment of reversible causes, and anticipating safety concerns for the patient. In addition, supportive reorientation and controlling the sensory environment (increasing stimuli for the sensory impaired and decreasing sensory stimuli for those who appear agitated by them) can be beneficial.

10. How common is fat embolism syndrome? Discuss its symptoms and treatment.

Clinically apparent fat embolism syndrome is infrequent after hip fracture repair but should be considered as a potential cause of postoperative respiratory distress. The condition is characterized by hypoxia, bilateral pulmonary infiltrates, and a change in mental status. Treatment is largely supportive; corticosteroid use is controversial.

11. Discuss orthopedic complications after surgery for hip fracture.

Specific orthopedic complications include infection of the wound, joint or bone, problems of fracture union (delayed union, malunion, and nonunion), avascular necrosis, compartment syndrome of the leg, and posttraumatic arthritis. Infection occurs in up to 5% of patients and is mainly treated with antibiotic therapy but may require surgical irrigation, debridement, or replacement. Loss of internal fixation occurs in up to 15% and usually requires additional surgery. Compartment syndrome occurs shortly after the injury or repair and results from increasing pressure (from edema, bleeding, infection, or an external brace or cast) within a confined anatomical compartment, causing uncontrollable pain out of proportion to the injury and findings of sensory preceding motor deficits. The threatened leg may require fasciotomy to relieve the pressure. Nonunion, avascular necrosis, and posttraumatic arthritis occur months to years after the injury.

12. How common is malnutrition? How can it be prevented or treated?

Severe malnutrition is identified in up to 20% of patients with hip fracture. Improving nutrition with oral protein supplementation has been shown to reduce postoperative complications, preserve body protein stores, and significantly reduce length of hospitalization. If oral intake is significantly inadequate, nocturnal nasogastric tube feeding has demonstrated similar improvement.

13. What about osteoporosis after surgery?

Evaluation for osteoporosis for all fall-related hip fractures should be done for both men and women. Bone density scanning, calcium and vitamin D supplementation, and bisphosphonate treatment may be appropriate to prevent future fractures.

14. How can falls be prevented?

Assessing fall risk in patients with hip fracture may help to reduce their high risk for recurrent fracture. Exercise and balance training can help to reduce fall risk. Home/environment safety modification can reduce fall risk. Recent studies of hip protectors have not shown reduction in fracture risk. (See Chapter 12 for assessment of fall risk and prevention treatment.)

BIBLIOGRAPHY

1. Brauer C, Morrison RS, Siu AL: The cause of delirium in patients with hip fracture. Arch Intern Med 160:1856–1860, 2000.
2. Cooper C, Campion G, Melton LJ III: Hip fractures in the elderly: A world-wide projection. Osteoporos Int 2:285–289, 1992.
3. Hannan EL, Magaziner J, Wang JJ: Mortality and locomotion 6 months after hospitalization for hip fracture: Risk factors and risk-adjusted hospital outcomes. JAMA 285:2736–2742, 2001.

4. Heit JA: The potential role of fondaparinux as venous thromboembolism prophylaxis after total hip or knee replacement or hip fracture surgery. Arch Intern Med 162: 1806–1808, 2002.
5. Huddleston JM, Whitford KJ: Medical care of elderly patients with hip fractures. Mayo Clin Proc 76:295–298, 2001.
6. Lawrence VA, Hilsenbeck SG, Carson JL: Medical complications and outcomes after hip fracture repair. Arch Intern Med 162:2053–2057, 2002.
7. Morrison RS, Chassin MR, Siu AL: The medical consultant's role in caring for patients with hip fractures. Ann Intern Med 128(12, Pt 1):1010–1020, 1998.

44. DEHYDRATION

John D. Cacciamani, MD, and Edna P. Schwab, MD

1. Is dehydration a significant cause of illness in the elderly?

Dehydration is a significant cause of mortality in the elderly. Studies have demonstrated that the mortality rate may exceed 50% in hospitalized dehydrated patients if they remain untreated. Other clinical studies have shown that as many as 50% of patients admitted with a primary diagnosis of dehydration die within 1 year after discharge. In addition, the incidence and social costs are significant. Data from the National Hospital Discharge Survey indicate that in 1991 189,000 elderly patients were discharged from short-stay hospitals with the primary diagnosis of dehydration; the average length of stay was 9.8 days. The cost to Medicare was estimated at $1,158,125,000.

2. Why are the elderly at greater risk for dehydration?

- Many elderly people have functional deficits that hinder access to water.
- Elderly patients generally have less total body water than younger patients and therefore less intracellular reserve.
- As one ages, many of the normal hormonal responses to dehydration are depressed.
- Many elderly people have an impaired central thirst mechanism.
- Elderly people are more likely to take medications that exacerbate or even cause dehydration.

3. What are the common signs of dehydration?

The most common physical findings of dehydration include dry mucus membranes, tachycardia, decreased skin turgor, constipation, and orthostatic hypotension. Confusion and disorientation also may be present. In elderly patients, such symptoms are generally more difficult to interpret, and confusion due to dehydration frequently is superimposed on a baseline dementia. Therefore, if dehydration is suspected, a thorough investigation to identify the possible underlying cause is justified.

4. How does one determine whether orthostatic hypotension is present?

Orthostatic hypotension is calculated by measuring the blood pressure and heart rate while the patient is sitting and standing. Wait at least 1 minute between each measurement. A drop in systolic blood pressure of 20 mmHg or a drop in diastolic blood pressure of 10 mmHg represents a positive test. An increase in heart rate of > 10 bpm also indicates a positive test. One must be cautious in interpreting this test for several reasons. Many elderly patients take medications that impair the natural compensatory response. Examples include most antihypertensive medications, particularly beta blockers, which usually diminish heart rate and vasoconstrictive response. Of note, several studies have indicated that 20–30% of community-dwelling elderly have orthostatic changes based on neurologic illness or prolonged bedrest—not on volume depletion.

5. Is there a difference between the normal extracellular volumes of young and elderly adults?

Extracellular volume levels are not significantly different in young and elderly adults of similar sizes. However, the total body water of elderly adults is lower because they have a higher percentage of fat than younger adults. The higher percentage of fat results in a lower percentage of intracellular water. When elderly patients experience dehydration, therefore, they have less intracellular water reserve and become dehydrated more quickly.

6. What are the hormonal differences in young and elderly adults?

Elderly patients have decreased renin activity and decreased aldosterone secretion. In addition, studies have shown that a pure volume stimulus results in lower vasopressin levels compared with younger adults, yet hyperosmolar stimuli of vasopressin are elevated. Despite the varied response of vasopressin, almost all elderly people demonstrate a relative end-organ resistance to vasopressin. This resistance is believed to have significant consequences, including decreased renal free water retention and impairment of thirst mechanisms. In general, dehydrated elderly adults take longer to correct volume depletion because they are unable to resorb free water and frequently are not thirsty.

7. How is dehydration most frequently categorized?

Dehydration frequently is divided into categories based on sodium status and osmolarity. Differentiating among these forms of dehydration is essential for appropriate treatment. Many clinicians believe that it is best not to simplify the presence of hypovolemia into the general category of dehydration but rather to describe the condition accurately. All forms of dehydration are found in elderly patients, but hypernatremic hypovolemia is more common than hyponatremic hypovolemia.

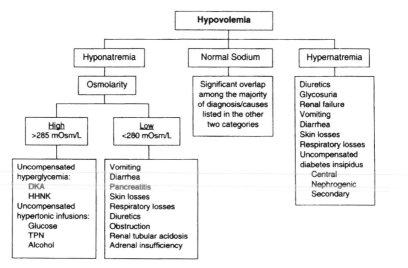

General conditions and causes associated with hypovolemia. DKA = diabetic ketoacidosis; HHNK = hyperglycemic hyperosmolar nonketotic coma; TPN = total parenteral nutrition.

8. What common medical conditions may cause hypernatremic dehydration?

The many causes of hypernatremic dehydration include renal failure, uncompensated diabetes insipidus, and gastrointestinal losses. But the most common cause in the elderly is insensible losses through the skin and lungs, which frequently are exacerbated by fever. If this condition is accompanied by inability to increase oral intake, dehydration results.

9. How should one correct the free water deficits of the elderly hospitalized hypernatremic patient?

The answer requires significant understanding of the patient's clinical condition and medical history. If a patient is in shock and hypotensive, pressure support with normal saline for volume repletion is the highest priority. If the patient is not in shock, other points need to be considered before volume repletion. A patient who has been hypernatremic for some time is at risk for cerebral edema if volume status and sodium status are corrected too quickly. The brain synthesizes idiogenic osmoles to help maintain intracellular volume. These intracellular osmoles counteract the high intravascular osmolarity caused by hypernatremia. Secondary cerebral edema occurs when the intravascular osmolarity is corrected too quickly, and fluid consequently moves into the cells of the central nervous system. This occurrence is rare, but congestive heart failure in elderly patients after rapid volume repletion is common. As a general rule of thumb for elderly patients, 30–50% of the free water deficit may be repleted in the first 24 hours. The key points:

- Treat symptomatic volume depletion with normal saline.
- Replete ongoing losses with the type of fluid lost.
- Continue to give fluid to cover normal daily requirements.
- Replete 30–50% of the free water deficit in the first 24 hours—no faster.
- Monitor the physical exam and serum sodium to confirm accurate and timely volume repletion.

10. When an elderly patient is dehydrated and has hypernatremia, how do you calculate the free water deficit?

$$FWD = (\text{baseline weight} \times 0.45) - (\text{baseline weight} \times 0.45 \times [140/\text{serum sodium}])$$
$$= (70 \times 0.45) - (70 \times 0.45 \times 140/160)$$
$$= 31.5 - 27.6$$
$$= 3.9 \text{ L}$$

where FWD = free water deficit, baseline weight = 70 kg, and serum sodium = 160. For elderly adults, 0.45 is used as the percentage of free water in the body, whereas in younger adults the percentage is 0.60. As mentioned before, this difference is due to the higher percentage of fat in older adults.

11. What conditions are most commonly associated with hypovolemic hyponatremia?

Hyponatremic dehydration frequently is associated with low serum osmolarity and often coincides with medical conditions such as renal tubular acidosis, adrenal insufficiency, partial renal obstructions, and, most commonly, diuretic effects. Other factors that may result in hyponatremic dehydration are diarrhea, vomiting, and skin losses. The last three also may present as hypernatremic dehydration and isotonic dehydration with normal serum sodium.

12. Is urine osmolarity a good measure for dehydration in elderly adults?

The normal renal response to dehydration is to retain water and thus to concentrate urine. This results in higher urine osmolarity, especially compared with plasma osmolarity. Yet in elderly adults, the kidney's response to vasopressin is often impaired. Thus the concentrating capacity is diminished. Therefore, the increase in urine osmolarity frequently underestimates the degree of dehydration.

13. Is measuring the blood urea nitrogen useful in measuring the volume status of elderly adults?

Measuring blood urea nitrogen helps to determine prerenal azotemia. In younger patients a ratio > 20:1 suggests prerenal azotemia. In general, the elderly have a decreased glomerular filtration rate and increased protein turnover; therefore, a ratio > 28:1 suggests dehydration. Other causes of an elevated ratio include renal vascular disease, gastrointestinal bleeding, obstructive uropathy, and steroid-induced catabolism, which may or may not be associated with concomitant dehydration.

14. Does incontinence contribute to dehydration?

Incontinence can indirectly result in dehydration. Because many elderly adults are fearful of having an incontinent episode in public, they severely restrict their fluid intake. Care should be taken to identify such patients. Encourage water intake; then diagnose and treat the incontinence.

15. What medications put patients at risk of dehydration?

The most common medications that cause dehydration are diuretics. Several psychiatric medications may result in dehydration. Lithium, in particular, may cause diabetes insipidus. Pain medications that alter mental status, such as opiates, are notorious for resulting in decreased oral intake and secondarily cause dehydration. In addition, the osmolarity and malabsorption associated with enteral tube feedings may result in diarrhea and dehydration.

16. What is hypodermoclysis (HDC)?

HDC is rehydration therapy in which fluid is infused directly into the subcutaneous tissue. This method usually is used for patients who are dehydrated but have poor IV access or are in a nursing home where IV access is not an authorized procedure. HDC was used more frequently in the 1950s and 1960s. During the 1960s a high incidence of infection and sepsis was noted; therefore, the practice was almost abolished. Since the advent of improved sterile methods and the creation of disposable catheters, the incidence of infection has decreased significantly. HDC is performed by inserting a catheter into the subcutaneous tissue of the abdomen, leg, or gluteal region and then infusing fluids. Normal saline is best tolerated, but 5% dextrose in water also may be given if it is supplemented with sodium. Maximal infusion rate is 1500 ml/day per site. No more than two concurrent sites are recommended. In the past hyaluronidase was added to the infusion solution to decrease pain and augment fluid resorption, but recent studies have shown that it does neither. Its use is no longer recommended.

17. Do patients with Alzheimer's disease have a greater risk of dehydration than other elderly patients?

Some studies suggest that patients with Alzheimer's disease have depressed vasopressin levels compared with age-matched controls. This finding was not always statistically significant and has not been directly associated with an increase in the incidence of dehydration. Nevertheless, this finding in combination with impaired mental status should alert the physician to monitor this type of patient carefully for dehydration.

18. Is the normal fluid volume of tube feedings adequate for most elderly patients?

In most cases enteral tube feedings do not have adequate amounts of free water. Free water needs to be supplemented to meet daily free water requirements. In general, total daily free water requirements range from 1.5–2 L/day.

19. What simple methods help to prevent dehydration during periods of extreme heat?

The most important factors are to drink at least 8 glasses of water per day during hot weather and to stay out of direct sunlight as much as possible. Because the elderly have diminished hormonal and central nervous system response to dehydration and temperature changes, they are at extreme risk for dehydration during hot and humid days. The best way to stay cool is to stay within an air-conditioned home. If this is not possible, fans should be used liberally. In addition, dampening clothes or adding moistened towels onto or over a fan can help to keep a room cool.

BIBLIOGRAPHY

1. Albert S, Nakra B, Grossberg GT, Caminal ER: Vasopressin response to dehydration in Alzheimer's disease. J Am Geriatr Soc 37:843–847, 1989.
2. Ferry M, Dardaine V, Constans T: Subcutaneous infusion or hypodermoclysis: A practical approach. J Am Geriatr Soc 47:93–95, 1999.
3. Lavizzo-Mourey R, Johnson J, Stolley P: Risk factors for dehydration among elderly nursing home residents. J Am Geriatr Soc 36:213–218, 1988.
4. Leaf A: Dehydration in the elderly. N Engl J Med 311:791–792, 1984.
5. Phillips PA, Rolls BJ, Ledingham JG, et al: Reduced thirst after water deprivation in elderly men. N Engl J Med 311:791–792, 1984.
6. Snyder N, Feigal DW, Arieff AI: Hypernatremia in elderly patients: A heterogeneous, morbid, and iatrogenic entity. Ann Intern Med 107:309–319, 1987.
7. Weinberg AD, Minaker KL: Dehydration: Evaluation and management in older adults. JAMA 274:1552–1556, 1995.

45. INFECTION CONTROL IN LONG-TERM CARE FACILITIES

Mary L. Fornek, RN, BSN, MBA, CIC, and
Kelly Henning, MD

1. What is an infection control program in a long-term care facility? Why is it needed?

Long-term care facilities (LTCFs) are covered by federal, state, and voluntary agency guidelines. Skilled nursing facilities are required by the Omnibus Budget Reconciliation Act of 1987 (OBRA) to have an active infection control program. Surveyor guidelines require LTCFs to establish and maintain an infection control program designed to provide a safe, sanitary, and comfortable environment and to help prevent the development and transmission of disease and infection. The infection control program must include definitions of infection, risk assessment, outbreak control, antibiotic monitoring, assessment of compliance with policies and procedures, and records of incidents and corrective actions related to infections. The written infection control program should be periodically (at least annually) reviewed by the facility and revised as indicated. The key components of an infection control program include:

- Infection surveillance
- Epidemic control program
- Education of employees for infection control methods
- Policy and procedure development and review
- Employee health program
- Resident health program and monitoring of resident-care practices
- Antibiotic usage and resistance
- Quality improvement
- Product evaluation

Infection control programs vary among LTCFs. An effective infection control program should have a small working group that is interdisciplinary and includes the medical director, administrator, director of nursing, and someone who specifically coordinates the various infection control functions as part of their job description. Secondary team members include employees from the nursing, dietary, housekeeping, and pharmacy departments and a representative from the laboratory that does the facility's cultures. An infection control practitioner (ICP) is not a regulatory requirement; however, most LTCFs employ one to direct the program. The group should meet regularly, and records of the meetings should be kept.

2. What is the prevalence of infections in LTCFs?

It is well known that the elderly population has a substantially increased incidence and severity of many infectious diseases. This vulnerability is due partly to an age-related decline in immunologic function, specifically cell-mediated immunity and antibody response. Numbers and function of T lymphocytes decline with age, as reflected in reactivation of latent infections in the elderly. Antibody production declines with age as well.

Elderly patients in a LTCF are particularly susceptible to infection on the basis of severity of underlying diseases and medications (steroids, antibiotics) that reduce patients' ability to fight infection. Incontinence, indwelling catheters, and other factors contribute as well. Although more studies are needed to determine the prevalence of infections in LTCFs, published infection rates range from 2–14 infections per 1000 resident days, or 1.6 to 3.8 million infections per year in the U.S. Respiratory infections, particularly pneumonias, are among the most common infections occurring in LTCF.

Endemic Infection Rates in Long-term Care Facilities, United States, 1978–1989[11]

CATEGORY OF INFECTION	RATE (NO. OF INFECTIONS/1000 RESIDENT CARE DAYS
All infections	1.8 to 13.5
Urinary tract infections (UTIs)	0.1 to 3.5
Respiratory tract infections	0.3 to 4.7
Skin and soft tissue infections	0.1 to 2.1

Endemic Infection Rates in 21 LTCFs in Canada for an 18-month Period (1998–2000)[7]

INFECTION SITE	LRI	URI	SKIN	EYE	GI	UTI	BSI
Rate/1000 res. days	1.40	1.33	0.61	0.57	0.41	0.20	0.03
% of infections	30.9	29.2	13.4	12.5	9.10	4.30	0.60

LRI = lower respiratory tract infection, URI = upper respiratory tract infection, GI = gastrointestinal infection, UTI = urinary tract infection, BSI = bloodstream infection.

3. When should I suspect an outbreak?

Surveillance data should be used to detect and prevent outbreaks in LTCFs. The occurrence of even a single verified case of disease of epidemiologic significance (such as nosocomial tuberculosis, influenza, or botulism) in the LTCF should prompt consideration of an outbreak, initiation of an investigation, and notification of appropriate administration and infection control personnel. Data accumulated by ongoing surveillance allow the detection of nosocomial outbreaks. When the monthly rate for a particular infection exceeds the 95% confidence interval based on the previous years' rates for that month, the possibility of an outbreak exists and an investigation is warranted. Nurses, physicians, or microbiology technologists who notice a cluster of infections may also detect outbreaks.

4. What steps do I implement if I suspect an outbreak?

- Promptly notify administrator or medical director.
- Institute temporary infection control measures.
- On-duty facility personnel should work only on their assigned floors for the duration of the outbreak.
- Isolation precautions may need to be implemented.
- Immediately assess exposed residents and personnel to detect additional cases.
- Notify the Department of Health.
- In some cases, a unit or the entire facility may be quarantined or new admissions halted.
- Symptomatic personnel should not provide direct resident care and should not work until symptoms have subsided.
- An outbreak is considered "over" when no new cases have been detected for the length of an incubation period.

The LTCF should have administrative protocols for outbreak investigations, which include the authority to relocate residents, confine residents to their rooms, restrict visitors, obtain cultures, isolate, and administer relevant prophylaxis or treatment.

5. Do I need an isolation/precaution system?

A variety of isolation systems may be appropriate for the LTCF. Every system should include standard precautions for the prevention of exposure to bloodborne pathogens. Masks, impervious gowns and gloves, and protective eyewear must be provided by the LTCF and used if contact with blood and/or body fluids is anticipated. Used needles, syringes, and other sharp objects must be disposed of in a puncture-resistant, leak-proof container. Three additional precautions are required for patients with suspected or documented contagious pathogens:

PRECAUTION CATEGORY	EQUIPMENT/ROOM	INDICATIONS
Airborne	A private room with negative pressure ventilation with a minimum of 6 air exchanges per hour Use of N-95 respirators if entering room	Measles Tuberculosis Disseminated herpes zoster Severe acute respiratory syndrome (SARS)
Droplet	A private room Wear masks upon entering room	Meningococcal pneumonia Pertussis Influenza
Contact	A private room Gowns*	MRSA *Clostridium difficile* VRE

MRSA = methicillin-resistant *Staphylococcus aureus*, VRE = vancomycin-resistant enterococci.
* Use of gowns is recommended for epidmiologically important microorganisms to reduce transmission.

For certain infections that have significant implications for the LTCF (such as TB, influenza, VRE), the facility should assess its isolation needs and capabilities before accepting a new admission case. Isolation/precaution policies and procedures should be developed, evaluated, and revised on a regular basis. The facility should have infection control policies for the acceptance and transfer of residents with infectious diseases.

6. What prevention programs are important in long-term care facilities?

Resident health programs are important in the prevention of nosocomial infections. Each resident should have an initial history (including past and present infectious diseases), immunization status evaluation, and a recent physical examination. All newly admitted residents should receive two-step mantoux/purified protein derivative (PPD) testing unless a physician's statement has been obtained that the resident had a past positive reaction to tuberculin. A PPD is considered positive and a chest radiograph is indicated when a resident has:

- ≥ 10 mm of induration
- ≥ 5 mm for residents with organ transplants, other immunosuppressed conditions, HIV positive, recent contact of an active TB case or fibrotic changes on chest radiograph

If chest radiographs are normal and no symptoms consistent with active TB are present, tuberculin-positive persons may be candidates for treatment of latent TB infection (LTBI). If radiographic or clinical findings are consistent with pulmonary or extrapulmonary TB, further studies (e.g., medical evaluation, bacteriologic examinations, comparison of the current and old chest radiographs) should be done to determine if treatment for active TB is indicated and an infectious disease or pulmonary specialist consult is advised. Such residents should be hospitalized and placed on airborne isolation until their TB status has been determined.

Single-step testing for TB of residents should be done on a regular basis (most facilities perform PPD skin testing annually) and after discovery of a new case of active TB in a resident or staff member.

One of the major functions of a resident health program is the immunization of the elderly resident. Each resident should receive:

- Tetanus and diphtheria vaccine every 10 years
- Pneumococcal vaccine at age 65 (see question 7)
- Influenza vaccine annually in the fall

All vaccinations must be recorded in the resident's medical record.

7. Why are the pneumococcal and influenza vaccines important?

Influenza and pneumonia combined represent the fifth leading cause of death in the elderly. The Federal Registrar (vol. 67, no. 191) states that "influenza and consequent respiratory diseases are common causes of morbidity and mortality in the United States each year with 20,000 to 40,000 deaths reported for each influenza epidemic. Over 90 percent of these deaths occur among those 65 or older." The report also states that influenza vaccination "has been shown to be efficacious in the elderly, decreasing hospitalizations by 27 percent to 57 percent and deaths by 27 percent to 30 percent." There are minimal adverse reactions or side effects related to influenza vaccines because, as the MMWR (vol. 46, no. RR-9) states, "inactivated influenza vaccine contains noninfectious killed viruses and cannot cause influenza." Influenza vaccine should be administered annually in the fall.

According to the Centers for Disease Control and Prevention (CDC), an estimated 40,000 deaths annually in the United States are attributed to *Streptococcus pneumoniae* (pneumococcal) infection. Immunization of high-risk persons (including persons aged 65 years and older) could prevent up to half of these deaths. The organism colonizes the upper respiratory tract and can cause the following types of illnesses: disseminated invasive infections, including bacteremia and meningitis; pneumonia and other lower respiratory tract infections; and upper respiratory tract infections, including otitis media and sinusitis. According to the MMWR (vol. 46, no. RR-8), the pneumococcal polysaccharide vaccine is both cost-effective and protective against invasive pneumococcal infection when administered to the following groups:

- Persons aged ≥ 65 years
- Persons aged 2–64 years with chronic cardiovascular disease, chronic pulmonary disease, or diabetes mellitus
- Persons aged 2–64 years with alcoholism, chronic liver disease, or cerebrospinal fluid leaks
- Persons aged 2–64 years with functional or anatomic asplenia
- Immunocompromised persons aged ≥ 2 years, including those with HIV infection, leukemia, lymphoma, Hodgkins disease, multiple myeloma, generalized malignancy, chronic renal failure, or nephritic syndrome; those receiving immunosuppressive chemotherapy (including corticosteroids); and those who have received an organ or bone marrow transplant.
- When indicated, vaccine should be administered to patients who are uncertain about their vaccination history.

In certain instances residents require repeat pneumococcal vaccination, particularly if the first dose was administered prior to 65 years of age. The national health goal is to immunize with influenza and pneumococcal vaccine at least 90% of the institutionalized population by 2010 through a national quality improvement program and to promote standing orders for immunization programs to ensure that all nursing facility residents are assessed for and offered influenza and pneumococcal vaccinations. Influenza and pneumococcal vaccines now can be administered per physician-approved facility or agency policy after an assessment for contraindications, without a physician signature. LTCFs can improve access to influenza and pneumococcal vaccine, as allowed by state law, by implementing a standing orders program similar to those used in community and physician's outpatient office settings.

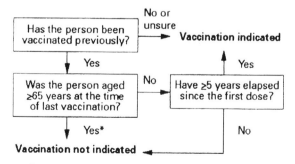

Pneumococcal vaccine algorithm for persons aged ≥ 65 years.

* Note: For any person who has received a dose of pneumococcal vaccine at age < 65 years, revaccination is definitely indicated. For any person over age 65 at first vaccination, it is not clear whether revaccination is necessary. Most physicians revaccinate at 6 years because of waning immunity.

8. What is the single most important factor in preventing infections in LTCF?

Hand hygiene is one of the most important measures for preventing infections in LTCFs. Hand hygiene is a general term that applies to handwashing, antiseptic handwash, antiseptic hand rub, or surgical hand antisepsis. The October 25, 2002 CDC Guidelines for Hand Hygiene in Health-Care Settings recommend the revised indications for handwashing and hand antisepsis:

- When hands are visibly soiled or visibly dirty with blood and/or other body fluids, wash hands with either a nonantimicrobial soap and water or an antimicrobial soap and water.
- If hands are not visibly soiled, use an alcohol-based hand rub for routinely decontaminating hands in the following clinical situations:

1. Before having direct contact with patients

2. Before donning sterile gloves when inserting a central intravascular catheter

3. Before inserting indwelling urinary catheters, peripheral vascular catheters, or other invasive devices that do not require a surgical procedure

4. After contact with a patient's intact skin (e.g., when taking a pulse or blood pressure, and lifting a patient)

5. After contact with body fluids or excretions, mucous membranes, nonintact skin, and wound dressings if hands are not visibly soiled

6. If moving from a contaminated-body site to a clean-body site during patient care

7. After contact with inanimate objects (including medical equipment) in the immediate vicinity of the patient

8. After removing gloves

Before eating and after using a restroom, wash hands with a nonantimicrobial soap and water or with an antimicrobial soap and water.

9. What factors put elderly people at risk for UTIs? How can they be prevented?

In most surveys, the leading nosocomial infection in LTCFs is UTI, generally related to an indwelling catheter. The prevalence of bacteriuria in the elderly is approximately 10% in men and 20% in women. In residents of LTCFs, bacteriuria is more common and the frequencies in men and women become similar. Asymptomatic bacteriuria is defined as the presence of a positive urine culture in the absence of new signs and symptoms of urinary tract infection. Asymptomatic bacteriuria in the elderly does not require antibiotic therapy. In contrast, symptomatic UTI should always be treated in the elderly.

One-third of UTIs or bacteriuria in residents of LTCF are caused by *Escherichia coli* and one third are caused by *Proteus* spp. The frequency of *Klebsiella* spp. and *Pseudomonas aeruginosa* UTIs are significantly higher among LTCF residents than elderly persons in the community. Twenty-five percent of bacteriuria in residents of LTCF are polymicrobial. Common risk factors that predispose the elderly to UTI include:

- Diabetic neuropathy
- Kidney stones
- Dehydration
- In older women, relaxation of the pelvic floor muscles leads to inefficient bladder emptying and allows bacteria to multiply in the residual urine
- Prostatic hypertrophy in elderly men may lead to bladder outlet obstruction and, consequently, increased residual urine
- In chronic prostatitis, the prostate may serve as a reservoir for pathogens
- Poor hygiene, which allows increased numbers of pathogenic bacteria in the periurethral area
- Incontinence of urine or feces
- Condom catheters are a potential factor in UTI in elderly men and may also lead to soft-tissue infection of the penis

The use of indwelling urinary catheters in long-term care facilities should be avoided. Most residents with indwelling urinary catheters for 30 days or more become bacteriuric, but only a small percentage become symptomatic. When symptomatic infections develop in patients with indwelling catheters, urine culture and sensitivity should be obtained and empirical antibiotics initiated.

10. The elderly are at risk for which types of respiratory infections?

Pneumonia is the third most common LTCF infection and the most costly of the common hospital-acquired infections. Common conditions that predispose the elderly to pneumonia include emphysema, chronic obstructive pulmonary disease, heart disease, and chronic bronchitis. The clinical presentation of pneumonia in the elderly is often atypical. Onset can be sudden with shaking chills, high fever, productive cough, acute pleurisy, and lung infiltrate. In 15–20% of the elderly, onset may be insidious; the main signs include confusion or general deterioration. Temperatures of elderly patients with bacteremic pneumococcal pneumonia are lower than those in younger patients, and cough and fever may be absent in the elderly with pneumonia. It is important to culture the blood and sputum of elderly patients with suspected pneumonia.

Streptococcus pneumoniae appears to be the most common etiologic agent. The elderly LTCF resident, with frequent underlying medical diseases, may develop pneumonia due to a variety of pathogens, including *Haemophilus influenzae, Staphylococcus aureus*, and gram-negative bacilli (Enterobacteriaceae, *Pseudomonas* spp., *Klebsiella pneumoniae, Legionella pneumophila*). Respiratory syncytial virus (RSV) is a more common cause of pneumonia in the older population. RSV is often of rapid onset; bronchospasm may be a frequent and prominent feature.

LTCF residents commonly have conditions that predispose to aspiration pneumonia, such as swallowing disorders, feeding tubes, and mental status abnormalities. Efforts to prevent pneumonia are important in the elderly population. They should include:
- Immunization with pneumococcal polysaccharide vaccine
- Immunization with influenza vaccine
- Limiting contact between patients or employees with respiratory illness and elderly individuals during an influenza outbreak
- Discouraging smoking
- Wearing gloves for suctioning
- Hand hygiene after contact with respiratory secretions
- Reducing the potential for aspiration by elevating the head of the bed 30° to 45° during tube feedings and for at least one hour after feeding.

11. Are LTCF residents at increased risk for tuberculosis?

Persons at increased risk for developing TB include residents and employees of high-risk congregate settings, such as LTCFs. Infected persons who are considered to be at high risk for developing active TB should be offered treatment of latent TB infection (LTBI), regardless of age. Before beginning treatment of LTBI, active TB should be ruled out by history, physical examination, chest radiography, and, when indicated, bacteriologic studies.

Baseline laboratory testing is not routinely indicated for all patients at the start of treatment for LTBI. Patients whose initial evaluation suggests a liver disorder should have baseline hepatic measurements of serum aspartate aminotransferase (AST/SGOT) or alanine aminotransferase (ALT/SGPT) and bilirubin. Baseline testing is also indicated for patients with HIV infection, persons with a history of chronic liver disease (e.g., hepatitis B or C, alcoholic hepatitis, cirrhosis), persons who use alcohol regularly, and persons at risk for chronic liver disease. Routine laboratory monitoring during treatment of LTBI is indicated for persons whose baseline liver function tests are abnormal and other persons at risk for hepatic disease. Testing may also be indicated for the evaluation of possible adverse effects during treatment (e.g., liver function studies for patients with symptoms compatible with hepatotoxicity or a uric acid measurement to evaluate complaints of joint pain).

Testing for and treating LTBI requires several steps, including administering a PPD test, reading the test, medically evaluating potentially infected persons, initiating treatment, and completing therapy. The local health department is available to serve as advisor, consultant, and facilitator to institutions that conduct testing and treatment programs.

For residents eligible for treatment of LTBI, the usual choice of therapy is isoniazid, 300 mg per day for 9 months, together with pyridoxine, 25–50 mg per day for 9 months. Consultation with infectious disease or pulmonary specialists is recommended for residents with underlying liver disease or other medical conditions that may complicate therapy.

12. What are the most common skin and soft tissue infections in LTCF residents?

Pressure sores are the second leading cause of LTCF infections. The prevalence of pressure ulcers ranges from 2% to 23% in LTCFs. Pressure sores are associated with increased mortality. Pressure sores occur primarily in residents with the following risk factors:

- Impaired mobility
- Poor nutrition
- Impaired circulation
- Incontinence
- Steroid use
- Diabetes
- Postcerebrovascular accident
- Moisture
- Friction
- Infection

A pressure ulcer may be associated with a number of infectious complications, which include, in order of frequency, local infection, cellulitis of surrounding tissue, contiguous osteomyelitis, and bacteremia. All pressure ulcers are colonized with bacteria; therefore, making an accurate bacteriologic diagnosis is difficult. Swabbing the wound often yields organisms that are colonizers and not actually causes of infection. To obtain a culture, the pressure ulcer must first be cleaned with sterile water or saline. Use a syringe to aspirate material from the margin or base of the ulcer, directing the needle through intact skin. Most pressure ulcers in the elderly yield multiple organisms when cultured. Aerobes that are commonly recovered include staphylococci, enterococci, *Proteus mirabilis*, *E. coli*, and *Pseudomonas* spp. In addition, anaerobic *Peptostreptococcus*, *Bacteroides fragilis*, and *Clostridium* spp. are frequently identified. Antibiotic therapy should be initiated only if the pressure ulcer is infected.

Scabies is the infestation of the skin caused by a mite, *Sarcoptes scabiei* subsp. *hominis*. Scabies mites are transferred by direct skin-to-skin contact. Indirect transfer from clothing, bedding, lotions or creams, walking belts, or upholstered furniture in close proximity to a patient may be a source of transmission. It may take 2–6 weeks after exposure before symptoms of scabies infestation are apparent. If the health care worker or resident has previously been infested, symptoms tend to develop sooner, within several days (1–4) after exposure. The most common symptom of scabies is extreme itching, especially at night or after bathing. Tiny vesicles or papular rash/lesions are usually seen between the fingers, on anterior surfaces of the wrists and elbows, axilla, belt line, abdomen, and thighs. The rash may resemble psoriasis or eczema; however, treatment with steroids will promote the infestation by suppressing the immune system. To confirm scabies, a health care worker proficient with the procedure should perform at least 6 skin scrapings from different sites. Contact precautions should be implemented until the diagnosis has been confirmed or ruled out. Residents with confirmed scabies should remain on contact isolation until they have received 24 hours of appropriate treatment.

13. What are the most common causes of outbreak-associated diarrhea?

Diarrhea is a significant cause of morbidity and mortality in the elderly. In the LTCF setting, outbreaks of diarrhea occur relatively commonly during the winter months. Both the norovirus (previously called Norwalk-like viruses) and the rotavirus have been implicated in these episodes. Viral diarrhea is usually abrupt in onset, lasts 24–72 hours, and produces malaise, anorexia, abdominal cramping, vomiting, and large watery stools without blood or mucous. Bacterial diarrhea (*Campylobacter jejuni*, *Salmonella*, *Shigella*, *E. coli*, *Vibrio parahaemolyticus*, *Yersinia enterocolitica*) usually has a gradual onset with fever, loose bloody stools or stools with occult blood; antibiotic therapy is recommended. *Clostridium difficile* is increasingly recognized as a cause of sporadic outbreaks in the LTCF. Diarrhea due to bacterial toxins, such as *C. difficile*, is abrupt in onset and usually accompanied by nausea without abdominal pain. Transmission of outbreak-associated diarrhea occurs from direct contact with the resident, the resident's environment, or health care worker's hands. Strict hand hygiene is very important to prevent ongoing transmission and widespread outbreaks of diarrhea.

14. Is conjunctivitis in the LTCF important?

Conjunctivitis in the LTCF is common and has been linked to transmission via hands of personnel. Conjunctivitis is an infection of the mucous membranes covering the eyelids and sclera.

It may be acute or chronic and sporadic or epidemic. Epidemic conjunctivitis may spread rapidly throughout a LTCF. Transmission may occur by contaminated eye drops or hand cross-contamination. Acute conjunctivitis may develop over several days and last several weeks; chronic conjunctivitis can lead to eyelid deformity. Many cases are viral, usually caused by an adenovirus. Most bacterial conjunctivitis is caused by *Staphylococcus aureus*, but a variety of other organisms have been implicated, including *Streptococcus* spp., *Proteus mirabilis*, *K. pneumoniae*, *Serratia* spp., and *E. coli*. Hand hygiene is the single most important factor in preventing transmission.

15. How do I prevent antibiotic resistance in my LTCF?

Antibiotic resistant bacteria cause colonization and infection in LTCFs. These bacteria include methicillin-resistant *Staphylococcus aureus* (MRSA), aminoglycoside (gentamicin, tobramycin, amikacin)-resistant gram-negative bacilli, and vancomycin-resistant enterococci (VRE). The widespread use of antibiotics is associated with the development of bacterial resistance in LTCFs. Antibiotics, both oral and parenteral, should be used to treat only patients with suspect or documented clinical infections. The infection control group should monitor all antibiotics administered, the indications for which the antibiotic was ordered, and the outcome of the resident receiving antibiotic therapy. Criteria for using specific antibiotics in defined clinical settings should be developed, and all physicians should be informed of the criteria. Antibiotics such as vancomycin and second- and third-generation cephalosporins should not be used when the clinical effectiveness of another class of antibiotics has been described in the literature.

Controlling the transmission of antibiotic resistant organisms is primarily the responsibility of those who have direct bedside contact with the resident. Handwashing and the appropriate use of gloves are the two primary transmission prevention measures. Private rooms or placing infected/colonized residents in a room together (cohorting) and the use of impervious gowns should be considered secondary infection control measures. Admission to an LTCF should never be denied based on the antibiotic resistance status of the resident.

BIBLIOGRAPHY

1. Allen J: Nursing Home Federal Requirements and Guidelines to Surveyors, 4th ed. New York, Springer, 2000.
2. Centers for Disease Control and Prevention: Guideline for hand hygiene in health-care settings. MMWR 51 (RR-16):1–45, 2002.
3. Centers for Disease Control and Prevention: Recommendations of the Advisory Committee on Immunization Practices: Prevention of pneumococcal disease. MMWR 46 (RR-8):1–24, 1997.
4. Centers for Disease Control and Prevention: Targeted tuberculin testing and treatment of latent tuberculosis infection. MMWR 49 (RR-6):1–53, 2000.
5. Crossley K, Peterson P: Infections in the elderly. In Mandell GL, Bennett JE, Dolin R (eds): Mandell, Douglas, and Bennett's Principles and Practice of Infectious Diseases, 3rd ed. New York, Churchill Livingstone, 2000, pp 3164–3169.
6. Federal Register: Medicare and Medicaid Programs; Conditions of participation: Immunization standards for hospitals, long-term care facilities, and home health agencies. (42 CFR Parts 482, 483, & 484) 67(19), 2002.
7. McArthur M, Liu B, Simore AE, et al: Infection rates in residents of long-term care facilities. Presented at Community and Hospital Infection Control Association Canada (CHICA) Conference, Toronto, Canada, 2000.
8. Rosenbaum P, Pass M, Roghmann M: Long term care. In APIC Text of Infection Control and Epidemiology. Association for Professionals in Infection Control and Epidemiology, 2000.
9. Smith PW, Rusnak PG: Infection prevention and control in the long term care facility: SHEA/APIC Position Paper. Infect Control Hosp Epidemiol 18:831–849, 1997.
10. Strausbaugh L, Sukumar S, Joseph C: Infectious disease outbreaks in nursing homes: An unappreciated hazard for frail elderly persons. Clin Infect Dis 36:870–875, 2003.
11. Strausbaugh L: Emerging health care-associated infections in the geriatric population. Emerg Infect Dis 7:268–270, 2001.
12. Vance J, Wilson K: Getting a handle on infection control in long-term care. Caring Ages 2(9):22–27, 2001.

46. PRESSURE ULCERS

Robert Goldman, MD

1. What are pressure ulcers? Where and how do they occur?

Pressure ulcers are areas of skin disruptions consisting of focal necrosis of epidermis, dermis, subdermis, fascia, muscle, or joint capsule. They are caused by excessive, prolonged pressure that produces ischemia to soft tissue over bony prominences (hot spots) such as the greater trochanter of the femur, sacrum, ischial tuberosity, or calcaneus. Injury may occur from prolonged sitting or lying without transient relief of pressure. Although commonly observed on patients that are bed-bound or bedfast, the term *pressure ulcer* is preferable to "bedsores" or "decubitus ulcers." Pressure ulcer better describes the cause, and because ulcers also occur on sitting patients, the other terms are not accurate descriptors.

2. What is the relationship of pressure to ulcer formation?

Unrelieved axial pressure of 4–6 times systolic blood pressure causes necrosis in as short as 1 hour, but pressure similar to systolic requires 12 hours to cause a similar lesion. Shear, defined as force tangential to the skin surface, causes ulceration at markedly lower axial pressure. Skin moisture aggravates both axial and shear forces and predisposes to breakdown; ischemic change occurs in response to compromised capillary perfusion. Periodic pressure relief increases resistance of tissue to breakdown. Therefore, sitting patients should be instructed to lift their buttocks from the seat at least 15 seconds every 15 minutes. Supine patients should be turned every 2 hours.

3. How are pressure ulcers assessed and classified?

The National Pressure Ulcer Advisory Panel (NPUAP) classification, which is partially based on the well-known Shea system, is recommended:

Stage I   Nonblanchable skin erythema (difficult to assess in patients with heavily pigmented skin)
Stage II   Breakdown into dermis, but not subcutaneous tissues (i.e., subdermis)
Stage III   Ulcer extends from subcutaneous depth to fascia
Stage IV   Ulcer extends from depth of the fascia to bone

Although not one of the NPUAP criteria, the following condition is clinically important:

Unstagable. Viable wound base is completely obscured by black or yellow eschar. Unstagable pressure ulcers are at least stage III. Unstagable pressure ulcers can appear deceptively shallow. Although shallow to the untrained eye, they can actually (after debridement) be very deep.

Serial reassessments of area and depth, at no longer than weekly intervals, quantify healing and assess the success of current treatment strategies. The simplest method is to measure the length along major and minor axes. A more quantitative technique is to trace the ulcer margin onto an acetate sheet (i.e., for photocopying transparencies) with a laundry marker, placing polyethylene film (e.g., acetate sheet) between the ulcer and the sheet. Photography assesses the ulcer's appearance and size. Depth should be documented with swabs. Be careful when using swabs to determine wound depth to avoid fragile structures (e.g., inferior gluteal artery). Wound is also assessed for color (red, yellow black), odor, and location (e.g., sacrum, coccyx, ischium, or heel).

From wound tracings on acetate sheet, area is derived accurately by computerized plainimetry. Multiplied by swab-determined wound depth, wound volume is over-estimated since pressure ulcers are not rectangular solids but spheroids. Volume is measured more accurately with Jeltrate dental mold material, or a Kundin gauge.

4. Are heel ulcers pressure ulcers?

Heel ulcers commonly occur in sedentary patients on the lateral outer surfaces of the heel (i.e., gravity positions legs by default in external rotation). Heel ulcers usually begin during hospitalization, such as during critical illness or associated with a surgical procedure. Heel ulcers are not simple pressure ulcers:

1. There is usually a component of arterial insufficiency or "small vessel" arterial disease—in fact, heel ulcers should be considered ischemic until proved otherwise (whereas pressure ulcers of the buttocks are typically well perfused).

2. Because they most often present with overlying black eschar, they are frequently unstagable.

3. Ambulation should be limited on an ischemic wound to reduce further "tissue damage," hypoxia, wound expansion, and possibly limb loss.

5. What interventions relieve pressure and shear?

- Placing pillows or other cushioning between trochanteric prominences and bed for side-lying patients
- Keeping the bed as horizontal as possible
- Using heel protectors
- Using special beds and mattresses

There is a wide spectrum of choice, with maximal efficiency of pressure and shear relief correlated with maximal cost. Geriatric patients with stage III or IV pressure ulcers, which exhibit dependent bed mobility, should receive an "active" mattress. Active mattresses include low air loss (SAR Low Air Loss Mattress System) or alternating air systems. Passive mattresses, including foam (Sof-care) or "egg-crate," are reserved for patients who can reposition themselves independently or on command. Less effective for pressure reduction and much lower in price are foam mattresses (e.g., "Sof-care" mattress). Seating systems for wheelchairs are issued to many patients who lack protective sensation or cannot shift weight. Examples are air-filled vinous (e.g., Roho), contoured foam with a gel insert (e.g., Jay), or contoured foam (e.g., polyurethane) with or without protective cover. A solid seat (rather than the usual sling seat) may be prescribed for stability. Doughnut-shaped air cushions are not recommended, because pressure at the margin of the cushion exceeds the safe limit.

The safe tissue pressure limit might be exceeded during sitting. A sitting human transmits trunk weight to the support surface across the ischial tuberosities. For a patient with an ischial pressure ulcer, enforced bed rest most of the day may be reasonable. Although activity limitation seems dramatic, the risks of wound expansion may outweigh complications of bed rest. Compliance with bed rest depends on buy-in by all stakeholders, including patient, family, and even other medical professionals. For instance, a patient with end-stage renal disease with an ischial pressure ulcer should not sit during hemodialysis.

6. Which patients are most likely to develop pressure ulcers?

The mnemonic **DECUBITUS** is suggested as a learning aid.

D Delirium, dementia, dependence. Only a patient with a clear mind can act purposefully to relieve a noxious stimulus. Therefore, patients with altered mental status, such as coma or severe dementia, are at risk for skin breakdown. Patients at risk of pressure ulcers are partially or completely dependent on others. Patients who require one or two persons to assist them in getting into bed are at high risk for ulceration.

E Elderly. Seventy percent of pressure ulcers occur in the elderly. Frailty, dependence, incontinence, chronic illness, and degenerative neurologic disease increase with age. Associated with aging are diminished pain perception and blunting of the inflammatory response. Histologic changes in skin include flattening of the dermal-epidermal junction and reduced elastin content, both of which increase susceptibility to shear and minor laceration. Ulcer closure is delayed because of reduced rates of both reepithelialization and contraction.

C Contractures. If severe, contractures prevent routine turning and positioning on most mattress types. Contractures increase point pressure. Thus they contribute to delayed healing and increased incidence.

U Urinary incontinence. Wet skin is easily macerated. If the urine is infected, the skin and any ulcers will be contaminated.

B Bowel incontinence. Soiling may lead to bacterial colonization or local infection. The wet skin associated with diarrhea also contributes to ulcer formation.

I Immobility. Chronic bed rest leads to a decrease in lean muscle mass of 5% per week and contributes to osteoporosis and contractures through collagen remodeling within tendons and joint capsules. Immobility feeds a vicious cycle of wasting, contractures, pressure "hot spots," and worsening ulceration.

T Tension O_2 low. Ischemia is related to ulcer formation. Anemia should be corrected (e.g., by iron supplementation). Edema impairs gas and nutrient exchange between healing tissue and the blood supply.

U Undernourishment. Inadequate caloric or protein intake may result in malnutrition and impaired ulcer healing. (See question 10.)

S Spasticity, sensory loss, spinal cord injury. By several mechanisms, neurologic injury predisposes to pressure ulcer formation:
- Spasticity (increased muscle tone) predisposes to contracture formation and poor mobility.
- Lack of protective sensation, which leads to pressure ulcer formation, may be dermatomal with spinal cord injury or hemisensory with stroke.
- Spinal cord injury, especially above T6, is related to sympathetic nervous system dysfunction and impaired skin perfusion at sites of pressure.

Employing most of the above elements, the Braden scale assesses predisposition to pressure ulcer formation.

7. What are occlusive or semiocclusive dressings? How are they used in pressure ulcer care?

Occlusive dressings create a barrier against moisture loss and a seal with normal skin around the ulcer. A moist environment results, with (semiocclusive) or without (occlusive) oxygen exchange. This moist milieu promotes formation of granulation tissue. The concern that an occluded environment brings about infection has not been substantiated for ulcers that are granulating. The choice to use one or the other is more a matter of personal preference than influence on wound-healing kinetics. Occlusive dressings form a better seal with skin outside the ulcer margin and thus resist contamination more effectively. Examples of occlusive dressings include polyurethane film (e.g., Tegaderm, OpSite), hydrocolloid (e.g., Duoderm), and hydrocolloid gel (e.g., Vigilon). The following treatment examples must be confirmed by experienced practitioners for specific cases:

Stage I: Cover with an occlusive dressing to prevent continued shear. Change every 3 days, when the dressing becomes dislodged, or when the ulcer seal is broken.

Stage II: If drainage is minimal, hydrocolloid wafers (e.g., Duoderm) are frequently effective and protective.

Stage III or IV: Treatment depends on appearance of ulcer base. A very clean, shallow stage III with minimal drainage can be managed with hydrocolloid wafer, but this is the exception. Most stage III pressure ulcers have some necrotic material and significant drainage, requiring bulk gauze dressing changes on at least a daily basis. The wound base should not be "too dry" or "too wet." Excessive moisture is always a concern since friction might abrade the fragile wound edge. Supply utilization and cost can be minimized with very absorptive dressings (e.g., alginate).
- Ulcers with a white to yellow film (i.e., fibrinous exudate) require debridement (see question 7).
  - Black, hard eschar (most often found about the heel) can be left exposed, although it is wise to protect an ischemic area from pressure and shear (e.g., DH walker, Multipodis or Proffo boots) to avoid inflammation and further hypoxia. Silver sulfadiazine

(Silvadine) can be applied to moisten and reduce bacterial count of eschar. Additionally, silver sulfadiazine softens the eschar to form a "pseudoeschar" that is straightforward to mechanically debride.

8. What types of debridement are used for ulcer care? What are their indications?

Devitalized tissue promotes infection and is a barrier to reepithelialization. Therefore, it should be debrided by mechanical, enzymatic, or autolytic means. Examples of **mechanical methods** include (1) manual (i.e., surgical or "sharps") debridement, (2) wet-to-dry dressings, and (3) irrigation. Sharp debridement is usually reserved for thick or adherent eschar or infected ulcers. Eschar (and, unfortunately, viable tissue) adheres to wet-to-dry dressings during removal; hence, the method is slower to work. Prepare by soaking gauze pads in saline, wringing out the liquid, completely unraveling, loosely packing all cavities of the ulcer, covering with dry gauze, and securing with paper tape. Irrigation can be done at the bedside with, for instance, a 50-ml syringe, 19-gauge Angiocath, and normal saline. Note that ischemic heel ulcers are fragile and must be debrided very carefully. **Enzymatic debridement agents** include Collagenase (Santyl; synthesized and refined from cultures of *Clostridium difficile*) and Papain-urea (Accuzyme). Enzymatic debridement is most appropriate between sharp debridements or when sharp debridement is not available. Disadvantages include nonselectivity (i.e., digesting both viable and nonviable tissue) and potential for increase in pain and drainage. **Autolytic debridement** is catalyzed by proteases in wound fluid beneath occlusive dressings. Although convenient, this method is not appropriate for wounds with large eschar burden, including unstagable pressure ulcers. Unstagable pressure ulcers must first be mechanically debrided to determine wound depth.

9. Should topical antiseptics, such as Betadine, peroxide, or sodium hypochlorite (i.e., Daken's) solution, be used routinely?

No, according to current guidelines. Overall, these agents retard epithelialization in animal models and are toxic to fibroblasts in vitro. However, this point is controversial. Some researchers point to animal studies suggesting that short-term, low-dose treatment may not delay healing. Some of the discrepancy may lie in how the agent is applied to the wound and the definition of healing. Animal studies that use daily application of topical agents and measure the time to 50% healing demonstrate reductions in healing rate. Studies that apply single doses of topical agent or measure time to 100% healing show no difference.

10. What is the role of adjunctive treatment?

- **Electrotherapy:** Both decubitus and leg ulcers reportedly heal more rapidly with electrotherapy. Short "high-voltage" pulsed electrotherapy, such as high volt pulsed current (HVPC), has been sanctioned to "promote local blood flow" by the Food and Drug Administration (FDA). However, the FDA has not specifically sanctioned electrotherapy for wound healing. This disparity has led to inconsistencies in Medicare reimbursement for this service. Nevertheless, there is good strength of evidence that HVPC, performed 1 hour daily, improves healing of pressure ulcers of the buttocks. Heel ulcers with mixed pressure-ischemic etiology also respond (i.e., in clinical case series and a phase I prospective trial).
- **Growth factor therapy:** Important wound healing phenomena include wound cell proliferation, extracellular matrix formation, and neoangiogenesis, which are all controlled by ubiquitous soluble proteins called growth factors. One of the best studied growth substances is platelet derived growth factor (PDGF). Rh-PDGF-BB (recombinant PDGF, BB isoform) has recently been FDA-approved for treatment of neuropathic, diabetic foot ulcers under the trade name Regranex®. Although randomized prospective trials have demonstrated improved healing relative to controls, control-healing rate in many of these studies has been slower than might be expected based on published benchmarks for healing rate. Therefore, the FDA has yet to approve PDGF-BB specifically to heal pressure ulcers. Still, results are promising.

11. What is the role of nutrition in the prevention and treatment of pressure ulcers?

A pressure ulcer might be a sign of malnutrition. For the geriatric population, the first sign of malnutrition might occur after a dramatic neurologic change (e.g., CVA, dysphagia) or critical illness. Because patients under the stress of critical illness require higher-than-normal protein to establish a positive "nitrogen balance," geriatric patients should be regarded as at risk for malnutrition. If malnutrition is likely, the team should consider total enteral or parenteral nutrition.

Indicators of poor nutrition include a serum albumin of < 3.5 mg/dl, total lymphocyte count of < 1,800 mm³, and body weight decrease of > 15%. Determining that the prealbumin is low is a sensitive measure of malnutrition, if available. Goals of nutrition therapy are correction of the above indices as well as a positive nitrogen balance (1.25–1.5 gm of protein/kg/day). Important vitamins for ulcer healing include vitamin C, vitamin A, and zinc. Supplementation of these substances is of questionable benefit if serum levels are normal.

12. How is an infected ulcer diagnosed and managed?

A foul smell, greenish or copious drainage, scant granulation, and dull whitish or pink base (rather than bright red granulation tissue) indicate local infection. Cellulitis is an invasion of organisms beyond ulcer margins, marked by erythema, warmth, swelling, or tenderness. Signs of bacteremia or systemic invasion include fever, elevated white count, change of mental status, or increasing insulin requirements in diabetics.

Bacteria colonize the surfaces of all ulcers; therefore, for uninfected wounds cultures have little meaning. If a wound appears locally infected in outpatient practice, oral broad-spectrum antibiotics are often empirically effective. However, for infection extending a few centimeters beyond wound borders and/or associated with systemic signs, bacterial culture is indicated. Culture techniques (in order of increasing sensitivity/specificity) include semiquantitative swab, quantitative swab, curettage, needle aspiration, and histologic bunch biopsy (for biopsy specimens, > 10⁵ colony forming units per gram of tissue suggest poor healing potential). Generally, the more accurate the culture method, the more invasive is the procedure and the more limited the availability outside specialized centers.

Clinical infection is almost always polymicrobial, including both facultative aerobes and strict anaerobes. Aerobic organisms are usually found in surface swabs, whereas anaerobes are more often isolated from deep tissue and blood. In one study deep tissue isolates included *Proteus mirabilis*, group D streptococci, *Escherichia coli, Staphylococcus aureus, Pseudomonas aeruginosa, Bacteroides fragilis,* and *Peptostreptococcus* species. Anaerobes are associated with ulcers having necrotic material and foul odor.

For locally infected ulcers, start a course of frequent ulcer inspection and mechanical debridement (e.g , wet-to-dry dressings and hydrotherapy). The Pressure Ulcer Advisory Panel recommends application of topical bactericidal agents only if infection does not resolve within 1 week. For systemic signs of infection, such as chills or sweats, fever or drop in body temperature, hypotension, or glucose intolerance (in diabetics), broad-spectrum coverage is recommended, because infection is usually polymicrobial. Urgent surgical debridement is required, because bacteremia doubtless will not clear without removal of necrotic material or drainage of abscess.

13. How is osteomyelitis in a pressure ulcer diagnosed and treated?

Osteomyelitis should be suspected in stage IV decubiti. However, the gold standard, a bone biopsy, is usually not done except as part of aggressive debridement. There is much controversy about the best noninvasive test for osteomyelitis. An elevated erythrocyte sedimentation rate, elevated white blood cell count, and positive plain x-ray, taken together, are 88% specific and 89% sensitive for osteomyelitis. (A plain film is positive in the presence of reactive bone formation and periosteal elevation.) For difficult cases, imaging studies with optimum diagnostic power include magnetic resonance imaging (MRI) and indium 111 leukocyte scanning. Indium leukocyte scanning has a sensitivity and specificity of 88% and 85%, respectively; in a review of 11 studies MRI has a sensitivity and specificity of 95% and 88%, respectively. In addition, MRI provides pathoanatomic detail (e.g., on location of sinus tracts or abscesses). In the presence of an infected ulcer and positive plain film, bone biopsy should be performed with needle aspiration through intact skin. The biopsy is positive if it shows a chronic inflammatory infiltrate (plasma cells, lymphocytes) and positive quantitative culture > 10^3 organisms/gm of bone.

14. When should surgical closure be considered?

Surgical closure should be done when the patient does not progress with optimal care, including available adjunctive care. In addition, the patient must agree to and be able to tolerate surgery, which may involve extensive blood loss, and osteomyelitis must be adequately treated. Usually stage IV ulcers require surgical evaluation. Musculocutaneous flaps are usually the treatment of choice. However, for the flap to be successful, pressure relief must be addressed; if inadequate pressure relief was the original cause of the ulcer, the skin is likely to break down again.

15. Should the goal of ulcer care always be complete healing?

Not all ulcers will heal, even with optimal care. Motivation of the patient and compliance with therapies are critical for a successful outcome. Factors associated with a high risk of non-healing include:

- Bacterial colonization by > 10^5 CFU/gm of tissue
- Osteomyelitis (25% of nonhealing ulcers)
- Chronic granulation for > 30 years (may indicate malignancy, with biopsies consistent with epidermoid cancer [Marjolin's ulcer])
- Moribund (i.e., preterminal) status

16. What is the differential diagnosis for pressure ulcers?

Skin conditions that cause erythema around perianal, perineal, or gluteal skin folds may be confused with stage I and stage II pressure ulcers. Examples include dermatophytosis (tinea cruris), *Candida albicans* (often associated with vaginal monilia), and intertrigo. Contact dermatitis also should be considered. Herpes zoster classically presents with vesicles and crusts and may occur around sacral dermatomes. Skin ulceration has a long differential diagnosis. However, subcutaneous and dermal ulcers at bony prominences at the ischium, gluteal fold, or sacrum usually are caused by pressure. In contrast, ulceration of the lower extremities may be vascular, arterial, infectious, or neoplastic. Neoplasms (although very unlikely) are included in the differential diagnosis of pressure ulceration of the buttocks. Buttock wounds in unusual locations (i.e., not on weight-bearing areas) that do not respond to a short course of optimal wound care should undergo biopsy to rule out basal or squamous cell carcinoma or cutaneous lymphoma.

17. Can a pressure ulcer be a marker for abuse?

Yes. A pressure ulcer is likely to occur in a neglected, bed-bound patient. Neglect can occur in the home or nursing home. In a nursing setting, neglect can take the form of alleged breaches of care regarding turning/positioning, nutrition, restorative care, support surface application, hygiene, or wound assessment with the result being disfigurement or death from pressure ulceration. Whether from inadequate staffing, reimbursement or other societal factors, allegations of neglect have increased over the past decade. This has resulted in litigation plus cost increases for the entire skilled care industry.

At home, unintentional abuse may result from inexperience, excessive caregiver burden, or lack of motivation. Elder abuse should be considered in the following settings:

- The caregiver has a history of mental illness or alcohol or drug abuse, is socially isolated, or has undergone recent stressful life events.
- The dependent patient presents with signs of dehydration, malnutrition, or poor personal hygiene in addition to the ulcer.

BIBLIOGRAPHY

1. Allman RM: Pressure sores among the elderly. N Engl J Med 320:850–853, 1989.
2. Berlowitz DR, Wilking SV: The short-term outcome of pressure sores J Am Ger Soc 38:748–752, 1990.

3. Bergstrom N, Bennett M, Carlson C: Treatment of Pressure Ulcers. Rockville, MD, Agency for Health Care Policy and Research, Public Health Service, US Department of Health and Human Services, 1994.
4. Cammer Paris BC, Meier DE, Fein ED: Elder abuse and neglect: How to recognize warning signs and intervene. Geriatrics 50(4):47–51, 1995.
5. Eaglstein WH: Occlusive dressings. J Dermatol Surg Oncol 19:716–720, 1993.
6. Garber S, Biddle A, Click C, et al: Pressure ulcer prevention and treatment following spinal cord injury: A clinical practice guideline for health care professionals. In Paralyzed Veterans of America, 2000.
7. Goldman R, Salcido R: More than one way to measure a wound: An overview of tools and techniques. Adv Skin Wound Care 15(5):236–243, 2002.
8. Goldman R: Update on growth factors and wound healing: Past, present and future. Adv Skin Wound Care [in press].
9. Lazarus G, Cooper D, Knighton D, et al: Definitions and guidelines for assessment of wounds and evaluation of healing. Arch Dermatol 130:489–493, 1994.
10. Lineaweaver W, Howard R, Soucy D, et al: Topical antimicrobial toxicity. Arch Surg 120:267–270, 1985.
11. Maklebust J: Pressure ulcer assessment. Clin Geriatr Med 13:455–471, 1997.
12. McGuckin M, Goldman R, Bolton L, Salcido R: The Clinical Relevance of Microbiology in Acute and Chronic Wounds. Adv Skin Wound Care [in press].
13. Salcido R, Goldman R: Prevention and management of pressure ulcers and other chronic wounds. In Braddom R (ed): Textbook of Rehabilitation, 2nd ed. Philadelphia, W.B. Saunders, 2000, pp 645–665.

47. DISCHARGE PLANNING

Jane Reitmeyer, MSW, LSW, and Charles Spencer, MD, PhD

1. What is discharge planning?

Discharge planning is a process in which an individualized plan is developed for a patient to ensure a safe discharge and appropriate aftercare. A proper discharge includes identification of patient needs, creation of an appropriate care plan that addresses those needs, and implementation of that care plan. These steps can be further divided into:
- Determination of patient needs and wishes
- Assessment of family resources and preferences
- Facilitation of communication between patients and family
- Selection of post-acute care facility
- Coordination of plans and necessary paperwork
- Assistance with insurance or reimbursement resources

Assessment and needs identification are the foundation of a proper discharge plan. Components of the assessment to consider are physical, mental, and social functioning (often referred to as a biopsychosocial assessment), support systems, family caregiving capabilities, financial situation and insurance coverage, patient and family preferences regarding possible transfer to a post-acute care facility (nursing home, rehabilitation hospital, or inpatient hospice), environmental barriers of patient's home, and services in place prior to hospitalization. *Appropriate discharge planning should result in a decreased length of stay, lower mortality, and a lower rate of readmission.*

2. What special considerations may be taken in discharge planning?

Other considerations include caregiver availability, cultural differences, age, sociodemographics, previous hospitalizations, and dependence on technology. This information is often obtained throughout the different phases of discharge planning. Integral to the successful implementation of a discharge plan is communication of the plan to the patient and family so that they are part of the decision-making process. Knowledge of the availability and eligibility requirements for community resources also contribute to successful discharge.

3. What special discharge planning needs arise in older patients?

Elderly patients have many factors that can complicate discharge planning:
- Living alone. A careful functional assessment can help determine service needs that will support the patient during the recovery period.
- Cognitive function. Mental status assessment during the hospitalization may identify early dementia which will compromise self-care after discharge.
- Multiple chronic diseases. Treatment of one dominant problem may aggravate other pre-existing problems.

Significant deficits in any of the above areas should prompt a referral to the social worker *early* in the hospitalization for successful discharge planning. Interdisciplinary teams of professionals such as physicians, nurses, rehabilitation therapists, and social workers meeting regularly throughout the hospitalization are ideal in the design of discharge plans.

4. Who provides discharge planning?

Social workers, discharge-planning nurses, or staff nurses can lead discharge planning, depending on the complexity of problems and staff availability at the hospital. For the patient with few aftercare needs, the staff nurse can complete paperwork and coordinate with family and physician to ensure a safe discharge. When a patient requires durable medical equipment or follow-up by visiting nursing services, a discharge-planning nurse may become involved. If the patient is discharged to a difficult environment or post-acute facility, a social worker may be needed to coordinate care.

5. How does discharge planning help families?

Proper support after a hospitalization benefits not only the patient but also the family. Consider the example of the family members of an elderly patient who will now need assistance with bathing, dressing, and food preparation. Many family members live in separate residences at some distance from the patient. The family members are usually employed in full-time positions; they often are involved in caring for their own families. Coordinating the care of an elderly family member may become an overwhelming responsibility. Discharge planning that offers community services such as home health aides or visiting nursing services can provide necessary personal care and alleviate some of the responsibility from the family.

6. Who makes a referral for discharge planning?

Any member of the health care team should be able to generate a referral for discharge planning. In older inpatients, discharge planning should begin at the time of admission (data gathering, family contacts and expectations). With the current emphasis on cost containment and shorter lengths of stays, discharge planners can find themselves in a position of trying to define a plan in a short period. This can lead to incomplete planning with inadequate support. Rapid readmissions can be the result. Proper discharge planning requires time to gather all required information from patient, family, and health care team. The potential for readmission diminishes. The patient receives effective aftercare, which allows higher patient satisfaction and better healthcare outcomes.

BIBLIOGRAPHY

1. Bull MJ, Roberts J: Components of a proper hospital discharge for elders. J Adv Nurs 35:571–591, 2001.
2. Hamilton M: Standards of practice for discharge planning. Contin Care Nov:33–36, 1995.
3. Naylor M, Brooten D, Jones R, et al: Comprehensive discharge planning for the hospitalized elderly: A randomized clinical trial. 129:999–1006, 1994.
4. Parkes J, Shepperd S: Discharge planning from hospital to home. Cochrane Database Syst Rev (4):CD000313, 2000.
5. Potthoff S, Kane RL, Franco SJ: Improving hospital discharge planning for elderly patients. Health Care Financ Rev 19(2):47–72, 1997.
6. Shepperd S: Review: Evidence of the effectiveness of discharge planning is equivocal. ACP J Club 135:19–21, 2001.

V. Alternative Sites of Care

48. NURSING HOMES

Joan Weinryb, MD, CMD

1. What is a nursing home? Describe its place in the continuum of long-term care.

A nursing home is a long-term care institution with at least three inpatient beds that offers round-the-clock nursing care as well as medical, social, and personal services to persons in need of rehabilitation, short-term nursing, or long-term maintenance. In the continuum of health services, nursing homes lie between the acute-care hospitals and assisted living/personal care homes. Nursing homes in the United States have their roots in

- Nineteenth century British workhouse infirmaries
- County poor houses
- State mental hospitals
- Voluntary homes for the aged
- Proprietary boarding houses
- Hospital-affiliated nursing homes

2. What types of nursing homes are available in the U.S.?

Nursing homes can be free-standing, associated with hospitals, part of chains of similar facilities, or linked with other facilities in a continuum of care.

- 68% are certified for provision of Medicare services.
- 56% of nursing home income comes from Medicaid payments.
- 73% are for profit.
- 22% are not-for-profit or have religious affiliation.
- 4% are government run.

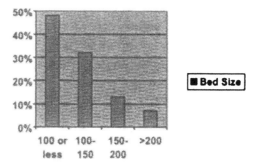

Breakdown of U.S. nursing homes by number of beds (bed size).

3. How do the epidemiology of the United States population and changes in social structure affect nursing home care?

The frail geriatric population is the most rapidly growing segment of our society. By the year 2030, the number of Americans over age 85 is expected to double. Almost half of those have some degree of dementia. Of those 75 years or older, 20% of men and 50% of women live alone. A third of these have no children. Elderly Americans have fewer children and tend to be more geographically separated from their children than previous generations. Much formal and informal care is arranged by daughters. More women now work outside the home, making care-giving for frail, elderly relations more stressful and difficult. Institutional care thus becomes a more frequently sought alternative.

It has been predicted that 52% of women and 33% of men turning 65 in 1990 will reside in a nursing home some time before they die. Twenty-five percent will spend at least 1 year and 9% will reside in a nursing home for 5 years or longer.

4. What elderly people are most often found in nursing homes?

Current rates of nursing home usage vary with age, sex, race, and bed availability, which differ from state to state. Chronically mentally ill, developmentally disabled and physically disabled Americans of all ages reside in nursing homes. Unavailability of community caregivers and decreased functional status are independent risk factors for nursing home admission. The proportion of each age group in the nursing home increases with age. More women than men in every age group live in nursing homes.

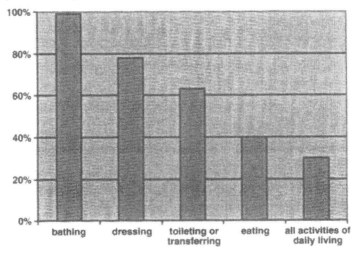

Proportion of patients residing in nursing homes who require assistance with activities of daily living.

5. Who uses the services of U.S. nursing homes?

Nursing homes contain short-term (< 6 months) and long-term (> 6 months) residents. Short-term residents are divided almost evenly between those who are admitted for terminal care and those admitted for rehabilitation or convalescence. Long-term residents may have physical and/or cognitive impairment, which precludes their continued management in the community. Most nursing home residents have a combination of physical and cognitive impairment. The prevalence of mental disorders including dementia, delirium, and psychiatric illness among nursing home residents is said to be about 90%.

6. What type of care is available in the nursing home?

Some nursing homes offer care for high-acuity, posthospital cases. Rehabilitation services including physical, occupational, and speech therapy for stroke, hip fracture, and other illness, intravenous therapy, wound care, and other skilled care are available. Ongoing care for those with disabling physical or cognitive impairments and specialized units for the demented and chronic ventilator patients as well as for developmentally delayed children are available in selected facilities.

7. How has the nursing home population changed in recent years?

The nursing home population has grown more dependent and more medically ill. Drastic shortening of hospital lengths of stay have created a demand for "subacute care." Managed care utilizes the nursing home setting as a more cost-effective alternative to expensive hospital care. Capitated systems have a strong financial incentive for treating acutely ill patients in less expensive settings such as nursing homes.

8. Which situations put elderly people at risk for nursing home admission?

Increasing age and frailty combined with:
- Mental, behavioral, or physical conditions that make management by a community care giver difficult
- Functional disabilities that preclude independent living
- Lack of a social support system
- Shortage of available, affordable, accessible community long-term care services

9. How expensive is nursing home care?

Generally, cost can be said to be $30,000–$45,000 per year per patient. Expenditures for nursing home care exceed $50 billion. Medicare pays less than 3% of nursing home cost; 68% is paid by Medicaid reimbursement; and 42% comes out of pocket. Twelve percent of elderly people live below the poverty line before nursing home admission and are already eligible for Medicaid grants. Others are forced to "spend down" their assets until they become impoverished and qualify for Medicaid. Long-term care insurance is being marketed but is not yet widely accepted.

10. How is medical care regulated and reimbursed in nursing homes?

Nursing home care is highly regulated by state and federal governments. Reimbursement for care given depends on compliance with regulations demonstrated during nursing home surveys and other oversight. The intent of nursing home regulations is to improve quality of care by requiring periodic comprehensive assessment of each resident, providing standards for training nurses aides, and reducing physical and pharmacologic restraint use. The Omnibus Budget Reconciliation Act of 1987 (OBRA 87) mandates that each resident be assisted to "attain or maintain the highest practicable physical, or mental and psychosocial well being." Nursing home oversight focuses on the process of care.

Formerly, nursing facilities billed Medicare, Medicaid, or private sources for services rendered to each resident. As of July 1998, nursing facilities are reimbursed under the prospective payment system (PPS) mandated by Congress. Patient acuity is classified according to resource utilization groups (RUGS), subdivided into 44 categories. Each RUG category is reimbursed at a specific level based on nursing/therapy staff time utilization. Reimbursement depends on electronic transmission of the MDS (minimum data set) that describes the resident's problems through objective behavioral observations rather than diagnoses. Analysis of patient care needs is based on:

- Rehabilitation requirements
- Cognitive function
- Distressed mood
- Ability to perform the activities of daily living
- Behavioral symptoms

A per-diem rate, based on the acuity of the residents, local employment costs, and rural vs. urban location is paid to the nursing home to cover all the costs of services expected as part of the patient's care plan.

PPS was designed to cut $9.5 billion per year from long-term expenses as part of the effort to reduce Medicare expenditures by $115 billion.

Nursing home surveys for quality of care are based on electronically transmitted MDS data. Such data identify the percentage of residents within a facility with conditions targeted as issues of care. Examples include:

- Pressure sores
- Dehydration
- Involuntary weight loss
- Untreated depression
- Use of psychotropic medications without appropriate indications
- Loss of ability to perform ADLs

Twenty-four quality indicators are evaluated monthly. Each nursing home can download a report comparing its performance with other, similar nursing homes. Incidence above a certain percentile may trigger a nursing home survey. Information about each nursing home's quality indicators and its surveys is available to the general public at such sites as <http://www.medicare.gov>.

11. How are nursing homes staffed?

Nursing homes are generally staffed by registered nurses (RNs) with supervisory responsibilities, licensed practical nurses (LPNs) who administer medications and treatments, and nurse's aides. Nursing home staffing does not resemble the staffing levels of the acute-care hospital. RN coverage may include only one person with supervisory responsibilities who must also assist in completing the minimum data set and other required paperwork, administer infection control programs, oversee the pharmacy, and manage wound prevention and care. Nurses' aides, often undereducated and poorly paid, do the bulk of the personal care and spend the most time observing the residents. "Burnout" and staff turnover rates as high as 90% for aides, 50% for LPNs and RNs, and 30–50% for directors of nursing can fragment care. The national nursing shortage has made staffing nursing homes even more difficult. The U.S. also has a shortage of physicians willing to provide care in nursing homes. At the same time as the elderly population most at risk for needing nursing care increases, a large number of the physicians attending nursing home patients are getting ready to retire. Regulatory agencies are currently deciding whether to allow "one-task staff" (e.g., feeding aides) to help allay the effect of staffing shortages.

12. How are the diagnosis and treatment of medical problems affected by nursing home residence?

Making an accurate diagnosis tends to be more difficult because of the effects of multiple chronic illnesses, multiple medications and their side effects and interactions, and the uncommon presentations of common illnesses in elderly patients. History taking is complicated by the cognitive disability of the patient and the failure of communication between different nursing shifts and ancillary personnel about the onset of pathologic signs and symptoms. The standard internal medicine approach of assessing all symptoms in search of a unifying diagnosis often fails to identify the acute problem, embedded as it is in a matrix of chronic symptoms. Atypical presentations (e.g., confusion or falls in urinary tract infection without dysuria) and nonspecific presentations (e.g., shortness of breath in pneumonia or myocardial infarction without cough or chest pain) may complicate decision-making. Delay may occur because nonspecific symptoms are overlooked by staff accustomed to cognitive dysfunction and dependency, especially those unfamiliar with the resident because of facility policy of "floating" assignments. There may be delay in physician evaluation or in diagnostic testing because of the facility's location, the facility's access to laboratories, radiologists, and the practitioner's other commitments. Some nursing homes are utilizing nurse practitioners to help improve timeliness and accuracy of medical care.

13. Are falls a problem in nursing homes?

Unintentional injury is the sixth leading cause of death in people 65 years or older. Falls are a frequent and serious problem in nursing homes. More than two-thirds of nursing home patients fall at least once a year. Falls may result in injury or in post-fall fear syndrome. A fall may cause well meaning nursing staff to encourage the resident to become more sedentary (leading to more deconditioning and more fall risk). Risk factors for falls include sedative drugs, antidepressants, antipsychotic medications, absolute number of medications taken, balance problems, hip weakness, poor functional status, and intermittent use of restraints. Nursing home financial constraints, leading to minimal staffing, suboptimal physical plants (e.g., slippery, hard floors, dim lighting, high beds), and increased utilization of the most highly trained staff to complete required paperwork, are contributing factors to fall risk in nursing homes. Customized seating, alarm devices, floor pads, and pharmacologic modifications can be used in mitigation. Physical therapy and exercise programs to increase strength and balance can be efficacious. Strength training and Tai Chi have been shown to decrease falls and injuries in even the frailest of nursing home residents. Aggressive treatment for osteoporosis in nursing home patients is only just beginning to be implemented.

14. Is urinary incontinence a problem in the nursing home?

Over 50% of nursing home patients are incontinent of bladder and/or bowel. Onset of incontinence is often the deciding factor leading to nursing home admission. Medical consequences of urinary incontinence include skin breakdown, falls, and use of urethral catheters (which may act as conduits for infection). Normal aging leads to decreased bladder capacity, increased detrusor irritability, decreased urethral length, and decreased closing pressure. The addition of immobility, cognitive impairment, medication effects, inaccessibility of toilet facilities, and chronic illnesses, such as diabetes mellitus, increases incontinence problems. The work-up for reversible conditions includes history, physical examination, urinary studies, and determination of postvoid residual. Cystometric evaluation can often be postponed while simple, ameliorative strategies are tried. Toileting schedules, treatment of impaired mobility, and removal of impediments to mobility such as bedrails and other restraints can often be helpful to nursing home patients. Pharmacologic treatment depends on the cause of the incontinence.

15. Is nutrition important in nursing homes?

Poor nutritional status alters susceptibility to infection, immune function, and wound healing, placing nursing home residents at higher risk for sepsis and death. Involuntary weight loss is considered a possible sign of poor quality of care by nursing home regulators. Loss of ≥ 5% of body weight in a month or > 10% in 6 months is considered significant. Nursing homes track body weight and laboratory indices such as albumin, plasma transferrin, and hemoglobulin to identify those at risk and intervene.

Risk factors for malnutrition
- Wasting conditions: cancer, pulmonary disease, heart disease, esophageal abnormalities, liver and biliary tract disease.
- Cognitive disabilities: anxiety, depression, psychosis, dementia.
- Infectious disease: AIDS, tuberculosis.
- Metabolic disorders: hypo- and hyperthyroidism, hyperparathyroidism, adrenal insufficiency.
- Movement disorders: essential tremor, tardive dyskinsia, Parkinson's disease.
- Mechanical problems: arthritis, dental problems, oral problems.

Metabolic abnormalities, chewing and swallowing difficulties, medication effects, and unpalatable diets (altered texture, low salt, low cholesterol) can be identified and corrected.

Regulatory guidelines suggest use of enteral feeding tubes for those with dysphagia or aspiration, decreased alertness, and malnutrition not attributable to a single reversible cause. Aspiration, diarrhea, electrolyte and fluid imbalance, gastric bleeding, and skin irritation or infection at the tube site can complicate tube feeding. Several medical professional organizations, including the AMA, consider tube feeding to be an invasive medical treatment that can be withheld or withdrawn. Some nursing home residents or their families may refuse enteral feeding as aggressive therapy not in keeping with the patient's wishes. This information must be carefully documented in the nursing home record. Studies of enteral feeding in advanced dementia have failed to demonstrate benefits in terms of weight gain, albumin normalization, wound healing, decrease in morbidity or mortality, or patient comfort.

16. Given the level of cognitive impairment of nursing home patients, are people commonly restrained?

Formerly, restraint was common. The past decade or so has shown tremendous progress toward restraint-free care. Federal regulation has contributed to the impetus to reduce both physical and chemical restraints. Before the passage of OBRA '87, use of restraints ranged from 25–85%. Despite widespread use, no studies demonstrated reduction of falls or injuries. Numerous complications (e.g., pressure sores, pneumonias, urinary tract infections, contractures, agitation, delirium) have been documented. Nursing home residents now have the legal right to be free of physical restraints or psychoactive drug administration not required for their safety or, in an emergency, the safety of others. Before restraints are used, the nursing facility must demonstrate that less restrictive measures were tried but proved ineffective. Restraints are to be used for the shortest time possible, and documentation must be provided to verify that the restraint enables the resident "to maintain the highest practicable physical, mental and psychosocial function." Psychoactive drugs, used to control mood, mental status, or behavior, are permitted only for specific conditions. Gradual dose reductions and behavioral interventions must be implemented, unless clinically contraindicated, and the absence of negative side effects must be documented. Since institution of the OBRA regulations, use of physical restraint has declined by 50% and use of psychoactive drugs unrelated to a psychiatric diagnosis by 25–36%. Many nursing homes are now considered restraint-free.

17. Is infection common in nursing homes?

Infection and infection control are important issues in the nursing home. Nursing home residents are more susceptible to infection because of their frailty, multiple medical problems, and close living quarters. Fifteen percent of nursing home residents suffer the effects at any one time. Clinical clues to acute infection include:

- Increase in temperature of 2.4°F above baseline
- Acute confusion
- Unexplained changes in behavior or functional status
- Loss of appetite or weight loss
- Weakness or lethargy
- Urinary incontinence
- Orthostatic hypotension or falls
- Tachypnea

18. Which infections are of particular concern in the nursing home?

Urinary tract infection: the leading cause of infection. Nursing home residents have rates of asymptomatic bacteriuria as high as 50%. Research has indicated no beneficial effect from treatment of asymptomatic bacteriuria. Nursing home patients often do not manifest the common symptoms of fever, dysuria, frequency, or hesitancy, presenting instead with confusion, hypotension, nausea, or anorexia from reactive intestinal ileus or worsened cognitive impairment. Interpretation of urine studies is affected by the presence of an indwelling catheter and the high rates of chronic asymptomatic bacteriuria.

Pneumonia: the second most common cause of infection in the nursing home, mainly caused by pneumococci, gram-negative bacilli, staphylococci, influenza and anaerobes. Complications include respiratory failure, bacteremia, and empyema. Mortality can be as high as 12–35%. Prophylactic immunization against influenza and pneumococcal infection have been shown to decrease infection.

Infected pressure sores: 10–15% of pressure sores become locally infected. Some develop contiguous osteomyelitis, and some progress to systemic infection. Chronic inflammation can exacerbate anorexia and weight loss, leading to non-healing.

Lower extremity cellulitis: related to peripheral arterial disease, chronic venous insufficiency, edema, and trauma occurs commonly.

Tuberculosis: Elderly persons have the highest risk for developing tuberculosis of any population group in the U.S. except AIDS patients. The case rate in nursing facilities is 4 times that of elderly community dwellers and 14 times that of the general population. Sixty percent of all TB deaths in the U.S. occur in nursing homes. Tuberculosis screening on admission and annual purified protein derivative tests and prophylactic treatment of recent converters with Isoniazid can limit morbidity and mortality.

MRSA, VRE: increasing numbers of nursing home residents return from the hospital colonized with MRSA (methicillin-resistant *Staphylococcus aureus*), VRE (vancomycin-resistant enterococci) and now gentamycin-resistant enterococci and resistant gram-negative bacteria. Advanced age, acuity, and frequent use of antibiotics in the nursing home increase antimicrobial resistance. Some nursing homes have the facilities to group colonized patients. Others are able to ensure that they do not share rooms with others who have enteral feeding tubes, indwelling urethral catheters, or tracheotomies and are at higher risk of infection. Isolation is not an appropriate strategy in the nursing home. Universal precautions, if exercised assiduously by the staff, limit spread of these organisms.

19. Is medication use different in a nursing home?

Nursing home residents use more medication than community elders—on average, over 8 concurrent prescriptions. This finding reflects the frailty of the population as well as the possibility of inappropriate prescribing practices. The more medicines and the more medical illnesses, the more likely an adverse drug event. Consensus about what constitutes appropriate medication use is poor. Medications such as sedative-hypnotics, antidepressants, antipsychotics, antihypertensives, NSAIDs, oral hypoglycemics, analgesics, dementia treatments, platelet inhibitors, histamine-2 blockers, decongestants, iron supplements, muscle relaxants, gastrointestinal antispasmodics, and antiemetics have come under scrutiny. Since it is often difficult for the nursing home to obtain medical information from hospitals, outpatient physicians, and family members, medications are often continued because of lack of information about the original prescribing purpose (e.g., H_2 blockers started in the hospital for "GI prophylaxis"). Good practice indicates that all medications should be related to particular diagnoses and reviewed monthly by the physician. Estimation of risk-benefit ratios and scrutiny for medications that should generally be avoided in the elderly as well as doses, frequencies, or durations not to be exceeded aid in appropriate prescribing. Diagnoses, disease severity, and symptoms and signs must be included in the analysis of medication appropriateness. CMS tracks the number of residents in each nursing home who use more than 9 medicines as indicative of a question about the quality of their care. With the current changes in the management of diseases common among nursing home residents such as congestive heart failure, diabetes mellitus, and hypertension, it may be that the conventional wisdom of minimizing the number of medications in elderly persons has become outmoded.

Other than number, there are several areas of medication management in nursing home patients that come under governmental scrutiny as quality indicators. For example, nursing home regulations require avoidance of long-acting benzodiazepines for people over 65 years old, unless there is documentation of the reason short-acting medications cannot be substituted. Anxiolytic/sedative drugs must be prescribed for particular indications in specified doses. Proof of symptoms, attempt to reduce or discontinue the medication, and efficacy of treatment must be documented. Antipsychotic medications must be used for specific psychotic symptoms. The patients must be followed for onset of abnormal involuntary movements, dyskinesia, and therapeutic effect. Other medications, such as digoxin, are reviewed for dose level appropriate to their narrow therapeutic range. Antibiotics should be prescribed for clear indications to avoid increasing levels of resistant organisms.

Pharmacy consultants review each nursing home resident's medications for efficacy, appropriateness, adverse drug effects, and interactions and advise the physician and nursing staff.

Knowledge of difference in geriatric pharmacokinetics and pharmacodynamics, combined with educated assessment by the nursing staff and review by the consultant pharmacist, mitigated by financial constraints and customary prescribing patterns, guides drug usage in nursing homes. Treatment of pain, depression, psychosis, agitation, infection, bowel problems, and other diseases can be managed appropriately.

20. Are pressure sores a consequence of nursing home residence?

Pressure sores, localized areas of tissue necrosis, are a serious consequence of immobility and debilitation. About 60% of pressure sores develop in the hospital, 18% in nursing homes, and 18% at home. The longer the nursing home stay and the older the patient, the more likely the patient is to develop a pressure sore. The four key factors involved in causing skin breakdown are pressure, shearing force, friction, and moisture. Immobility, malnutrition, fecal and urinary incontinence, and altered level of consciousness are risk factors common among nursing home patients. Efforts to limit pressure sore development in nursing homes include risk assessment with standardized instruments (e.g., Braden or Norton scale), nutrition evaluation by following body weights, and laboratory tests (e.g., cholesterol, albumin, total lymphocyte count). Repositioning schedules and assistive devices (including cushions, mattresses, splinting devices) to counteract immobility and pressure are useful. Strategies for prevention were formalized into clinical guidelines published by the U.S. Department of Health and Human Services. It has been estimated that

29–79 minutes of nursing time per day is needed to implement these guidelines. Little reimbursement is available for preventative strategies, even though development of pressure sores causes much suffering, may lead to serious complications, including cellulitis, osteomyelitis, infection of adjacent structures like joints, sepsis, and death. Capitated systems have a financial incentive to prevent pressure sores since prevention is much less expensive than healing.

21. What quality-of-life issues are involved in nursing home residence?

The nursing resident has the legal right to dignity, self-determination, and communication with and access to persons and services outside the nursing home.

Areas that have become protected by law
- Privacy and respect
- Medical care and treatment
- Right to refuse treatment
- Freedom from abuse and restraint
- Freedom of association and communication in privacy, activities, work, personal possessions, grievances and complaints, financial affairs
- Transfer and dismissal from the nursing home

Facilitating personal autonomy for physically and mentally impaired nursing home patients requires identifying what is appropriate and eliminating impediments. Nursing home residents are most often women, many of whom have cared for ailing husbands and other relatives. Moving to a nursing home often means sharing a room for the first time in many years. Personal space is reduced to an area around the bed. Possessions must fit into this limited space or be stored or given away. The routine of the nursing home is often inflexible, since a limited staff must get through bathing, toileting, meals, medication administration, and other treatment. People with varying levels of mental acuity are often housed together. Entertainment is often geared to the lowest common denominator. On one hand, there may be long idle periods; on the other hand, residents who prefer to be solitary may be cajoled into social activities so that the home avoids the quality indicator of "little or no activity." Rules designed to avoid injuries often restrict the activities of the less impaired residents. The need to provide medical and nursing care to a diverse population, while complying with multiple regulations, makes maintaining a home-like setting increasing difficult.

Many cognitively impaired patients have lost the capacity for medical decision-making. The physician must judge whether the patient, in the context of each individual decision, understands the consequences of his/her decision. When the patient appears to be unable to make an informed decision, a hierarchy of decision-making is to be followed. Advance directives, made when the patient was competent, can help to guide treatment. Advance directives often include a durable power of attorney for health matters, which empowers a surrogate decision-maker to make decisions when the individual is no longer able. If no advance directive exists, the physicians may seek advice from family or friends, often according to a hierarchy decided upon by state law. A court may be asked to appoint a guardian to act for the incapacitated patient.

Conflict may exist between family members or between family and physician about what treatment is in the patient's best interest. Resuscitation decisions and decisions connected with feeding and hydration are highly emotionally charged and often the subject of disagreement. Physicians and other nursing home staff can decrease the stress of decision-making at crisis times by discussion in advance of crucial decisions about resuscitation, invasive treatments, and enteral nutrition. The intervention of an ethics committee or a hospice may help to achieve the most comfortable end of life for a nursing home resident.

BIBLIOGRAPHY

1. Avorn J, et al: Drug use in the nursing home. Ann Intern Med 123:195–204, 1995.
2. Beers MH, et al: Explicit criteria for determining inappropriate medication use in nursing home residents. Arch Intern Med 151:1825–1832, 1991.
3. Capitano B: Evolving epidemiology and cost of resistance to antimicrobial agents in LTC facilities. JAMDA 3(Suppl), 2003.

4. Evans J: Medical care of nursing home residents. Mayo Clin Proc 70:694–702, 1995.
5. Evans JM, et al: Pressure ulcers: Prevention and management. Mayo Clin Proc 70:789–799, 1995.
6. Kane R: Everyday Ethics: Resolving Dilemmas in Nursing Home Life. New York, Springer Publishing, 1990.
7. Levenson S: Medical Direction in Long Term Care. Durham, NC, Carolina Academic Press, 1993.
8. Norton D, et al: An investigation of Geriatric Nursing Problems in Hospital. Edinburgh, Churchill Livingstone, 1974, pp 193–236.
9. Ouslander J: Medical Care in the Nursing Home. New York, McGraw-Hill, 1997.
10. Panel for the Prediction and Prevention of Pressure Ulcers in Adults: Clinical Practice Guidelines, No. 3. Rockville, MD, Agency for Health Care Policy Research, 1992 (Pub. no. AHCPR 92-0047).
11. Smith D: Pressure ulcers in the nursing home. Ann Intern Med 123:433–442, 1995.
12. Thomas: Nutritional deficiencies in long-term care. Ann Long-term Care III 6(10):325–332; 250–258, 1998.
13. Schrier RW: Geriatric Medicine. Philadelphia, W.B. Saunders, 1990.

49. HOME CARE

*Hollis Day, MD, MS, Bruce Kinosian, MD, and
Jean Yudin, MSN, RN, CS*

Mrs. W.

Mrs. W. is a patient introduced in the first chapter of this book. She is a 68-year-old female with complications of diabetes mellitus that included peripheral neuropathy and autonomic nervous system dysfunction. Mrs. W. is the beneficiary of the interdisciplinary team approach that includes physicians, nursing staff, social workers, and family members to coordinate the patient's care, improve her quality of life, and decrease her need for hospitalizations for poor glycemic control. As Mrs. W.'s diabetes progresses, she will be one of many patients who benefit from home health care services that allow her to remain at home, in the community and not in a nursing home, while still receiving excellent medical and social support.

1. What is home health care?

Home health care is a subset of the broad range of health and social services that are provided to an individual living in the community. Care provided to the patient in the home environment could be either health-related in the sense that a patient is receiving skilled therapy (e.g., speech, occupational therapy or nursing services, or physical therapy, wound care, medication monitoring), or social services, as in assistance with instrumental activities of daily living (e.g., meals-on-wheels, household chores, paying bills, personal care).

2. What is the purpose of home care?

The purposes of home care vary in accordance with the perspectives of society, providers, payors, and consumers. Medicare-funded home health care is designed to be post-acute care, intended to restore individuals to their pre-illness level of functioning. Historical (pre-Medicare) home care had a substantial public health function, with a focus on infants, children and communicable diseases. More recently, attention has focused on the ability of home health care to allow individuals to avoid institutionalization. Care at home can enable individuals to live with their families, instead of in institutions (e.g., patients on home ventilators). Long-term care (LTC) services in the community range from highly technical medical supports, such as chronic parenteral infusions, to meeting nonmedical needs such as cooking, shopping, and cleaning. Consequently, maximizing a patient's functional status and allowing him or her to live in the least restrictive environment possible becomes an important goal of long-term home care.

3. Why should physicians consider home care as an option for patients?

Patient preferences are very important when instituting a plan of care. If a patient is more invested in his or her care, the plan is more likely to be thoroughly implemented. Many patients prefer to remain in their homes as long as possible. While an institution can effectively provide physical ADL support, it is difficult to provide the caring bonds, and many people prefer to receive their care at home.

4. Does home care improve survival?

Studies have demonstrated that home care improves survival and morbidity. Although past data are inconsistent, more recent data support the belief that home care is cost-effective for discharge planning and preventing re-hospitalization.

5. Who is eligible for home care?

The most common consumers of home care are the geriatric population. Patients appropriate for home care may be recovering from an acute illness that required hospitalization, patients with a disability that prevents them from coming into the office, patients with a terminal illness, and patients with an acute exacerbation of a chronic illness. These subpopulations represent distinct forms of home health care programs: post acute, long term care, primary care, hospice, home hospital, and urgent care.

Generally, home care is reserved for patients who are considered homebound. The current definition of a homebound individual according to the Center for Medicaid and Medicare Services (CMS) is one for whom the "ability to leave home creates a considerable/taxing effort and when [the patient] leaves home it is for infrequent or short time periods (e.g., to receive medical treatment)." Proposals have been made to more quantitatively define the term *homebound* but to date have not been adopted. However, managed care plans have taken a more restrictive view of medical home care, restricting skilled services to those specifically required for post-acute recovery and disallowing provision of nonskilled services that individuals need to remain in the community. Other programs provide aides and nonskilled services to individuals residing in the community in order to maintain them independently at home.

Eligibility does not equal need. Individuals with a chronic, relapsing condition, such as class IV congestive heart failure, may need a daily home health aide to maintain function. However, Medicare and most HMOs will not pay for assistance in maintaining function but only for assistance with progression toward a "goal of therapy." Once the goal has been met, these types of insurance no longer will pay for assistance.

6. Who provides care for homebound patients?

In the ideal setting, an interdisciplinary group provides medical and social care for a patient. They often are linked to providers of durable medical equipment. A patient's primary care physician is considered part of a "team" of home health agency (HHA) personnel, the physician, the family, and the patient, because the physician is required by CMS to authorize all care provided by the HHA.

The core team provided by HHAs consists of physicians, nurses, nurse practitioners, social workers, home health aides, physical and occupational therapists, and sometimes speech therapists as well. A few home health agencies separately have physicians and advance practice nurses. In settings with strong community based long-term care programs, such interdisciplinary groups may include members from the local community agencies (i.e., the local area agency on aging), which provides much of the nonskilled services for a care plan. The importance of communication is never lessened; however, in settings with less interdisciplinary structure, communication burdens, particularly upon the primary physician, primary nurse, and primary aide, are heightened.

The implementation of a successful home care plan depends on frequent, clear, well-documented communication among the members of the team. Equally, the success of a home care plan depends not only on the team members but on the ability of the patient and informal caregivers (family, friends) to execute the plan.

7. What is the role of the physician in providing home care?

Historically, the physician routinely made house calls and provided primary care in the patient's home. Over the past few decades, this practice has declined as the emphasis on either acute hospital care or outpatient office practice increased. More recently, however, there has been a resurgence of interest in physicians seeing patients at home, and some physicians have made this a full-time practice. Home visits are highly rewarding for the physician: a special bond develops when patients realize that the physician has made an effort to see them in their natural setting. Similarly, the physician can enjoy getting to know the patient in a more social context, learning about the family and seeing what the patient truly values. Still, in general, the office-based physician's role is to be actively involved in the interdisciplinary plan of care that has been jointly developed with the nursing provider directing the case, the patient, and the patient's caregivers; to participate in team meetings; and to facilitate changes in the care plan as circumstances demand.

8. What new or different information can be gained through a home assessment that may not be achieved through a routine history and physical in the office?

An assessment of the patient in his or her home environment can be highly educational. A patient's functional status depends on the interaction between his or her physical and cognitive capacities and the environment in which he or she lives. In the office the physician can test physical and cognitive ability, but he or she cannot fully appreciate the patient's functional capacity until the demands that the patient's environment make upon these abilities (and vice versa) are seen. For example, the physician can see what medications the patient actually is taking including any over-the-counter, outdated, or duplicate medications. New light may be shed on a patient's complaint of incontinence when you see that the bathroom is unable to be reached easily. Equally important, a home visit provides a thorough comprehension of the caregiver's burdens and a clearer understanding of why a particular care plan is difficult to implement.

For the physician who does not make home visits, CMS now requires the home health agency to record a standardized, detailed assessment of the person's function at the beginning and termination of home care. This detailed functional information is recorded in the OASIS instrument (Outcome and ASsessment Information Set) and can be provided by the assessor to the physician if requested.

9. List services that can be provided in the home.
- A complete geriatric assessment with an emphasis on physical/basic and instrumental activities of daily living
- Physical (PT), speech, and occupational therapy (OT)
- Phlebotomy and home monitoring of specific measures such as INRs
- X-rays, including ultrasound, echocardiography, sleep studies, nerve conduction/electromyography (EMG), Doppler blood flow studies, pulmonary function testing
- Nutrition support services, such as total parenteral nutrition or enteral feeding using g-tubes, jejunostomy tubes
- Home infusion services, such as parenteral antibiotics, transfusions, chemotherapy, and hydration
- More advanced therapies, such as home dobutamine infusions and home ventilators
- Social services, including evaluation of abuse or neglect, need for home-delivered meals
- Home safety evaluations
- Assessment of caregiver's burden

10. What are some conditions that can be treated as safely in the home as in the hospital?
- Deep venous thrombosis (DVT)
- Uncomplicated community-acquired pneumonia
- Cellulitis
- Uncomplicated urinary tract infection

These conditions have been extensively studied and offer relatively easy medication administration, do not require intensive monitoring of laboratory values (e.g., with low–molecular-weight heparin in DVT you do not have to monitor prothrombin times), and do not require close monitoring of vital signs. Families and patients are instructed how to administer many of the treatments, and nurses are sent to the home to administer intravenous medications and monitor a patient's progress. Treatment of these conditions at home is both cost-effective and more comfortable for the patient.

11. Describe the elements of a home safety evaluation.

A home safety evaluation is designed to evaluate a patient's ability to function safely in the home both in the routine setting and in the event of an emergency. Often individuals are more stable in a familiar home setting than they appear to be when evaluated in an unfamiliar hospital or office site.

One portion of a home safety evaluation includes the search for potential environmental factors that contribute to falls. Environmental factors that may precipitate falls include:

- Throw rugs or carpeting that may not be tacked down
- Uneven steps or flooring that may cause a person to trip
- Shaky or absent handrails that do not extend far enough at the ends of the stairs
- Poor lighting
- Beds and toilets from which it is difficult to arise
- Bathtubs and showers that are difficult to enter and exit and do not have non-skid surfaces
- An extremely cluttered environment that provides no access to an immediate exit in the case of an emergency

Other elements of the home safety evaluation:

- Check the temperature setting on the water heater to prevent scalding
- Assess safety features on doors and windows to prevent forced entry
- Survey the kitchen for potential fire hazards
- Test fire alarms to ensure their proper functioning
- Guarantee easy access to a telephone

12. Why is the assessment of caregiver burden important?

Informal caregivers, usually a spouse or other family member, provide the bulk of care for most homebound patients. When they become stressed, the patient is affected, often leading to hospitalizations or ultimately to placement in a long-term care facility. An assessment of the caregiver in the home can reveal how many hours a day the caregiver is attending to the needs of the patient, what type of tasks they are performing, and the obstacles (physical, mental, and social) that may prevent adequate implementation of the care plan. It also may reveal who the actual caregivers are.

13. How do patients gain access to home care?

In the post-acute model, patients commonly enter the home care system at the time of discharge from the hospital. In this situation, case managers develop a plan of care with the help of the physician and make referrals to home care agencies that then follow a patient's progress. They are followed for a brief period of time and services are subsequently discontinued after all goals have been met.

More commonly, however, home care services are being used to provide long-term care in the community. Patients often are referred from the physician's office when they frequently fail to arrive for their appointments or are known to have significant difficulty in leaving the house. One recent study demonstrated that 78% of home care visits occurred more than one month after a patient had been discharged from the hospital and that 61% of visits were to patients who received home care for 6 or more months. These often are patients who gain access to nonmedical home services through their area agency on aging or other community sources.

14. What are the different levels of care that are available at home?

The highest level of care available is skilled nursing care, often designated as home *health* care. Skilled professional or nursing services focus on assessment and management of medical problems and provide family education and recommendations for additional support services (e.g., social work, physical therapy). Other professional services include physical, occupational, and speech therapy.

An additional level of home care is that provided by paraprofessionals known as home health aides, or personal care assistants. These assistants help patients with activities of daily living (ADLs), taking medication at the appropriate time, and maintaining a safe environment. Homemakers provide chore services, such as cooking, cleaning, and shopping. They are provided by payors for community-based LTC services, but not (officially) by CMS. However, many HHAs will provide homemaker services for clients who require such assistance.

15. Who pays for these services?

Medicare will pay for home care if a patient has a skilled nursing need. Payment is dependent on constant reassessment and ongoing improvement in the patient's condition. Medicare will not pay for daily skilled services unless they are of finite duration. Medicare may not pay for a patient's medications. For example, if a patient is receiving antibiotic therapy at home, he or she must pay for it privately or have another type of insurance that will cover the medication. A physician must supervise the patient's progress and adequately document the patient's need for ongoing care so that all parties involved can receive payment. Medicare will pay for a limited amount of personal care services (maximum of 20 hours/week) and again, only if the patient has a skilled nursing need. These home care services are therefore generally paid for by the individual or family and can lead to substantial expense. Beginning in 2000, CMS began to pay for home health care prospectively for a 60-day period if the individual requires more than 4 skilled visits at home. This has given agencies greater discretion in the mix and duration of services that can be provided to a patient.

For individuals who require assistance with ADLs for chronic conditions, the short "post-acute" period may often leave them without needed services after their skilled need ends. Through the use of allowed services—that is, skilled nursing to monitor changes in therapies, new diagnoses, to teach families about aspects of care, manage a complex care plan, or through subsequently requiring PT for mobility or OT to help with ADL performance, aide services can be maintained for individuals with chronic conditions for extended periods. However, annual caps on total home health services require that such services be viewed as stop-gap measures until waiting lists for community-based services can be negotiated and community based LTC services can begin.

No standardized system is in place for long-term care of the frail patient in the community, except in communities that have PACE, a program for all inclusive care of elders. It is a Medicare benefit that pools the individual's long-term care (Medicaid) and acute-care (Medicare) funds. Thus, it is important that every physician be aware of local resources through which services— both medical and nonmedical—can be obtained to allow as many patients as possible to function safely and at maximum capacity outside of an institution. Further, as a patient advocate, it is important for the primary care physician to challenge agency assertions of "Medicare doesn't allow . . ." or "Medicare requires. . . ." Often local agency policy is portrayed to ordering physicians as federal regulation, an inaccuracy that does disservice to needy, frail elders.

16. What is the difference between home care, palliative care, and hospice?

Hospice is care of the terminal patient whose life expectancy is 6 months or less. Although hospice care can be provided in the home, it also can be provided in more institutional settings. Hospice care has traditionally been associated with oncology, although recently criteria have been promulgated for individuals with a number of other terminal conditions, such as congestive heart failure, chronic obstructive pulmonary disease, renal failure, and dementia. In addition to the services that HHAs provide, hospices often provide augmented volunteer support services and pastoral and social work counseling services. Providers from HHAs and hospices, however, may apply principles of **palliative care**. These principles are generically focused on relief of symptoms and attention to individual patient's spiritual, emotional, and physical concerns, rather than resolving specific illness episodes. Some hospices have affiliated HHAs for individuals not yet willing to accept all the restrictions of hospice (e.g., many hospices require that individuals renounce treatment of infections or hospitalizations, no matter how transitory).

Home care, however, is for any patient who meets the criteria previously mentioned, not just for someone who is terminally ill.

17. Where can I go for more information about home care?

More information can be found through the American Academy of Home Care Physicians at www.aahcp.org/aahcp/ or by calling 410-676-7966.

BIBLIOGRAPHY

1. American Medical Association Home Care Advisory Panel: Guidelines for the medical management of the home-care patient. Arch Fam Med 2:194–206, 1993.

2. Boling PA: Home care physicians in the interdisciplinary team. In The Physician's Role in Home Health Care. New York, Springer, 1997, pp 42–69.

3. Health Care Financing Administration: The Home Health Agency Manual, publication number 11. Revised. Washington, D.C., Department of Health and Human Services, 1996.

4. Leff B, Burton JR: The future history of home care and physician house calls in the United States. M603–M608.

4. Ramsdell JW, Swart JA, Jackson JE, Renvall M: The yield of a home visit in the assessment of geriatric patients. J Am Geriatr Soc 37:17–24, 1989.

5. Repetto L, Granetto C, Venturino A: Home care in the older person. Clin Geriatr Med 13:403–413, 1997.

6. Van Gerpen BS, Scott CB: Home care: What is it? J Med Assoc Ga 86:119–120, 1997.

7. Vladeck BC, Miller NA: The Medicare home health initiative. Health Care Financing Rev 16:7–16, 1994.

8. Welch HG, Wennberg DE, Welch WP: The use of Medicare home health care services. N Engl J Med 335:324–329, 1996.

50. HOSPICE CARE

Jennifer M. Kapo, MD, and David Casarett, MD, MA

1. What is hospice?

Hospice is a multidisciplinary program of service that is designed to provide care for patients near the end of life and their families. Hospice recognizes that the dying process is a natural and important stage of life, and its goal is to optimize comfort and quality of life while diminishing suffering. Hospice neither seeks to prolong life nor to hasten death. Instead, hospice provides supportive care while addressing spiritual, social, psychological, and physical suffering in an effort to maximize quality of life.

2. Who provides hospice services?

In the United States, hospice services are provided by over 3,000 hospice organizations. Hospices can be Medicare-certified or independent of Medicare. Although the majority (72%) of hospices operate as not-for-profit facilities, 24% are for profit and 4% are funded by the government.

3. Who is eligible for hospice?

In general, patients are eligible to receive hospice care if they have a prognosis of 6 months or less if the patient's illness follows its natural course, as certified by two physicians, and if they choose to forgo life—sustaining treatment. Additional criteria are established by the payer. For instance, to qualify for the hospice Medicare benefit, patients must be eligible to receive Medicare Part A benefits. These patients must also meet disease-specific prognostic criteria developed and promulgated by Medicare fiscal intermediaries.

4. When are patients generally referred to hospice?

In general, patients are referred to hospice late in the course of their illnesses. Currently, the median length of stay in hospice is 21 days, and one-third of patients spend less than a week in hospice before death. These patients and their families receive hospice care only briefly and often do not benefit from the full range of services that hospice can provide.

Late referrals to hospice may be related to the well-documented propensity of physicians to overestimate prognosis and lack of reliable prognostic indicators to serve as guides. Predicting prognosis is particularly difficult for noncancer diagnoses such as end-stage heart disease, end-stage renal disease (ESRD), chronic obstructive pulmonary disease, and dementia. Compared to cancer, which has a relatively predictable illness trajectory, the illness trajectory of end-organ failure is typically marked by a series of illness exacerbations, and stabilizations. There may never be a time when the patient is clearly dying of his or her illness. Referral patterns to hospice reflect this finding. In 2000, 52% of patients in hospice had cancer, 10% heart disease, 6% dementia, 6% COPD, 3% ESRD, and 2% end-stage liver disease. To improve clinicians' ability to prognosticate, guidelines were developed by the National Hospice and Palliative Care Organization for determining when patients with noncancer disease would be appropriate for hospice referral. Although they were intended as guidelines to facilitate referrals, they have been implemented by fiscal intermediaries as criteria that must be met.

5. When should patients be referred to hospice?

Clinicians should use broad prognostic criteria in determining hospice eligibility. A reasonable heuristic is to consider whether one would be surprised if a patient were to die in the next 6 months. A negative answer should prompt consideration of hospice for that patient. In general, this single criterion is much easier to apply than are the fiscal intermediary requirements. Indeed, it is usually impractical to expect generalist clinicians to remember hospice eligibility criteria for a variety of illnesses. Instead, clinicians should estimate prognosis using the question above and allow the hospice intake department to establish medical eligibility. It is important to note that there are no penalties for clinicians who underestimate prognosis and refer a patient to hospice who does not die within 6 months. Both the Centers for Medicare and Medicaid Services and its fiscal intermediaries acknowledge that prognostication is inexact and that errors are expected. Next, clinicians should consider whether a patient's goals for care are consistent with the goals of hospice. In general, this means that patients should want to focus on comfort rather than on treatments to prolong life. However, it is important to note that these goals need not be absolute. For instance, it is appropriate to refer a patient to hospice who still desires an attempt at resuscitation even in the event of a cardiac arrest. These patients may still benefit from the support that hospice can provide.

6. How are hospice organizations reimbursed?

Medicare is the single largest payer for hospice care in the U.S. However, many private insurance and managed care programs offer hospice services. In addition, Medicaid provides some hospice service coverage in 42 states and the District of Columbia.

Hospice organizations are reimbursed on a capitated, per-diem basis, contingent on the level of care that the hospice provides. Most care is reimbursed as regular home care, acute care, and intensive home care (i.e., 24-hour home nursing). In general, the payer reimburses the hospice organization directly, regardless of where care is being provided. If care is provided in a nursing home or hospital, the hospice subcontracts with that facility to provide the physical care setting and some aspects of care.

The hospice per-diem payment does not include services of nonhospice physicians, who can still bill Medicare or, in most cases, a private insurer. The per-diem payment also does not cover the costs of medications and treatments that are not related to the admitting hospice diagnosis.

7. What services does hospice provide?

Core hospice services are required of hospices that are Medicare-certified. In theory, noncertified hospices can provide fewer services, and some do. Core services include:
• Home visits by registered nurses and licensed practical nurses
• Evaluation and counseling by a social worker
• Oversight by a physician, with home visits as necessary
• Home health aide services
• The support of a volunteer who can provide companionship and/or assistance
• Physical, occupational, and speech therapy if indicated
• Durable medical equipment, medications, and medical supplies related to the hospice admitting diagnosis
• Bereavement services up to a year after the patient's death
• Chaplain visits

8. How does hospice help family members?

Many of the core hospice services described above, such as home health aide services, social work, and spiritual support, offer clear benefits to family caregivers. For instance, by coordinating all of the services, medications, and supplies, hospice offers a valuable case management or "concierge" function that families may find to be very valuable. Hospice also offers respite care for the patient up to a maximum of 6 consecutive days. Additionally, volunteers can attend to the patient when the caregiver needs to leave the home for errands and/or personal reasons. Home health aides and trained volunteers can help with the personal care of the patients and household chores.

9. Where can hospice provide care?

The majority of patients receive hospice care in the home with a friend or family member acting as the primary caregiver. The hospice staff makes regular home visits and is available 24 hours a day, 7 days a week for urgent calls. If the patient has an acute exacerbation of a symptom that needs continuous care, care can be provided in the patient's home by a visiting nurse, or by admission to a hospital or a designated hospice care unit, if one is available. Patients who can no longer remain at home can also receive care in an acute care setting or, more commonly, in a long term care facility. Placement may be permanent or may provide respite care for caregivers. In all of these settings, the patient's hospice team retains primary caregiving responsibilities.

10. Do patients ever leave hospice?

Yes. A patient can leave hospice voluntarily by revoking the hospice benefit. For example, a cancer patient may decide that he or she wants to have more chemotherapy with the goal of cure and/or life prolongation. While the patient is pursuing this therapy, he or she cannot receive hospice care covered by Medicare. If the patient decides in the future to cease life-extending therapies, he or she can re-elect the hospice benefit at any time without a penalty.

There are patients whose medical conditions improve after receiving the comprehensive care hospice delivers. If they improve to the extent that they no longer have a prognosis of 6 months or less, hospice can decertify the patient and discharge him or her from hospice. Hospices may feel constrained to discharge a patient who no longer meets enrollment criteria out of concerns about denials of payment. However, patients who are discharged from hospice can be re-admitted in the future without penalty when they meet prognostic criteria once more.

11. What happens if a patient lives longer than 6 months?

For the first 180 days of admission, a patient's case is reviewed twice, at 90-day intervals. The patient must be re-certified for continuing care at each review. After the first 180 days, the patient is eligible for an unlimited number of 60-day recertification periods. That is, as long as the patient still meets the criteria of a prognosis of 6 months or less, theoretically he or she can remain in hospice indefinitely.

12. What are some common misperceptions of hospice by physicians, patients, and their families?

- *Myth:* Hospice is unaffordable. *Truth:* Hospice is covered by many payers, and most hospices will accept patients without insurance.
- *Myth:* Hospice is for cancer patients only. *Truth:* Almost half of hospice patients have non-cancer diagnoses.
- *Myth:* Hospice patients can no longer see their primary care providers. *Truth:* Primary care providers can and should continue to follow their patients and can bill under Medicare Part B.
- *Myth:* Hospice is for those who are imminently dying. *Truth:* Although it is true that many patients die soon after enrollment, this is a function of late referral, not of hospice's goals for care.
- *Myth:* Patients cannot disenroll from hospice. *Truth:* Patients can leave hospice whenever they wish and can return later if they choose.

USEFUL RESOURCES

1. American Academy of Hospice and Palliative Medicine: www.aahpm.org
2. Berger A et al: Palliative Care and Supportive Oncology, 2nd ed. Philadelphia, Lippincott Williams & Wilkins, 2002.
3. National Hospice and Palliative Care Organization: www.nhpco.org
4. Storey P: Primer of Palliative Care, 2nd ed. Gainsville, FL, American Academy of Hospice and Palliative Medicine, 1996.

51. ALTERNATIVE LONG-TERM CARE

Thomas Lawrence, MD

1. What is alternative long-term care?

In past years, long-term care most often referred to care provided in the nursing home setting. Nursing homes had two designated levels of care: skilled nursing care and intermediate care. Skilled nursing referred to caring for the most frail nursing home residents who often were completely dependent in activities of daily living (ADLs), were unable to ambulate, and had medical needs that required a registered nurse. Included in the skilled care group of nursing home residents are patients with needs such as wound care, use of gastrostomy tubes, and intensive treatment of medical conditions such as diabetes. Intermediate care encompassed higher-functioning residents who did not have major nursing needs and were able to ambulate and self-feed.

Although long-term care continues to have a heavy institutional bias, most Americans demonstrate a clear preference for care in the home setting. Many services previously available only in an institutional setting are now available in the home. If care at home is not appropriate or available, the setting that is the least institutional and most home-like is desirable. In addition, the Olmstead decision of the U.S. Supreme Court (1999) arose out of the Americans with Disabilities Act and has promoted the placement of care-dependent people who receive public funding to community settings.

The long-term care needs of the elderly are increasingly met outside nursing homes. Non-traditional long-term care, also called alternative long-term care, includes a wide variety of programs, most of which have developed and become widely available in the past 15–20 years in the United States. Like traditional long-term care services, alternative long-term care refers to longitudinal supportive services and health care designed to meet the care needs of frail dependent people, the majority of whom are elderly and often would be eligible for nursing home placement.

2. What are the most commonly used institutional sites of alternative long-term care?

1. Assisted-living facilities which, in some states, are also known as personal care facilities or senior housing with services

2. Retirement communities, which include continuing care retirement communities (also known as life-care communities)

3. Adult day-care programs, often augmented with in-home support services

4. Home-based community care (services in this area are growing at a rapid rate)

Less commonly used sites of care include long-term care hospitals and community-based continuing care programs. Day hospitals, which provide multidisciplinary patient assessment and rehabilitation services, are common in England and elsewhere but are not widely available in the United States.

3. Explain continuum of care.

As a wide variety of alternative institutional and community-based long-term care options have become available, continuous care with minimal disruption during times of health transitions has become a reality. Complete continuum of care refers to a spectrum of services designed to provide all of the social and health care needs of people as they age. This spectrum ranges from independent living to acute hospital-based care and nursing home-based long-term care. Many community facilities in the U.S. currently house the two most commonly utilized long-term care alternatives, assisted living and nursing care, within one facility. Within this model, one important goal is to accomplish transitions from one setting to another with a minimum of disruption in care.

A broader definition of the continuum of care includes caregiver continuity and continuity within an individual's health domains. This concept promotes the continuance of a patient's care-giving team, medical care, and physician services, including primary care physicians and consultants, as the patient moves from office-based care to home care services, assisted living, and nursing home care. Continuity of health domains involves creating links among issues relating to health promotion, disease prevention, treatment of acute disease, and the management of chronic diseases and conditions. Creating linkages in care between physical health domains and spiritual and psychosocial health also is receiving increasing attention.

The continuing care retirement community (see question 5) is an example of a long-term care continuum that covers the full spectrum of individual needs. The challenge in the future will be for health care providers to develop fully functioning continuums of care in community settings that are accessible and affordable to those in greatest need.

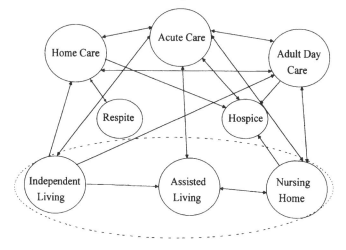

The long-term care continuum. Arrows indicate transitions in care. Dotted lines indicate continuing care retirement community.

4. What are assisted-living facilities?

Assisted-living facilities provide a combination of housing, personalized support services, and health care services. They are among the fastest growing markets in senior housing, and currently there are over 36,000 assisted-living residences in the U.S., housing more than 1 million Americans. The typical assisted-living resident is age 83 or older, widowed or single, and most often female. These facilities range in size from a few beds to several hundred; typical facilities have between 25 and 120 beds. They may be freestanding or part of a retirement community, nursing home, or residential care home. The term *assisted living* encompasses the older designations of personal care home, residential care home, domiciliary care home, and group home.

Typical services provided in assisted living include support with the instrumental activities of daily living (IADLs) of meal preparation, transportation, shopping, housekeeping, laundry, and activities. Support with ADLs, such as bathing, dressing, eating, toileting, and ambulation, is more variable and depends on the specific facility and the population. The number of services usually reflects increasing charges to residents.

Assisted-living facilities are extremely heterogeneous; of this form of senior housing it has been said, "When you've seen one assisted-living facility, you've seen one assisted-living facility." Nonetheless, one common finding is that resident acuity (level of infirmity) is continuing to climb as residents from intermediate care nursing home units are placed in assisted-living sites. Some assisted-living or personal care facilities provide on-site nursing care for all or part of the day, but, unlike nursing homes, they are not required to provide this service according to state licensure. Health care services are generally supervised by most assisted-living facilities, including medication assistance and emergency call systems. Many provide on-site physician care, especially those that are part of a retirement community or nursing home. Some facilities are specialty-based; the most common type serves residents with Alzheimer's disease and other dementias. Assisted-living dementia units frequently provide care with greater attention to resident dignity, autonomy, safety, and quality of life than is ordinarily available in a nursing home dementia unit.

5. What is a continuing care retirement community?

Continuing care retirement communities (CCRCs) are retirement communities that provide a spectrum of services ranging from independent living to assisted living or nursing facility care. These programs are also called life care communities, because the long-term contract provides for housing, community services, nursing care, and other health care programs for the duration of the recipient's life. There are three common types of CCRC contracts. The first may offer nursing care with little or no increase in monthly payments. The second may place a cap on the amount of nursing care that is covered; beyond the cap additional payments are made. The third type of contract may require full per-diem rates for all nursing care. CCRCs generally require a one-time entrance fee that may or may not be partially refundable. Monthly fees generally depend on the size and amenities of the resident's housing.

The average age at entry of CCRC residents is about 77 years, younger than with assisted living. About 23% of CCRC residents are married couples, whereas most assisted-living residents are single or widowed. Many CCRCs contract with primary care physicians who then manage the care and health care services provided in all settings. Most CCRCs have on-campus assisted living and nursing care, but some have one or both levels available off site, although they still are covered by contract.

6. What is adult day care?

Adult day care offers a variety of supportive and social services and health care in a community-based environment during daytime hours. Services may be utilized part-day or full-day, usually 1–5 days weekly. The clients of adult day programs typically have a mix of physical and cognitive impairments for which they need assistance. Most but not all clients live with caregivers who are unable to provide full daytime care because of work schedules or the need for daytime respite care. Typically one meal and a schedule of activities are the focus of the program. Some programs offer specialized services, including dementia programs, incontinence management, and pain management. Some offer more extensive services, including rehabilitation therapies and physician services. Transportation often is coordinated by the center, and some centers offer transportation services directly for a fee.

7. What other community-based alternative long-term care programs are available?

The most commonly used alternative to nursing home care for frail elders in need of assistance with daily functioning is informal caregiver services in the home setting. Most older Americans prefer to live independently in their own homes for as long as possible, and although this is not possible for all dependent elders, most are able to remain in the community, often living with family or other caregivers, while receiving community-based services. For every older person being cared for in an institutional long-term care setting, at least three or four with equal impairment are cared for in the community.

In recent years, community-based services are being financed increasingly through public funding for Medicaid recipients. The federal government has expanded the Home and Community-Based Service (HCBS) Waiver program to allow states to develop creative alternatives to nursing home care. The program specifically lists seven services to be covered: case management, homemaker and home health aide services, personal care services, adult day health, rehabilitation services, and respite care. HCBS programs are available in essentially all states and are expanding each year. The viability of the program is based on the requirement that the alternatives to nursing home-based care must be less costly than nursing home care on an average per-capita basis.

8. What is respite care?

Respite care provides relief for usual caregivers. Most often it involves a short admission, ranging from a few days to a few weeks, to a nursing home or assisted-living facility. Respite care has become widely available in recent years at most community long-term care facilities and is financed on a per-diem rate paid by the patient. The cost of this service may be less than half the cost of nursing home care; however, most insurance plans, including Medicare and Medicaid, do not cover the costs of respite care. Respite care may be needed to provide caregiver relief for vacation, provision of personal health needs, or periodic relief to prevent caregiver stress and exhaustion. It generally is believed that the availability of respite care delays or prevents the need for institutionalization for many functionally impaired elders living in community settings.

9. What is PACE?

One unique community-based program covered by Medicare is the Program for All Inclusive Care for the Elderly (PACE). PACE is an optional benefit under both Medicare and Medicaid that provides comprehensive community-based care for people who qualify for nursing home care according to state standards. The PACE program uses a case management approach to provide medical, rehabilitation, social, and personal services to its enrollees. Services are available 7 days per week; usually an adult day health center serves as the base of operations. PACE care may include care at the day center as well as in-home care. Primary care physicians and nurses provide continuous care, including treatment of acute illness. The PACE program currently operates nationally in over 40 centers with plans for annual expansion. Since its beginning in 1986, the PACE program has proved to be successful in providing high-quality community-based long-term care as well as preventing nursing home placement and reducing hospitalization. At the same time, most programs have demonstrated cost savings in caring for extremely frail and chronically ill elderly patients compared with usual options.

10. What factors determine which level of care an individual requires?

The two most important factors that determine level of care are functional status and medical needs (see Chapter 3). **Functional assessment** is the process through which an individual's ability to perform basic and instrumental activities of daily living is evaluated. The pattern of functional deficits predicts what services the person will need. For example, unmanaged bowel incontinence, complete feeding dependency, and requirement of two persons for transfers are functional problems that frequently predict the need for nursing home care rather than alternative types of long-term care. Assisted-living facilities often will not accept residents with unmanaged urinary incontinence, any degree of feeding dependency, or inability to transfer independently and ambulate with minimal assistance. The two IADLs indicating that an independent elder with basic ADLs may be safely left alone for brief periods in a community setting are the ability to provide meals and hydration and the ability to use a telephone to call for emergency assistance.

Medical needs that may predict nursing home care rather than alternatives include extensive wound care needs in bed-bound patients and management of complex comorbid active diseases (e.g., diabetes, congestive heart failure, chronic obstructive pulmonary disease, coronary heart disease) that require close monitoring and adjustment of treatment regimens.

11. What principles of preventive health care apply to alternative long-term care?

Typical health promotion and disease prevention activities that are appropriate for independent, high-functioning elderly people may not be effective or desired by frail older populations in need of long-term care. Examples include cancer screening and cardiovascular risk reduction in people without known cardiovascular disease. There are, however, several areas in which prevention is quite important. Depression is extremely prevalent in long-term care populations (50–60% of nursing home residents have symptoms of depression). Periodic screening for depression can be accomplished with such tests as the 15-item Geriatric Depression Scale. Frail, functionally impaired elders also are at high risk for weight loss with subsequent malnutrition. Monitoring monthly weights and checking baseline serum albumin levels are effective measures for early diagnosis of protein malnutrition. Prevention of infectious disease by maintaining vaccination with pneumo-coccal, influenza, and tetanus vaccines is recommended for elders in all long-term care settings. Residents in long-term care programs generally are at high risk for falls and fall-related injuries, including hip fracture. Prevention of falls is best achieved by implementing a formal program to identify risk factors and to design specific interventions that reduce or eliminate those risks.

12. What role do physicians play in the care of patients in alternative long-term care settings?

Physicians have a central role in the care of nursing home residents, in part due to extensive state and federal regulations that mandate regular visits by physicians to nursing home residents. Although regular on-site physician visits are not required by regulations in other settings, the role of physicians and mid-level practitioners is vital to the delivery of high-quality care in alternative long-term care settings. Physicians see residents in assisted-living facilities at a growing rate, partly because reimbursement recently has been improved and partly because the boom in the de-velopment of larger assisted-living facilities makes them an efficient site for physician practice. The physician's role in home care visits to chronically ill elderly people is also a growing trend nationally. On-site physician services usually are an integral part of continuing care retirement communities. Most adult day programs do not incorporate on-site physician services.

13. What factors indicate the need for hospitalization to manage acute illness among people in long-term care programs?

Hospitalization for long-term care residents usually is indicated by the need for medical ser-vices that are not available in the current setting or by the development of barriers to services, such as poor coordination of care or financing problems. Common medical conditions that lead to hospitalization include inadequate oral intake, dehydration, infections, acute respiratory fail-ure, unstable angina, gastrointestinal bleeding, and fractures of the lower extremity. Inadequate intake of food and fluid causing dehydration, due to either acute illness or progressive dysphagia, may result in the need for hospitalization for intravenous fluid or to establish access for enteral nutrition. Infections that require intravenous antibiotics are a common cause for hospitalization. However, many currently available broad-spectrum antibiotics have good oral bioavailability and have reduced the need for hospitalization to treat infection. Hospitalization for more intensive treatment or closer monitoring often is needed in patients with acute respiratory failure, unstable angina, and gastrointestinal bleeding. In addition, people who have multiple chronic comorbid conditions, such as chronic obstructive pulmonary disease, coronary heart disease, and diabetes, may have acute problems that require hospitalization.

Barriers to the management of acute illness in long-term care settings may involve lack of diagnostic or therapeutic services or delays in accessing these services; examples include labora-tory, radiology, and pharmacy services. Long-term care settings may have nursing staffs that are less experienced or are not as highly trained in the management of acute illness as hospital nurs-ing staffs. Lack of physician availability for diagnosis and treatment of acute illness may result in hospitalization of long-term care residents. In addition, there is the financial incentive of higher reimbursement for physicians for hospital-based care. Poor information transfer from prior health care settings in the long-term care continuum or between consultants and primary care physician may result in unnecessary hospitalization due to incomplete medical information upon which to make treatment decisions.

BIBLIOGRAPHY

1. Eng C, Pedulla J, Eleaser GP, et al: Program of all-inclusive care for the elderly (PACE): An innovative model of integrated geriatric care and financing. J Am Geriatr Soc 45:223–232, 1997.
2. Goldberg TH, Chavin SI: Preventive medicine and screening in older adults. J Am Geriatr Soc 45:344–354, 1997.
3. Gordon M: On-site acute care for residents of long-term care facilities. J Am Geriatr Soc 44:606–607, 1996.
4. Kane RA: Expanding the home care concept: Blurring distinctions among home care, institutional care, and other long-term-care services. Millbank Q 73:161–185, 1995.

5. Krothe JS: Giving voice to elderly people: Community-based long-term care. Public Health Nurs 14:217–226, 1997.
6. Markle-Reid M, Brown G: Explaining the use and non-use of community-based long-term care services by caregivers of persons with dementia. J Eval Clin Pract 7:271–287, 2001.
7. Mollica R: Coordinating services across the continuum of health, housing, and supportive services. J Aging Health 15:165–188, 2003.
8. Petty S: What does the Olmstead decision mean for LTC? Caring Ages 2:8–11, 2001.
9. Phillips-Harris C, Fanale JE: The acute and long-term care interface: Integrating the continuum. Clin Geriatr Med 11:481–501, 1995.
10. White M: Eligibility in the ever-changing continuum of care. Ann Long-Term Care 7:112–114, 1999.

INDEX

Page numbers in **boldface type** indicate complete chapters.